A Clinician's Guide to
Prenatal and Postnatal Care

A Clinician's Guide to Prenatal and Postnatal Care

Edited by Nicola Morse

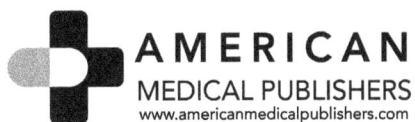

AMERICAN
MEDICAL PUBLISHERS
www.americanmedicalpublishers.com

American Medical Publishers,
41 Flatbush Avenue,
1st Floor, New York,
NY 11217, USA

Visit us on the World Wide Web at:
www.americanmedicalpublishers.com

ISBN: 978-1-63927-149-8

Cataloging-in-Publication Data

A clinician's guide to prenatal and postnatal care / edited by Nicola Morse.
p. cm.
Includes bibliographical references and index.
ISBN 978-1-63927-149-8
1. Prenatal care. 2. Postnatal care. 3. Maternal health services. 4. Preconception care. I. Morse, Nicola.
RG801 .C55 2022
618.6--dc23

Table of Contents

Permissions

List of Contributors

Index

Preface

The main aim of this book is to educate learners and enhance their research focus by presenting diverse topics covering this vast field. This is an advanced book which compiles significant studies by distinguished experts in the area of analysis. This book addresses successive solutions to the challenges arising in the area of application, along with it; the book provides scope for future developments.

The field of obstetrics is concerned with the care of women through the period of pregnancy until after delivery. An important objective of this field is to provide adequate prenatal and postnatal care. Prenatal care is a form of preventive healthcare, which ensures that potential health problems are prevented and treated throughout the course of pregnancy by promoting a healthy lifestyle which benefits the mother and the child. Physical examinations comprising of blood and urine tests, blood pressure measurements, Doppler fetal heart rate monitoring, pelvic exam, weight and height measurements as well as obstetric ultrasounds provide insights into prenatal development and the health of the mother. Post delivery, the uterus size and hormone levels gradually return to a non-pregnant state. It is a critical period, as several complications can arise in the mother and the child during this period. The 6-12 hours after childbirth carry risk of postpartum bleeding, and hence frequent assessments of the fundus and the bleeding, and uterine massages are required. This book studies, analyzes and upholds the pillars of prenatal and postnatal care, and their utmost significance in the modern day. It elucidates the concepts and innovative models around prospective developments with respect to pregnancy care and childbirth. The topics covered in this book offer the readers new insights in the field of obstetrics.

It was a great honour to edit this book, though there were challenges, as it involved a lot of communication and networking between me and the editorial team. However, the end result was this all-inclusive book covering diverse themes in the field.

Finally, it is important to acknowledge the efforts of the contributors for their excellent chapters, through which a wide variety of issues have been addressed. I would also like to thank my colleagues for their valuable feedback during the making of this book.

Editor

Preferred prenatal counselling at the limits of viability: a survey among Dutch perinatal professionals

R. Geurtzen[1*], Arno Van Heijst[1], Rosella Hermens[2], Hubertina Scheepers[3], Mallory Woiski[4], Jos Draaisma[1] and Marije Hogeveen[1]

Abstract

Background: Since 2010, intensive care can be offered in the Netherlands at 24^{+0} weeks gestation (with parental consent) but the Dutch guideline lacks recommendations on organization, content and preferred decision-making of the counselling. Our aim is to explore preferred prenatal counselling at the limits of viability by Dutch perinatal professionals and compare this to current care.

Methods: Online nationwide survey as part of the PreCo study (2013) amongst obstetricians and neonatologists in all Dutch level III perinatal care centers ($n = 205$).The survey regarded prenatal counselling at the limits of viability and focused on the domains of organization, content and decision-making in both current and preferred practice.

Results: One hundred twenty-two surveys were returned out of 205 eligible professionals (response rate 60%). Organization-wise: more than 80% of all professionals preferred (but currently missed) having protocols for several aspects of counselling, joint counselling by both neonatologist and obstetrician, and the use of supportive materials. Most professionals preferred using national or local data (70%) on outcome statistics for the counselling content, in contrast to the international statistics currently used (74%). Current decisions on initiation care were mostly made together (in 99% parents *and* doctor). This shared decision model was preferred by 95% of the professionals.

Conclusions: Dutch perinatal professionals would prefer more protocolized counselling, joint counselling, supportive material and local outcome statistics. Further studies on both barriers to perform adequate counselling, as well as on Dutch outcome statistics and parents' opinions are needed in order to develop a national framework.

Keywords: Counselling, Decision-making, (extreme) prematurity, (limits of) viability

Background

The anticipated delivery of an extremely premature infant at the limits of viability confronts parents as well as perinatal professionals with medical, ethical and emotional issues; especially when a decision on the initiation of care has to be made. Since the first publication in 2002 by the American Academy of Pediatrics several (albeit different) guidelines and, recommendations and comments on periviability counselling have been published [1–13]. However, there is no universally accepted way of performing prenatal counselling and, consequently, studies describe heterogeneous counselling practices worldwide [14–25].

Some guidelines on resuscitation at the limits of viability have included recommendations on the parental involvement in the decision-making process. However, both the extent of involvement of parents, as well as the range of gestational ages (GA) at which parents should be involved, varies between countries [8, 9, 11, 26].

In 2010, the Dutch guideline on perinatal practice in extremely premature delivery lowered the limit offering intensive care from 25^{+0} to 24^{+0} weeks GA. Just as some international guidelines which include a role for parents the Dutch guideline explicitly requires informed consent of parents when initiating intensive care at 24 weeks GA

* Correspondence: Rosa.Geurtzen@radboudumc.nl
[1]Amalia Children's Hospital, Department of Pediatrics, Radboud university Medical Center, PO Box 9101, 6500HB Nijmegen, The Netherlands
Full list of author information is available at the end of the article

[27]. Although this guideline acknowledges the importance of prenatal counselling, recommendations on organization, content or decision-making of the counselling are very limited. A pilot-study exploring prenatal counselling in a simulated setting in a Dutch and American cohort (2010), showed heterogeneity in content and decision-making [28]. Although there are some recommendations on counselling [1–11], they may not be generally applicable in the Netherlands since cross-cultural differences in perinatal practices, healthcare organization, and physician and patient views are likely to exist [8, 9, 11, 26–31].

To compose a national framework on prenatal counselling at the limits of viability (currently 24 weeks GA in the Netherlands), the nationwide PreCo study (Prenatal Counselling in Prematurity) was designed, examining both professional and parental views. High quality of care originates when no differences exist between preferred and current counselling with uniformity between the involved caregivers (obstetricians and neonatologists) and specified to the needs of those receiving counselling [17, 21, 22].

The views of parents are at least as important as the view of the professionals in the topic of prenatal counselling at the limits of viability, and they will be studied separately. The primary aim of this study is to explore preferences amongst Dutch perinatal professionals on prenatal counselling at the limits of viability on three domains: *organization*, *content*, and *decision-making-process*. The secondary aim is to study differences between preferred and current counselling and between counselling preferences of neonatal and obstetrical professionals.

Methods
Study design
Cross-sectional study (PreCo survey) using an online survey.

Setting and study population
This study is part of the PreCo study, evaluating Dutch care in (imminent) extremely preterm birth including current and preferred counselling, barriers and facilitators for preferred counselling from both obstetrician and neonatologist, as well as parents' views on this (clinicaltrials.gov, NCT02782650 & NCT02782637). The results of the studies in parents are described [32] and will be described separately.

The care for extreme preterm births is centralized in the Netherlands in 10 level III centers for perinatal care which all participated in this study. Surveys were sent to all fellows and senior staff members in both obstetrics and neonatology. Data were collected from July 2012 through October 2013, approximately two to 3 years after the introduction of the new Dutch guideline on perinatal practice in extreme premature delivery.

Survey design and data collection
We developed the current survey in three stages just as described elsewhere. The first version was based on a combination of literature on prenatal counselling, several prenatal counselling surveys that were kindly shared with us [5, 16, 17, 33–35], observations from previous Dutch studies [28], and on public discussions generated by the Dutch guideline on perinatal practice in extreme premature delivery [27]. This survey was improved in two Delphi rounds containing both four team members and two independent professionals. The entire PreCo-survey required ~20 min to complete. The survey was adapted for both professional groups to exclude irrelevant questions and to optimize the participation rate.

The content of the PreCo survey included two topics on the care for children born at the limits of viability: prenatal counselling (preferred and current) and treatment decisions [36]. For this substudy we were interested in the first: both preferred and current prenatal counselling. We defined three domains of interest to investigate this: 1) *organization* 2) *content* and 3) the *decision-making-process*. We used a fictitious case of an 'uncomplicated' extreme premature delivery at 24 weeks to examine the three domains (textbox). The survey questions were designed to ask for both the preferred and current practice (Additional files 1 and 2).

Characteristics of the fictitious case

A consultation for prenatal counselling with an impending extreme premature delivery, singleton fetus, unremarkable history of pregnancy, average estimated fetal birth weight, unknown gender, no known congenital abnormalities, unremarkable social and medical history of parents, antenatal corticosteroids have been administered and normal fetal heart rate recording.

An individual link to the online survey was sent to all participants. Three reminders were sent to non-responders. Survey results were anonymized before analysis. This study was exempt from IRB approval.

Data analysis
Summary statistics were given as proportions of the respondents for that specific question. To compare preferred counselling with current counselling McNemars χ^2, Bowker McNemars χ^2 or Wilcoxon-signed-rank test were used when applicable. For comparison of the counselling methods of obstetricians and neonatologists χ^2, Fisher exact test (F.ex) or Mann Whitney U test (MWU) were used when applicable. Exact p values were provided, values <0.05 were considered significant. Statistical analyses were conducted using IBM SPSS Statistics (Version 20.0. Armonk, NY: IBM Corp).

Results

Demographics

We received 122 surveys from 205 eligible perinatal professionals[1]; a response rate of 60%. Of those, 45 were from obstetricians and 77 from neonatologists. Each Dutch perinatal center was represented by at least five respondents. Of all 122 returned surveys, eight were partially completed. Obstetricians had fewer years of experience than neonatologists (Table 1).

Organization of prenatal counselling

With respect to the person who should conduct the counselling of the prospective parents, perinatal professionals (91%) preferred this done by the obstetrician and neonatologist jointly, but it occurred in 61% of current practice (Table 2).

Perinatal professionals would preferably like a protocol on several aspects of prenatal counselling (Table 3); who should be counselling (94%) and at which GA (98%), which topics should be discussed (85%), and the GA at which intensive care can be offered (98%) and comfort care accepted (84%). In current practice, some of these aspects were already put into protocols.

Neonatologists wanted to use more supporting material in their consultation ($p < 0.01$); either written (93%) or online (65%) information or a decision-aid (DA) (42%). This was different from the current situation where only 38% of the neonatologists used written information. Other modalities were used less (website 7%, video 3%, DA 1%, other 7%).

Starting at $24^{+0/7}$ weeks of GA, obstetricians preferred to ask the neonatologist often or always (98%) to provide counselling to parents in imminent preterm delivery (Fig. 1). At 22 weeks of GA, neonatologists should never or rarely be asked according to 86% of the obstetricians. At 23 weeks of GA, there was no consensus.

Of the neonatologists, 58% preferred to have more than one prenatal counselling meeting with the parents, significantly different from current practice (only 18% had more than one meeting) ($p < 0.01$). Preferably counselling should take between 15 and 45 min,

Table 2 Person(s) who generally conduct(s) the prenatal counselling with the parents

	Preferred	Current
Neonatologist	3%	22%
Gynecologist	0%	1%
Obstetrician + neonatologist jointly	91%	61%*
Obstetrician + neonatologist not jointly	3%	15%
Other	3%	2%

* p 0.01 (McNemar Bowker)

comparable with current practice. The content of the consultation should be documented in both the mother's and the infant's medical record (76%) which was different from the current situation where it was documented only in the mother's file (58%) ($p < 0.01$).

Content of prenatal counselling

An overview of topics (from a predefined list) that neonatologists think should be discussed during prenatal counselling is given in order of frequency in Table 4. The most important topics were: mortality, morbidity, intubation/ventilation and intraventricular hemorrhage.

When providing outcome statistics, perinatal professionals preferred to use national (48%) or hospital-specific (22%) outcome statistics. Only 21% preferred international data, which was used by the majority in current practice (74%) (p < 0.01). Not every neonatologist did provide outcome statistics in current practice: the 'mortality rate for the unborn fetus' was provided by 38%, the 'mortality rate for live-born infants' was provided by 66% and the 'survival rate without severe disabilities' was provided by 76%. When providing prognostic statistics, there was a wide range in the used percentages by neonatologists (Fig. 2).

Table 1 Characteristics of perinatal professionals

	Obstetricians (n = 84 sent)	Neonatologists (n = 121 sent)
Response rate	54%	64%
Gender, % male	32%	69%
Having children (parent)	91%	83%
Of those: parent of premature child (<27 weeks)	0%	2%
Median age in years (q25-75)	40 (38-47)	45 (37-50)
Median years of experience (q25-75)	5 (1-10)	9 (4-17)*

*p 0.02 (MWU)

Table 3 Existence of protocols for the different aspects of prenatal counselling mentioned

	% of perinatal professionals that do have a protocol	
	Preferred	Current
The GA at which the obstetrician or gynecologist has to ask a neonatologist or pediatrician to provide prenatal counselling to the parents	98%	80% *
The professional who conducts the consultation with the parents	94%	76% *
The topics that should at least be discussed during prenatal counselling	85%	41% *
The minimal GA for offering intensive treatment at birth	98%	88% **
The GA (upper/lower limit) at which the parents' opinion can be decisive in whether or not to initiate intensive treatment at birth	84%	60% *

* p < 0.01 ** p = <0.05 (McNemar) comparing preferred and current practices

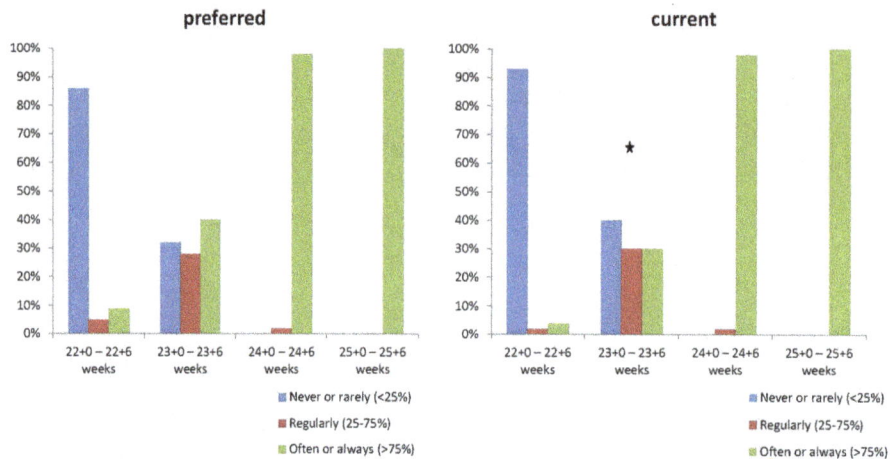

Fig. 1 Percentages of obstetricians that ask the neonatologist for prenatal counselling in threatened preterm delivery

Table 4 Topics preferably addressed during prenatal counselling

Topics to be discussed (preferred)	(% of neonatologists)
The chance the baby will have disabilities (morbidity)	96%
The chance the baby will die (mortality)	94%
Intubation and/or ventilation	93%
Intraventricular hemorrhage	91%
Cognitive impairment (e.g. mental retardation)	90%
Motor impairment (e.g. cerebral palsy)	88%
Susceptibility for (nosocomial) infections	85%
Who will be present during the delivery	82%
RDS and/or surfactant administration	78%
Expected duration of the hospital stay	75%
Breast milk and/or pumping	74%
Total Parental Nutrition (TPN)	70%
Long term pulmonary impairment	67% (*)
Non-invasive respiratory support	60%
Vision problems and/or ROP	58% (*)
Tube feeding	58%
Necrotizing enterocolitis	54%
Infection as a cause of premature delivery	49%
Social services that are available	47%
Hearing problems	47% (*)
Apneas and/or caffeine	25%
Visiting hours	17%
Hygienic rules	13% (*)
Financial consequences for the family	11% (*)

(*) $p < 0.05$ compared to current practice

Decision-making in prenatal counselling

The decision to initiate intensive care treatment should, according to perinatal professionals, preferably be made using the shared decision making (SDM) model 95% strongly agreed (Fig. 3). There was less preference for the other models, of all perinatal professionals 27% agreed with the informed and 13% with the paternalistic model as preferred decision-model. There was a significant disagreement within the informed model; obstetricians mainly agreed and neonatologists mainly disagreed with this model.

Current decisions were mostly made by the parents and doctor together (99%). Of those decisions, 28% stated that the professional opinion is decisive, 24% said parents and professional were equally decisive and for 47% the parental opinion was decisive. In these, there were no differences between obstetricians and neonatologists.

Other

Six potential indicators of high quality of prenatal counselling were rated. In order of importance, the indicator *health care professional and parents take the decision together equally (shared-decision making)* scored highest (86% of the participants thought this was a fairly good or very good indicator), followed by *when the parents are very satisfied with the consultation* (78% fairly good or very good) and *when the content and percentages are medically accurate* (68% fairly good or very good). Lower scores were found for *when the health care professional is very satisfied with the consultation* (44% fairly good or very good), *when all possible complications of premature delivery are discussed* (37% fairly good or very good) and *the length of the consultation – the longer, the better/more accurate* (4% fairly good or very good).

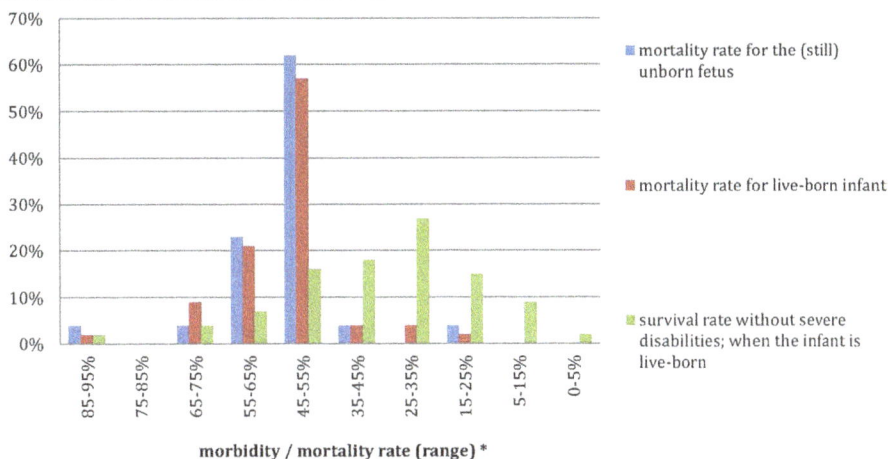

Fig. 2 Morbidity and mortality rates currently provided by neonatologist during prenatal counselling (24 weeks GA)

Discussion

This nationwide study on prenatal counselling includes both obstetricians and neonatologists from all level III perinatal care centers. In the domain of *organization*, perinatal professionals preferred joint counselling by both the obstetrician and neonatologist, protocols for several aspects of prenatal counselling, supportive material, and the neonatologist to join counselling starting at 23-24 weeks GA. In the domain of *content*, the most important topics to discuss were: mortality, morbidity, intubation/ventilation and intraventricular hemorrhage. Perinatal professionals wanted national or hospital based outcome statistics. In the domain of *decision-making*, perinatal professionals preferred the SDM-model to decide whether or not to initiate treatment. Results of this study can be used when developing a national framework, combined with the results from parental preferences and qualitative explorations.

Organization of prenatal counselling

Prenatal counselling done together by the neonatologist and obstetrician was preferred just as recommended internationally [1, 2]. Further qualitative research is required to study why this is not usually done in current care, but a hypothesis is that caregivers are simply not simultaneously available at all hours of the day.

The content of the consultation should be documented in both mother's and infant's file instead of just in the mother's file. It is known that records of antenatal consultations were often lacking important information [37]. A technical barrier might be the absence of a medical record for an unborn baby.

A preference for more guidance of prenatal counselling at the limits of viability was reported. In other countries several guidelines and recommendations have been suggested to support professionals performing this difficult task [1–3, 6, 11]. However, disadvantages were

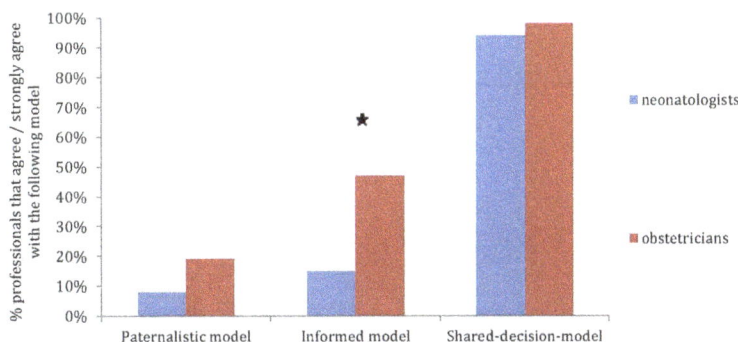

Fig. 3 Preferred decision-making-model at 24 weeks GA on initiating intensive treatment at birth or not. Answer options: •The decision to initiate intensive treatment at birth should only be made by a health care professional (paternalistic model). •The decision to initiate intensive treatment at birth should be made by the parents, after prenatal counselling (informed model). •The decision to initiate intensive treatment at birth should be made by the health care professional and parents together (shared-decision model)

mentioned by Janvier [38], who advocates for an approach where doctors should personalize their information and distinguish what specific information parents need. An individual approach and a guideline might not necessarily conflict: a framework on certain aspects of counselling can be of additional value without standardizing prenatal counselling sessions, especially when it's not too rigid and incorporates solutions to help professionals personalizing the counselling.

Dutch neonatologists wanted to use more supportive material. Grobman found that 60% of parents asked for written material, in contrast to 15% of the physicians who were concerned that clinical conditions could change so rapidly that static resources would not be effective [19]. In 2012, Muthusamy showed in a randomized controlled trial that supplementation of face-to-face verbal counselling with written information improved knowledge and decreased anxiety in women expecting a premature delivery [39]. Guillen and Kakkilaya suggest benefit by the use of a DA [40, 41].

Currently, at a nonviable GA the neonatologist was not considered to take part in counselling in the Netherlands. This in contrast to e.g. California (survey from 1996) and the Pacific Rim (survey from 1999 to 2000) in which at 22 and 23 weeks GA neonatologists were asked to counsel parents [14, 42] The presence of a neonatologist might be helpful, even to explain the rationale of non-active management and to offer comfort care in live-born, immature infants, although a barrier is present since only neonatologists in tertiary centers are trained to counsel these parents.

Content of prenatal counselling

Many topics were considered important to discuss. However, time might be limited due to an impending delivery and parents will not remember everything when overloaded with information [43]. Therefore, parents' view on which content should be discussed is essential. From a caregivers perspective, a vast majority preferred to discuss two of the major disabilities (motor and cognitive impairment), but the other two major disabilities (blindness and deafness) were considered less important. We hypothesize that this might be explained by the higher incidence of impaired mental development and cerebral palsy compared to blindness and deafness [44].

Variable morbidity and mortality rates were communicated in prenatal counselling. It is difficult to pinpoint *the* correct percentages for the Dutch situation since during this survey no Dutch outcome data were available, and international statistics vary. A considerable number of neonatologists did not even mention prognostic statistics. Statistics may not always be of additional value to parents. Boss found that physicians' predictions of morbidity and death are not central to

parental decision-making regarding delivery room resuscitation [33]. Janvier rightly appoints the disadvantages of using statistics, i.e. that percentages might not be understood, that its interpretation is framing-dependent and that percentages do not predict the outcome for the individual baby [38]. Nevertheless, Partridge found that *"more data on outcomes"* was recommended for NICU counselling by parents, suggesting that parents want to be informed about prognostic statistics [35].

Decision-making in prenatal counselling

SDM was the preferred decision-model at the threshold of viability, which is consistent with other studies [2, 4, 11, 34, 35, 45]. Although in current prenatal counselling 99% of the decisions are made by doctor and parent together, 28% of the caregivers state that *their* decision is decisive. It is likely that caregivers might not be fully aware of the way they perform both their current counselling nor that they understand what SDM actually means. SDM is defined as clinicians and patients making decisions together using the best available evidence. This definition states that patients are encouraged to think along and benefits and harms are discussed together [46]. For the implementation of SDM, ready access to evidence based information about treatment options must be met, as well as guidance on how to weigh up the pros and cons of different options and a supportive clinical culture that facilitates patient engagement. Although neonatologists agreed that a DA could be helpful, earlier studies suggested a paternalistic approach [28] and even in this current survey, some of the participants did endorse the informed and/or paternalistic model as well as SDM.

Other

Participants regarded the implementation of SDM a good indicator for a high quality consultation. Furthermore, they thought an important indicator is *when parents were very satisfied with the consultation* – more important than the satisfaction of the professional. Therefore it is of utmost importance to reveal the preferences of parents in the prenatal counselling. Especially since it is known that views of professionals and parents might differ [47, 48]. Input of professionals and parents should be used for the development of (local) recommendations for prenatal counselling in extreme prematurity.

Strengths and limitations

The strongest aspect of this study is its nationwide character, together with an adequate response rate. Part of the survey was directly related to content of the Dutch guideline on perinatal practice, making it relevant for daily practice. This guideline recommends counselling but without giving tools to do so. Our nationwide PreCo study has been set up to examine this counselling, starting with this first exploration of preferred and current counselling.

The limitation of the survey methodology is a potential discrepancy between answers given and actual practice. Besides, direct observations of the counselling conversations could potentially reveal other strengths and weaknesses than we have questioned in this survey, especially interpersonal communication is not easily highlighted in a survey. Due to the inclusion period, effects of experience or learning cannot be ruled out. Furthermore, these Dutch results may not be generalized to an international population. However, both guidelines and a 'gray zone of viability' exist worldwide, and although these are not exactly similar to the Dutch counterpart, general conclusions might be applicable.

Conclusion

This first study on prenatal counselling in the Netherlands revealed differences between preferred and current counselling, and between obstetricians and neonatologists, suggesting a potential for improvement. Further studies looking into the barriers of preferred prenatal counselling [49] could be used to make improvements. Also, preferences of parents will be investigated.

Variation in prenatal counselling is in the best interest of the patient when due to individual (maternal or fetal) characteristics or parental beliefs. When, however, variation is due to unclear background information, insufficient organizational support or incorrect personal habits of healthcare providers, it is not in the best interest of the patient. The use of a nationally developed and supported framework might improve quality of prenatal consultation and even give more scope for individualization.

Endnotes

[1]When in this manuscript the *perinatal professionals* were mentioned: both obstetricians and neonatologists are meant. Since some in-depth questions were asked only to one of the disciplines, we then noted the applicable discipline (either neonatologists or obstetricians)

Additional files

Additional file 1: Survey neonatologists. Survey presented to the neonatologists, translated from Dutch to English. *Note: The actual survey was sent out online, with a different lay-out.*

Additional file 2: Survey obstetricians. Survey presented to the obstetricians, translated from Dutch to English. *Note: The actual survey was sent out online, with a different lay-out.*

Abbreviations
DA: decision-aid; F.ex: Fisher exact test,; GA: gestational age; MWU: Mann Whitney U test; SDM: shared-decision-making,

Acknowledgements
The authors would like to thank all participating Dutch obstetricians and neonatologists. Also, the authors would like to thank all authors who shared their survey with us [5, 16, 17, 33–35].

Funding
No external funding for this manuscript. All authors have indicated they have no financial relationships relevant to this article to disclose.

Authors' contributions
RG conceptualized the study, designed the survey, carried out the data collection and initial analysis, interpreted the results, drafted the initial manuscript and approved the final manuscript as submitted. AvH and JD conceptualized the study, helped designing the survey, interpreted the results, critically reviewed and revised the manuscript and approved the final manuscript as submitted. RH and MW helped designing the survey, interpreted the results, critically reviewed and revised the manuscript and approved the final manuscript as submitted. HS interpreted the results, critically reviewed and revised the manuscript and approved the final manuscript as submitted. MH conceptualized the study, helped designing the survey, supervised data collection and analysis, interpreted the results, critically reviewed and revised the manuscript and approved the final manuscript as submitted. All authors have read and approved the final version of this manuscript.

Competing interests
All authors declare that they have no competing interest.

Author details
1Amalia Children's Hospital, Department of Pediatrics, Radboud university Medical Center, PO Box 9101, 6500HB Nijmegen, The Netherlands. 2Scientific Institute for Quality of Care, Radboud university medical center, Nijmegen, The Netherlands. 3Department of Gynecology, Maastricht UMC+, Maastricht, The Netherlands. 4Amalia Children's Hospital, Department of Gynecology, Radboud University Medical Center, Nijmegen, The Netherlands.

References
1. Batton DG, Committee on F, newborn. Clinical report–antenatal counseling regarding resuscitation at an extremely low gestational age. Pediatrics. 2009; 124(1):422–7.
2. Griswold KJ, Fanaroff JM. An evidence-based overview of prenatal consultation with a focus on infants born at the limits of viability. Pediatrics. 2010;125(4):e931–7.
3. Jefferies AL, Kirpalani HM, Canadian Paediatric society F, newborn C. Counselling and management for anticipated extremely preterm birth. Paediatr Child Health. 2012;17(8):443–6.
4. Janvier A, Barrington KJ, Aziz K, Bancalari E, Batton D, Bellieni C, Bensouda B, Blanco C, Cheung PY, Cohn F, et al. CPS position statement for prenatal counselling before a premature birth: simple rules for complicated decisions. Paediatr Child Health. 2014;19(1):22–4.
5. Kaempf JW, Tomlinson M, Arduza C, Anderson S, Campbell B, Ferguson LA, Zabari M, Stewart VT. Medical staff guidelines for periviability pregnancy counseling and medical treatment of extremely premature infants. Pediatrics. 2006;117(1):22–9.
6. Kaempf JW, Tomlinson MW, Campbell B, Ferguson L, Stewart VT. Counseling pregnant women who may deliver extremely premature infants: medical

care guidelines, family choices, and neonatal outcomes. Pediatrics. 2009;123(6):1509–15.

7. Raju TN, Mercer BM, Burchfield DJ, Joseph GF Jr. Periviable birth: executive summary of a joint workshop by the Eunice Kennedy Shriver National Institute of Child Health and Human Development, Society for Maternal-Fetal Medicine, American Academy of Pediatrics, and American College of Obstetricians and Gynecologists. Obstet Gynecol. 2014;123(5):1083–96.

8. Gallagher K, Martin J, Keller M, Marlow N. European variation in decision-making and parental involvement during preterm birth. Arch Dis Child Fetal Neonatal Ed. 2014;99(3):F245–9.

9. Pignotti MS, Donzelli G. Perinatal care at the threshold of viability: an international comparison of practical guidelines for the treatment of extremely preterm births. Pediatrics. 2008;121(1):e193–8.

10. MacDonald H, American Academy of Pediatrics. Committee on F, Newborn. Perinatal care at the threshold of viability. Pediatrics. 2002;110(5):1024–7.

11. Cummings J, Committee On F, Newborn. Antenatal counseling regarding resuscitation and intensive care before 25 weeks of gestation. Pediatrics. 2015;136(3):588–95.

12. Guillen U, Weiss EM, Munson D, Maton P, Jefferies A, Norman M, Naulaers G, Mendes J, Justo da Silva L, Zoban P, et al. Guidelines for the Management of Extremely Premature Deliveries: a systematic review. Pediatrics. 2015;136(2):343–50.

13. Ohlinger J, Kantak A, Lavin JP Jr, Fofah O, Hagen E, Suresh G, Halamek LP, Schriefer JA. Evaluation and development of potentially better practices for perinatal and neonatal communication and collaboration. Pediatrics. 2006;118(Suppl 2):S147–52.

14. Martinez AM, Partridge JC, Yu V, Wee Tan K, Yeung CY, JH L, Nishida H, Boo NY. Physician counselling practices and decision-making for extremely preterm infants in the Pacific Rim. J Paediatr Child Health. 2005;41(4):209–14.

15. Mulvey S, Partridge JC, Martinez AM, VY Y, Wallace EM. The management of extremely premature infants and the perceptions of viability and parental counselling practices of Australian obstetricians. Aust N Z J Obstet Gynaecol. 2001;41(3):269–73.

16. Bastek TK, Richardson DK, Zupancic JA, Burns JP. Prenatal consultation practices at the border of viability: a regional survey. Pediatrics. 2005;116(2):407–13.

17. Chan KL, Kean LH, Marlow N. Staff views on the management of the extremely preterm infant. Eur J Obstet Gynecol Reprod Biol. 2006;128(1-2):142–7.

18. Govande VP, Brasel KJ, Das UG, Koop JI, Lagatta J, Basir MA. Prenatal counseling beyond the threshold of viability. J Perinatol. 2013;33(5):358–62.

19. Grobman WA, Kavanaugh K, Moro T, DeRegnier RA, Savage T. Providing advice to parents for women at acutely high risk of periviable delivery. Obstet Gynecol. 2010;115(5):904–9.

20. Mehrotra A, Lagatta J, Simpson P, Kim UO, Nugent M, Basir MA. Variations among US hospitals in counseling practices regarding prematurely born infants. J Perinatol. 2013;33(7):509–13.

21. Taittonen L, Korhonen P, Palomaki O, Luukkaala T, Tammela O. Opinions on the counselling, care and outcome of extremely premature birth among healthcare professionals in Finland. Acta Paediatr. 2014;103(3):262–7.

22. Duffy D, Reynolds P. Babies born at the threshold of viability: attitudes of paediatric consultants and trainees in south East England. Acta Paediatr. 2011;100(1):42–6.

23. Tucker Edmonds B, McKenzie F, Panoch JE, Barnato AE, Frankel RM. Comparing obstetricians' and neonatologists' approaches to periviable counseling. J Perinatol. 2015;35(5):344–8.

24. Keenan HT, Doron MW, Seyda BA. Comparison of mothers' and counselors' perceptions of predelivery counseling for extremely premature infants. Pediatrics. 2005;116(1):104–11.

25. Tucker Edmonds B, Krasny S, Srinivas S, Shea J. Obstetric decision-making and counseling at the limits of viability. Am J Obstet Gynecol. 2012;206(3):248 e241-245.

26. Brunkhorst J, Weiner J, Lantos J. Infants of borderline viability: the ethics of delivery room care. Semin Fetal Neonatal Med. 2014;19(5):290–5.

27. de Laat MW, Wiegerinck MM, Walther FJ, Boluyt N, Mol BW, van der Post JA, van Lith JM, Offringa M, Nederlandse Vereniging voor K, Nederlandse Vereniging voor Obstetrie en G. Practice guideline 'Perinatal management of extremely preterm delivery'. Ned Tijdschr Geneeskd. 2010;154:A2701.

28. Geurtzen R, Hogeveen M, Rajani AK, Chitkara R, Antonius T, van Heijst A, Draaisma J, Halamek LP. Using simulation to study difficult clinical issues:

29. prenatal counseling at the threshold of viability across American and Dutch cultures. Simul Healthc. 2014;9(3):167–73.

29. Cuttini M. Neonatal intensive care and parental participation in decision making. Arch Dis Child Fetal Neonatal Ed. 2001;84(1):F78.

30. Lorenz JM, Paneth N, Jetton JR, den Ouden L, Tyson JE. Comparison of management strategies for extreme prematurity in New Jersey and the Netherlands: outcomes and resource expenditure. Pediatrics. 2001;108(6):1269–74.

31. Lantos JD. International and cross-cultural dimensions of treatment decisions for neonates. Semin Fetal Neonatal Med. 2015;20(5):368–72.

32. Geurtzen R, Draaisma J, Hermens R, Scheepers H, Woiski M, van Heijst A, et al. Prenatal (non) treatment decisions in extreme prematurity: evaluation of decisional conflict and regret among parents. J Perinatol. 2017;37(9):999-1002.

33. Geurtzen R, Draaisma J, Hermens R, Scheepers H, Woiski M, van Heijst A, Hogeveen M. Perinatal practice in extreme premature delivery: variation in Dutch physicians' preferences despite guideline. Eur J Pediatr. 2016;175(8):1039–46.

34. Kavanaugh K, Savage T, Kilpatrick S, Kimura R, Hershberger P. Life support decisions for extremely premature infants: report of a pilot study. J Pediatr Nurs. 2005;20(5):347–59.

35. Partridge JC, Martinez AM, Nishida H, Boo NY, Tan KW, Yeung CY, JH L, VY Y. International comparison of care for very low birth weight infants: parents' perceptions of counseling and decision-making. Pediatrics. 2005;116(2):e263–71.

36. Boss RD, Hutton N, Sulpar LJ, West AM, Donohue PK. Values parents apply to decision-making regarding delivery room resuscitation for high-risk newborns. Pediatrics. 2008;122(3):583–9.

37. Janvier A, Barrington KJ. The ethics of neonatal resuscitation at the margins of viability: informed consent and outcomes. J Pediatr. 2005;147(5):579–85.

38. Janvier A, Lorenz JM, Lantos JD. Antenatal counselling for parents facing an extremely preterm birth: limitations of the medical evidence. Acta Paediatr. 2012;101(8):800–4.

39. Muthusamy AD, Leuthner S, Gaebler-Uhing C, Hoffmann RG, Li SH, Basir MA. Supplemental written information improves prenatal counseling: a randomized trial. Pediatrics. 2012;129(5):e1269–74.

40. Guillen U, Suh S, Munson D, Posencheg M, Truitt E, Zupancic JA, Gafni A, Kirpalani H. Development and pretesting of a decision-aid to use when counseling parents facing imminent extreme premature delivery. J Pediatr. 2012;160(3):382–7.

41. Kakkilaya V, Groome LJ, Platt D, Kurepa D, Pramanik A, Caldito G, Conrad L, Bocchini JA, Jr., Davis TC: Use of a visual aid to improve counseling at the threshold of viability. Pediatrics 2011, 128(6):e1511-e1519.

42. Partridge JC, Freeman H, Weiss E, Martinez AM. Delivery room resuscitation decisions for extremely low birthweight infants in California. J Perinatol. 2001;21(1):27–33.

43. Kessels RP. Patients' memory for medical information. J R Soc Med. 2003;96(5):219–22.

44. Lorenz JM. The outcome of extreme prematurity. Semin Perinatol. 2001;25(5):348–59.

45. Haward MF, Kirshenbaum NW, Campbell DE. Care at the edge of viability: medical and ethical issues. Clin Perinatol. 2011;38(3):471–92.

46. Elwyn G, Laitner S, Coulter A, Walker E, Watson P, Thomson R. Implementing shared decision making in the NHS. BMJ. 2010;341:c5146.

47. Roscigno CI, Savage TA, Kavanaugh K, Moro TT, Kilpatrick SJ, Strassner HT, Grobman WA, Kimura RE. Divergent views of hope influencing communications between parents and hospital providers. Qual Health Res. 2012;22(9):1232–46.

48. Zupancic JA, Kirpalani H, Barrett J, Stewart S, Gafni A, Streiner D, Beecroft ML, Smith P. Characterising doctor-parent communication in counselling for impending preterm delivery. Arch Dis Child Fetal Neonatal Ed. 2002;87(2):F113–7.

49. Geurtzen R, van Heijst A, Draaisma J, Ouwerkerk L, Scheepers H, Woiski M, Hermens R, Hogeveen M. Professionals' preferences in prenatal counseling at the limits of viability: a nationwide qualitative Dutch study. Eur J Pediatr. 2017;176(8):1107–19.

2

The role of community-based health services in influencing postnatal care visits in the Builsa and the West Mamprusi districts in rural Ghana

Evelyn Sakeah[1*] [iD], Raymond Aborigo[1], James Kotuah Sakeah[2], Maxwell Dalaba[1], Ernest Kanyomse[1], Daniel Azongo[1], Dominic Anaseba[1], Samuel Oladokun[1] and Abraham Rexford Oduro[1]

Abstract

Background: Globally, maternal mortality is still a challenge. In Ghana, maternal morbidity and mortality rates remain high, particularly in rural areas. Postnatal Care (PNC) is one of the key strategies for improving maternal health. This study examined determinants of at least three PNC visits in rural Ghana.

Methods: We conducted a cross-sectional study at the Community-Based Health Planning and Services (CHPS) Zones in the Builsa and West Mamprusi Districts between April and June 2016. We selected 650 women who delivered within 5 years preceding the survey (325 from each of the two sites) using the two-stage random sampling technique.

Results: Of the 650 respondents, 62% reported attending postnatal care at least three times. In the Builsa district, the percentage of women who made at least three PNC visits were 90% compared with 35% in the West Mamprusi district. Older women and those who attended antenatal clinics at least four times (AOR: 5.23; 95% CI: 2.49–11.0) and women who had partners with some secondary education (AOR: 3.31; 95% CI: 1.17–9.39) were associated with at least three PNC visits.

Conclusions: Men engagement in maternal health services and the introduction of home-based PNC services in rural communities could help health workers reach out to many mothers and children promptly and improve PNC visits in those communities.

Keywords: Community-based health service delivery-Ghana- maternal mortality-women service utilization-postnatal care

Background

Despite the establishment of a number of global and national initiatives to improve maternal health, maternal mortality is still a major concern in sub-Saharan Africa [1]. Every year in Africa, at least 125,000 women and 870,000 newborns die in the first week after birth [2]. In 2015, global maternal mortality was 303,000 with sub-Saharan Africa accounting for the highest number of deaths (201,000) [1]. In 2015, Ghana recorded 2800 maternal deaths which is high when compared with other sub-Saharan Africa countries [1]. Ghana is one of the countries that failed to achieve the targets set for the fourth and fifth Millennium Development Goals [3].

Postnatal care (PNC) is the care given to the mother and her newborn baby immediately after the birth and for the first 6 weeks of life [2]. The PNC period is crucial for both the mother and the newborn [2, 4, 5]. The first 6 weeks after birth is known as the PNC period [2]. The first day after birth is associated with the highest risk for both mother and baby [2]. Most deaths occur during the first 24 h after childbirth and half of maternal and neonatal deaths occur during the first week after birth [4]. Postpartum haemorrhage is the main cause of maternal mortality [4, 5]. Other causes include complications

* Correspondence: esakeah@yahoo.co.uk
[1]Navrongo Health Research Centre, Post Office Box 114, Navrongo, Upper East Region, Ghana
Full list of author information is available at the end of the article

from unsafe abortion, hypertensive disorders during pregnancy, postpartum infections, obstructed labor [6] puerperal sepsis [5] and HIV [4].

For babies, many of them die due to birth asphyxia during the first day after birth and a lot more because they are born preterm [2]. In the second week after birth, about 38% of them in sub-Saharan Africa die due to infections [2]. Long term disability and poor development of both the child and the mother is reported to be associated with the early postnatal period [2].

Recognizing the role of PNC during this critical period for mothers and babies, the WHO recommended at least three PNC visits for all nursing mothers to ensure their survival and that of their newborns [7]. PNC is important to identify and manage complications that arise as a result of child birth and to provide health information that is beneficial to both mother and baby [2, 4, 5]. It ensures monitoring of women and their newborns in the pueperium so as to reduce morbidity and mortality risks. PNC also ensures prompt access to family planning services to prevent poorly spaced pregnancies [2].

In the national safe motherhood service protocol of Ghana, it is specified that all pregnant women attend PNC at least three times for uncomplicated pregnancies with more visits recommended in case of complications [8]. The first PNC visit is within 48 h, the second by day 7 and the third, 6 weeks after birth [9]. PNC is high (78%) across the country but the proportion of women receiving a PNC check-up within 2 days of delivery is higher in urban than rural settings [10]. Also, the number of women receiving the three recommended PNC visits in rural Ghana is low [10], thus necessitating an enquiry into the factors that are associated with such low attendance.

A number of studies have examined factors that influence utilization of PNC services by mothers [11–20]. Some have highlighted important linkages between demographic factors such as parity, birth rank, number of pregnancies, religion, mother's education and utilization of PNC services [14–17, 20]. Studies in developing countries such as Ethiopia and Nepal show that access to economic resources ensures that women are able to finance their deliveries in health facilities and are able to obtain subsequent services such as PNC [15, 17]. Besides, women with better financial resources have a better chance of benefiting from health education campaigns through media outlets like television, and newspapers because they are able to afford them [17]. Also, physical access as well as the geographical location of the mother have been shown to influence the use of PNC services [15, 19]. At the individual and social levels, factors like ANC attendance, skilled attendant during child birth, place of delivery, previous use of PNC services, and experience of medical complications have had

significant influence on utilization of PNC services as observed by several studies [13, 15, 16, 19].

UNICEF together with the Ghana Health Service pilot-tested a package of interventions that focused on maternal, neonatal and child health (MNCH) within the framework of the life cycle approach in the Builsa Districts from 2012 to 2017 aimed at reducing maternal, newborn and child health mortality in the Builsa Districts [21]. As part of the intervention strategies UNICEF/Ghana Health Service implemented home-based postnatal care in the Community-based Health Planning and Services (CHPS) zones. The health providers visited women, who resided far away or were unable to come to the health facilities for care to provide postnatal services at their doorsteps [21]. This study evaluates the effectiveness of the intervention program comparing PNC service access in CHPS zones in two rural communities, one with home-based postnatal care (Builsa) and one without this service (West Mamprusi).

Primary health care

Primary health care in Ghana is delivered through the CHPS Program and the health centres. After many years of investigation into appropriate strategies for service delivery in rural settings, the CHPS Initiative has adapted strategies tested in the successful Navrongo experiment to guide national health reforms that mobilize volunteerism, resources and cultural institutions for supporting community-based primary health care [22]. In 2000 the Ghana Health Service began training Community Health Officers (CHOs) to provide basic services in rural areas through the CHPS program [22]. The CHPS initiative is a community-based health program aimed at increasing availability and access to basic health services including maternal and child health services to rural communities in Ghana [22]. It is a government initiative that brings together CHOs and community members to deliver health services to rural communities [22, 23]. The overall strategic goal of CHPS is to improve the health status of the population by strengthening the health system and empowering communities and households for service delivery and utilization [24]. This study was conducted in CHPS zones to ascertain the percentage of women who have had at least three PNC visits and determine factors associated with at least three PNC visits.

Methods

Study setting

The study was carried out in the Builsa and the West Mamprusi Districts of the Upper East and Northern Regions of Ghana. The population estimate for the 2010 census for the Upper East region was 1,046,545 with 79% being rural while that of the Northern region was 2,479,461 with 70% rural dwellers [25].

The Builsa district which is located in the Upper East Region of Ghana, has a population of 92,991 [25]. In 2012, the district was divided into two-Builsa North and South Districts -but for the purposes of this study, the old demarcation and name of the district would be maintained. The Builsas constitute about 83% of the entire population and the remaining 17% is made up of minor ethnic groups [25]. The district is served by a district hospital located at Sandema, the district capital, four health centres, two private clinics and twenty functional CHPS zones with resident CHOs [26].

The West Mamprusi District was carved out of the Gambaga District in 1988 under the Government of Ghana's decentralization and local government reform policy. The district's administrative capital is Walewale, which lies on the Tamale-Bolgatanga trunk road, approximately 68 miles away from Tamale. The West Mamprusi District has a population of 117,821 made up of mostly Mamprusis who constitute about 75% of the total population [25]. There are three main ethnic groups (Mamprusis, Kantosis and Comas) mixed with settlers such as Frafras, Kassenas, Bulisas, Zambarmas and Hausas. The most widely spoken language is Mampruli [26]. The districts' health infrastructure is made up of one hospital in Walewale, one polyclinic, one health centre, two clinics and six functional CHPS zones with resident CHOs [26].

The study was conducted in the two districts because of the vast differences in health infrastructure, particularly the number of CHPS compounds and human resources.

Study design

This was a cross-sectional household survey with women who had ever given birth in the 5 years prior to the study in the Builsa and the West Mamprusi Districts.

Sample size and sampling

The sample size was calculated based on the average proportion of skilled delivery (50%) in the Upper East and Northern Regions with 5 year annual average of skilled delivery (2005–2009) of 1250 in the two districts (Builsa and West Mamprusi Districts) and 95% confidence interval as well as a corresponding $p < 0.05$ for significance. We used the formula for sample size $n = \{DEFF*Np (1-p)\}/ \{(d^2/Z^2_{1-\alpha/2}*(N-1) + p*(1-p)\}$ [27] and this gave a sample size of 295 women. We assumed a refusal rate of 10%, which brought the total sample size for each district to 325 women.

A two-stage sampling method was used and the primary sampling unit was the enumeration area (EA), defined as the geographic area canvassed by one census representative. Sampling EAs and households was based on the assumptions that: [1] CHOs were working in these EAs in the two districts and [2] there is homogeneity in the provision of CHO services across the EAs.

The first stage involved selecting geographical clusters or EAs, from an updated master sampling frame constructed from the 2000 Ghana Population and Housing Census. A total of 50 clusters were selected from the master sampling frame of 323 (West Mamprusi-197 and Builsa Districts-144). The clusters were randomly selected from the list of EAs in each district. The selection was based on a simple random technique. In the second stage of selection, we listed all households in the selected enumeration areas (clusters) and used the simple random sampling method to sample 50 of them from each selected cluster. We compiled the list of women with children less than 5 years in each household and randomly selected one of them for the interview. For the random selection process, each eligible member of the household was assigned a unique number, then each number was placed in a bowl and mixed thoroughly. The fieldworker then randomly picked numbered tags from the bowl and interviewed the selected women. A total of 1623 eligible women were on the household list compiled for the study.

Data collection

Data was collected using a structured questionnaire, which included items concerning social and demographic characteristics, such as age, religion, marital status, education and partner's education, the wealth of the woman, ethnicity, religion, ANC attendance during previous pregnancy, skilled attendant at birth and PNC visits. Age represented the woman's age at the time of interview, marital status reflected the type of union the respondents were involved in. Woman and partner's education reflected the educational levels of respondents and their partners, respectively. Wealth index reflected their financial status, which was based on household assets. The questionnaire was developed in the English language, but the research team translated it into Buli and Mampruli-the major languages of the study areas. The questionnaire was pretested in communities outside the study sites. We trained six senior high school graduates as fieldworkers and two university graduates as supervisors for the data collection. The fieldworkers had a two-week training prior to the survey and visited households to interview eligible women. We started fieldwork on the 14th of April and ended on the 13th of June, 2016.

Data analysis

We performed descriptive statistics, bivariate and multivariable analysis. All p-values were two-tailed, and a value of $p < 0.05$ was considered significant. The outcome

Table 1 Socio-demographic characteristics of respondents

Characteristics	Builsa District ($n = 325$) N (%)		West Mamprusi District ($n = 325$) N (%)		Both Districts ($n = 650$) N (%)		p-value[†]
Age group							< 0.001
15–24	108	(33.7)	63	(19.6)	171	(26.7)	
25–34	133	(41.6)	182	(56.7)	315	(49.1)	
35–49	79	(24.7)	76	(23.7)	115	(24.2)	
Religion							< 0.001
Traditional	70	(21.6)	13	(4.0)	83	(12.8)	
Christianity	249	(76.9)	79	(24.3)	328	(50.5)	
Islam	5	(1.5)	233	(71.7)	238	(36.7)	
Ethnicity							< 0.001
Builsa	324	(99.7)	2	(0.6)	326	(50.2)	
Mamprusi		NA	188	(57.9)	188	(28.9)	
Other	1	(0.3)	135	(41.5)	136	(20.9)	
Marital status							
Married	309	(95.4)	317	(97.5)	626	(96.5)	0.135
Single/widowed/separated	15	(4.6)	8	(2.5)	23	(3.5)	
Education							
None	165	(50.8)	175	(53.9)	340	(52.3)	
Primary	69	(21.2)	73	(22.5)	142	(21.9)	
Middle/JSS/JHS	64	(19.7)	46	(14.1)	110	(16.9)	
Secondary/SSS/SHS and above	27	(8.3)	31	(9.5)	58	(8.9)	0.305
Partner's Education							
None	223	(68.8)	187	(57.5)	410	(63.2)	< 0.001
Primary	42	(13.0)	35	(10.8)	77	(11.9)	
Middle/JSS/JHS	31	(9.6)	36	(11.1)	67	(10.3)	
Secondary/SSS/SHS and above	28	(8.6)	67	(20.6)	95	(14.6)	
Number of children alive							
1	67	(20.6)	58	(17.9)	125	(19.2)	0.876
2	54	(16.6)	54	(16.6)	108	(16.6)	
3	64	(19.7)	70	(21.5)	134	(20.6)	
4	63	(19.4)	60	(18.5)	123	(18.9)	
5 or more	77	(20.7)	83	(25.5)	160	(20.6)	
Distance to health facility							
Less than 30 min	204	(62.8)	192	(59.1)	396	(60.9)	0.002
30 mins – 2 h	119	(36.6)	116	(35.7)	235	(36.2)	
2 h – 4 h	2	(0.6)	17	(5.2)	19	(2.9)	
Wealth Index							
Poor	40	(16.1)	117	(52.5)	157	(33.4)	< 0.001
Middle	75	(30.3)	82	(36.8)	157	(33.3)	
Rich	133	(53.6)	42	(10.7)	157	(33.3)	
ANC attendance							< 0.001
≥ 4 attendance	298	(93.1)	257	(80.8)	555	(87.0)	
≤ 3 attendance	22	(6.9)	61	(19.2)	83	(13.0)	

Table 1 Socio-demographic characteristics of respondents *(Continued)*

Characteristics	Builsa District (*n* = 325) N (%)		West Mamprusi District (*n* = 325) N (%)		Both Districts (*n* = 650) N (%)		*p*-value[†]
Skilled delivery							< 0.001
Yes	245	(75.4)	186	(57.2)	431	(66.3)	
No	80	(24.6)	139	(42.8)	219	(33.7)	
PNC visits							< 0.001
≥ 3 visits	293	(90.1)	112	(34.5)	405	(62.3)	
≤ 2 visits	32	(9.8)	213	(65.5)	245	(37.7)	

variable for the analysis was at least three PNC visits (Yes or No). This was ascertained by the question: How many times did you receive PNC after your last child birth? We included explanatory variables such as age of the woman, marital status, geographical location, women's education, husband's education, wealth index, religion, ANC attendance and type of delivery. The wealth index consisted of 23 household-related items. These independent variables were selected based on previous studies [28–31]. We generated quintile ranks for wealth status using principal component analysis.

All statistical analyses were performed using Stata Version 12 (Stata Corp., TX).

Results

Respondents' socio-demographic characteristics

Table 1 shows the characteristics of 650 women from the Builsa and the West Mamprusi districts that participated in the study. The number of respondents from these districts were 325 and 325 respectively. Of all the respondents, 50% were Builsa, 29% were Mamprusi, and 21% were other tribes living in the West Mamprusi district. Half of the respondents were Christians, 37% practiced Islam and 28% worshipped ancestral religion (Table 1). Slightly over half of the women and nearly three quarters of their husbands had no education. However, more of the men attained secondary or higher education than the women.

About 87% of the women reported having had at least four ANC attendance, and 66% of them were supervised by a skilled attendant during child birth and 62% had attended PNC at least three times.

The significant difference in the PNC attendance rate between the two districts indicates the need for a stratified analysis and presentation of the data.

Factors associated with PNC visits by Study District

Table 2 presents the results of a regression analysis for at least three PNC visits according to selected characteristics, in the West Mamprusi district. The results revealed that, women who attended ANC four times (AOR: 8.88; 95% CI: 2.94–26.8), aged 36–49 (AOR: 12.33; 95% CI: 2.94–51.9), and whose partners had some

secondary education (AOR: 3.66; 95% CI: 1.57–8.51) were more likely to attend PNC at least three times relative to those who attended ANC three or less times and whose partners had no education respectively.

Table 3 presents regression analysis for at least three PNC visits by selected characteristics in the Builsa district. Adjusted odd ratios revealed that ANC attendance, age, women's education, religion, marital status, partner's education, parity, and distance to health facility, wealth and type of delivery were not associated with PNC visits.

Discussion

The study revealed that 62% of women made at least three PNC visits, despite the wide difference between the two sites. Women attendance of four or more ANCs, age and partner's education were associated with at least three PNC visits in the West Mamprusi district.

In the Builsa district, the percentage of women who made at least four ANC attendance, skilled delivery and at least three PNC visits were 90, 75 and 90% respectively. On the other hand, in the West Mamprusi district, the percentage of women having four ANC attendances, skilled delivery and at least three PNC visits were 81, 57 and 35% respectively. However, our results showed that the differences in use of ANC and skilled delivery in the West Mamprusi District compared to that of Builsa are not as low as that for PNC. The community engagement component of the CHPS program ensures that community health volunteers are able to identify all pregnant women and nursing mothers within their locations and monitor their use of health services [23]. This could have contributed to improved utilization of PNC services in the Builsa district. In addition, the introduction of home-based postnatal care in the Builsa district helped health workers to reach out to many mothers and children promptly and that improved PNC visits in those communities [21]. Home-based care is an integral part of health service delivery, particularly in the Builsa district. The relevance of this approach to health care delivery lies in the wide coverage of services to both mothers and children in the comfort of their homes. The approach brings health services to the doorsteps of

Table 2 Regression Analysis Results for Postnatal Care Attendance in the West Mamprusi District

Characteristic	OR	(95% CI)	AOR	(95% CI)
ANC attendance				
≤ 3 attendance		1		1
≥ 4 attendance	**5.00**	**(2.19–11.41)**	**8.88**	**(2.94–26.8)**
Age group				
15–24 (r)		1		1
25–35	0.81	(0.44–1.48)	2.54	(0.84–7.66)
36–49	1.36	(0.68–2.70)	**12.3**	**(2.94–51.9)**
Woman's education				
None (r)		1		1
Primary	0.97	(0.44–2.16)	1.45	(0.39–5.36)
Some secondary	1.40	(0.55–3.58)	2.95	(0.76–11.5)
Husband's education				
None (r)		1		1
Primary	1.58	(0.74–3.36)	2.82	(0.89–8.95)
Some secondary	**2.33**	**(1.41–3.85)**	**3.66**	**(1.57–8.51)**
Religion				
Traditional		1		1
Christianity	3.74	(0.78–18·0)	8.03	(0.70–92.9)
Islam	2.77	(0.60–12.0)	10.5	(0.92–12.1)
Marital status				
Divorced/widowed/ never married (r)		1		1
Married	0.87	(0.20–3.72)	1.01	(0.09–11.6)
Number of children alive				
1 (r)		1		1
2 + 3	0.84	(0.44–1.60)	0.60	(0.19–1.86)
4+	0.83	(0.44–1.55)	0.76	(0.20–2.86)
Distance to health facility				
Less than 30 min		1		1
30 mins – 2 h	1.19	(0.75–1.89)	0.75	(0.36–1.57)
Wealth Index				
Poor (r)		1		1
Middle	**0.55**	**(0.31–0.99)**	0.63	(0.30–1.31)
Rich	0.56	(0.22–1.42)	1.01	(0.29–3.54)
Skilled delivery				
No		1		1
Yes	1.05	(0.66–1.67)	1.31	(0.65–2.65)

Bold values are significant (*p < 0.05; **p < 0.01; ***p < 0.001) AOR: adjusted odds ratio; CI: confidence interval; JHS: junior high school; JSS: junior secondary school; OR: odds ratio; SHS: senior high school; SSS: senior secondary school

Table 3 Regression Analysis Results for Postnatal Care Attendance in the Builsa District

Characteristic	OR	(95% CI)	AOR	(95% CI)
ANC attendance				
≤ 3 attendance		1		1
≥ 4 attendance	1.46	(0.41–5.25)	3.01	(0.64–14.2)
Age group				
15–24 (r)		1		1
25–35	1.93	(0.85–4.35)	1.44	(0.42–4.90)
36–49	2.57	(0.90–7.35)	1.24	(0.24–6.33)
Woman's Education				
None (r)		1		1
Primary	**4.00**	**(1.34–12.0)**	2.84	(0.55–14.6)
Some secondary	2.33	(0.70–7.02)	2.35	(0.46–12.1)
Husband's Education				
None (r)		1		1
Primary	0.57	(0.19–1.65)	0.74	(0.20–2.75)
Some Secondary	**0.34**	**(0.15–0.77)**	0.60	(0.18–2.02)
Religion				
Traditional		1		1
Christianity	1.04	(0.43–2.53)	1.51	(0.46–4.95)
Marital status				
Divorced/widowed/ never married (r)		1		1
Married	0.64	(0.08–5.04)	0.45	(0.04–5.26)
Number of children alive				
1 (r)		1		1
2 + 3	1.42	(0.58–3.43)	1.01	(0.27–3.76)
4+	2.55	(0.98–6.62)	1.14	(0.21–6.16)
Distance to health facility				
Less than 30 min		1		1
30 mins – 2 h	1.88	(0.82–4.33)	1.65	(0.61–4.50)
Wealth Index				
Poor (r)		1		1
Middle	2.01	(0.54–7.37)	1.22	(0.29–5.14)
Rich	1.04	(0.36–3.05)	0.59	(0.16–2.16)
Skilled delivery				
No		1		1
Yes	0.84	(0.35–2.03)	0.85	(0.26–2.73)

Bold values are significant (*p < 0.05; **p < 0.01; ***p < 0.001)

the people and might have impacted positively on maternal health outcomes in the Builsa district (32). Thus, the home-based postnatal care strategy could have contributed to the difference in the PNC uptake between the two districts. This observation suggests that where health services are brought closer to the people, it could improve the uptake of the services including PNC as reported in other studies in Ethiopia and Tanzania [15, 32, 33].

Women who attended ANC at least four times were more likely to make three or more PNC visits. ANC offers women the opportunity to access health information and to appreciate the importance of PNC. In addition, women who make at least four ANC attendances are more likely to be those who adhere to health recommendations and therefore would make the required number of PNC visits. Evidence from other studies show that ANC attendance strongly predicts utilization of PNC services [17, 32–35].

Older women were associated with at least three PNC visits in the West Mamprusi district. These findings contradict those of Workineh and Hailu (2014), Neupane and Doku (2012) and Rwabufigiri et al. (2016) who said that women with multiple pregnancies usually perceive themselves as having acquired enough experience to handle subsequent pregnancies, hence they fail to use PNC services [20, 36, 37]. The long interaction between women and CHOs through the CHPS program and other community engagement strategies [23, 38] could have contributed to the older women knowing the importance of PNC and therefore utilizing the services. The findings suggest that, previous reproductive health activities such as ANC, skilled delivery, PNC and family planning services offered an important avenue for older women to establish contact with health services and develop a good relationship with health care providers which ultimately leads to an increase in utilization. Also, past experience of medical complications could have influenced the use of PNC services by older women as observed in other studies [15, 16, 19].

Higher educational level of partner was positively associated with at least three PNC visits in the West Mamprusi district. In northern Ghana, men as heads of their lineages have power and authority to make decisions pertaining to their families including maternal health care [39–42]. Although research has shown men's involvement in maternal health services [43, 44], they could do more to improve the health seeking behaviour of their partners by reminding them about appointment days, encouraging them to seek skilled care and accompanying them to the health facility for maternal health services. Also, in patriarchal societies where women lack autonomy, their partners should be given information on the need for routine visits to health care providers during pregnancy as well as the postpartum period to improve maternal and newborn survival.

Study limitations

This study had some limitations. First, recall bias was a potential limitation because some participants could have forgotten about past events involving PNC services, but to minimize this bias, past events were limited to the 5 years preceding the interview. Using different local languages to collect the data could also have distorted the presentation of the questions to the respondents. However, the standard training for fieldworkers and supervisors and the in-depth translation and back translation of the questions minimized the language bias.

Conclusions

Women who have had four ANC visits and those whose partners received some secondary education are more likely to have at least 3 PNC visits. The availability and access to PNC services in rural communities, particularly at the home-based level and male involvement in maternal health care could improve the use of PNC services in rural settings.

These key recommendations could help improve the use of PNC services:

- The Ghana Health Service needs to scale-up the CHPS program to give all community members, particularly pregnant women and nursing mothers in rural communities, the opportunity to access health services at their doorsteps.
- The Ghana Health Service needs to roll out the home-based PNC services, beginning with rural communities where distance from care may be a challenge for women with newborn babies.
- Health professionals could use more innovative approaches to reach out to women in the West Mamprusi district to increase the use of PNC services.
- Health professionals need to educate and engage men in maternal health programs.

Abbreviations
ANC: Antenatal Care; AOR: Adjusted Odd Ratio; CHOs: Community Health Officers; CHPS: Community-based Health Planning and Services; CI: Confidence Interval; EA: Enumeration Area; HIV: Human Immunodeficiency Virus; MDGs: Millennium Development Goals; NHIS: National Health Insurance Scheme; PHC: Primary Health Care; PNC: Postnatal Care

Acknowledgements
The authors are grateful to the Navrongo Health Research Centre, The World Health Organization-TDR, the Ministry of Health in Ghana and the Ghana Health Service. We also appreciate the District Health Management Teams of the Builsa North and South Districts and the West Mamprusi District for contributing to this study. We are also grateful to the data collectors and supervisors for collecting the data. The authors also thank the study communities for their cooperation during the data collection.

Author' contributions
ES conceptualized the idea, designed the study, conducted the data collection, performed the data analysis, interpreted the results, and drafted the manuscript. RA, JKS, MD, EK and ARO contributed to the study design and interpretation and critical revision of the manuscript. DAz, DAn and SO contributed to the study design and interpretation and critical revision of the manuscript. All authors read and approved the final manuscript.

Funding
This work was funded by the UNICEF/UNDP/World Bank/WHO Special Programme for Research and Training in Tropical Diseases (No.B40118).

Competing interests
The authors declare that they have no competing interests.

Author details
[1]Navrongo Health Research Centre, Post Office Box 114, Navrongo, Upper East Region, Ghana. [2]Department of Medicine, University of Calgary, Alberta, Canada.

References
1. WHO Trends in Maternal Mortality: 1990 to 2015. WHO. [cited 2016 May 13]. Available from: http://www.who.int/reproductivehealth/publications/monitoring/maternal-mortality-2015/en/.
2. Warren C, Daly P, Toure L, Mongi P. Opportunities for Africa's newborns. "Postnatal care.". Geneva, Switzerland: WHO; 2006.
3. UNDP. Ghana Millennium Development Goals, 2015 Report [Internet]. Accra, Ghana; 2015 [cited 2016 Jul 14]. Available from: http://www.gh.undp.org/content/ghana/en/home/library/poverty/2015-ghana-millennium-development-goals-report.html.
4. Ronsmans C, Graham WJ. Maternal survival series steering group., maternal mortality: who, when, where, and why. Lancet. 2006;368(9542):1189–200.
5. Say L, ChouD Gemmill A, Tunçalp O, Moller A, Daniels J, Gülmezoglu MA, Temmerman M, Alkema L. Global causes of maternal death: a WHO systematic analysis. Lancet Glob Health. 2014;2:e323–33.
6. GBD 2013 Mortality and Causes of Death Collaborators. Global, regional, and national age-sex specific all-cause and cause-specific mortality for 240 causes of death, 1990–2013: a systematic analysis for the Global Burden of Disease Study 2013. Lancet. 2015;358(9963):117–71.
7. WHO. WHO Recommendations on Postnatal Care of the Mother and Newborn. Geneva, Switzerland; 2013 [cited 2016 Aug 5]. Available http://www.who.int/maternal_child_adolescent/documents/postnatal-carerecommendations/en/.
8. Ghana Health Service. Ghana National Safe Motherhood Service Protocol [Internet]. Accra, Ghana Health Service; 2008 [cited 2016 Apr 7]. Available from: http://mtshohoe.edu.gh/library/index.php?keywords=National+Safe+Motherhood+Service+Protocol&search=search.
9. Ministry of Health. Ghana National Newborn Health Strategy and Action Plan 2014–2018. 2014. Available from: https://www.ghanahealthservice.org/downloads/Ghana_National_Newborn_Strategy_Final_Version_March_27.pdf.
10. Ghana Statistical Service (GSS), Ghana Health Service (GHS), and ICF Macro. Ghana Demographic and Health Survey 2014 Key indicators. Accra, Ghana: GSS, GHS, and ICF Macro; 2015.
11. Chakraborty N, Islam MA, Chowdhury RS, Bari W. Utilization of postnatal care in Bangladesh: evidence from a longitudinal study. Health Soc Care Community. 2002;10(6):492–502.
12. Ciceklioglu M, Soyer MT, Öcek ZA: Factors associated with the utilization and content of prenatal care in a western urban district of Turkey. Int J Qual Health Care. 2005;17(6):533–9.
13. Dhaher E, Mikolajczyk RT, Maxwell AE, Krämer A. Factors associated with lack of postnatal care among Palestinian women: a cross-sectional study of three clinics in the West Bank. BMC Pregnancy Childbirth. 2008;8(1):1–9.
14. Dhakal S, Chapman GN, Simkhada PP, van Teijlingen ER, Stephens J, Raja AE. Utilisation of postnatal care among rural women in Nepal. BMC Pregnancy Childbirth. 2007;7:19.
15. Hordofa MA, Almaw SS, Berhanu MG, Lemiso HB. Postnatal care service utilization and associated factors among women in dembecha district, Northwest Ethiopia. Sci J Public Health. 2015;3(5):686–92.
16. Hove I, Siziya S, Katito C, Tshimanga M. Prevalence and associated factors for non-utilisation of postnatal care services: population-based study in Kuwadzana Peri-urban area, Zvimba District of Mashonaland West Province. Zimbabwe Afr J Reprod Health. 1999;3(2):25–32.
17. Khanal V, Adhikari M, Karkee R, Gavidia T. Factors associated with the utilisation of postnatal care services among the mothers of Nepal: analysis of Nepal demographic and health survey 2011. BMC Womens Health. 2014;14(1):1–13.
18. Mrisho M, Obrist B, Schellenberg JA, Haws RA, Mushi AK, Mshinda H, Schellenberg D. The use of antenatal and postnatal care: perspectives and experiences of women and health care providers in rural southern Tanzania. BMC Pregnancy Childbirth. 2009;9(1):1–12.
19. Titaley C, Dibley M, Roberts C. Factors associated with non-utilisation of postnatal care services in Indonesia. J Epidemiol Community Health. 2009; 63(10):827–31.
20. Workineh G, Hailu DA. Factors affecting utilization of postnatal care service in Jabitena district, Amhara region, Ethiopia. Sci J Public Health. 2014;2(3):169–76.
21. UNICEF. Project for Improving Access to Quality Health and Education Services in the Northern and Upper East Regions of Ghana-An Endline Evaluation. Ghana; 2017. Report No.: 9127709
22. Nyonator FK, Awoonor-Williams JK, Phillips JF, Jones TC, Miller RA. The Ghana community-based health planning and services initiative for scaling up service delivery innovation. Health Policy Plan. 2005;20(1):25–34.
23. Sakeah E, McCloskey L, Bernstein J, Yeboah-Antwi K, Mills S, Doctor HV. Is there any role for community involvement in the community-based health planning and services skilled delivery program in rural Ghana? BMC Health Serv Res. 2014;14(1):340.
24. Ghana Health Service. Community-Based Health Planning and Services (CHPS)-Operational policy document. Policy Document No. 20 [Internet]. Ghana; 2005 [cited 2016 Sep 15]. Available from: http://www.moh.gov.gh/wp-content/uploads/2016/02/CHPS-Operational-Policy-2005.pdf.
25. Ghana Statistical Service. 2010 Population and Housing Census: Summary Report of Final Results. In Accra, Ghana: Ghana Statistical Service; 2012 [cited 2013 Dec 16]. Available: http://www.statsghana.gov.gh/docfiles/2010phc/2010_POPULATION_AND_HOUSING_CENSUS_FINAL_RESULTS.pdf.
26. Ministry of Local Government. Ghana Districts - A repository of all Local Assemblies in Ghana. 2014. Available from: http://ghanadistricts.com/Home/Reader/6932736-59fd-4a13-be.
27. Dean AG, Sullivan KM, Soe MM. OpenEpi: Open Source Epidemiologic Statistics for Public Health. 2011 [cited 2013 Dec 19]. Available from: http://www.openepi.com.
28. Pell M, Meñaca A, Were F, Afrah AN, Chatio S, Manda-Taylor L, Hamel JM, Hodgson A, Tagbor H, Kalilani L, Ouma P, Pool R. Factors affecting antenatal care attendance: results from qualitative studies in Ghana, Kenya and Malawi. PLoS One. 2013;8(1):e53747.
29. Overboscha GB GB, NNN N-N, Van den Booma GJM GJM, Damnyag L. Determinants of antenatal care use in Ghana. Ournal Afr Econ. 2004;2(13):277–301.
30. Browne JL, Kayode GA, Arhinful D, Fidder SAJ, Grobbee DE, Klipstein-Grobusch K. Health insurance determines antenatal, delivery and postnatal care utilisation: evidence from the Ghana demographic and health surveillance data. BMJ Open. 2016;6(3):e008175.
31. Abekah-Nkrumah G, Abor PA. Socioeconomic determinants of use of reproductive health services in Ghana. Health Econ Rev. 2016;6(1):9.
32. Kanté AM, Chung CE, Larsen AM, Exavery A, Tani K, Phillips JF. Factors associated with compliance with the recommended frequency of postnatal care services in three rural districts of Tanzania. BMC Pregnancy Childbirth. 2015;15:341. Available from: https://www.ncbi.nlm.nih.gov/pmc/articles/PMC4687308/.
33. Abor AP, Abekah-Nkrumah G, Sakyi K, Adjasi KC, Abor J. The socio-economic determinants of maternal health care utilization in Ghana. Int J Soc Econ. 2011;38(7):628–48.
34. Dahiru T, Oche MO. Determinants of antenatal care, institutional delivery and postnatal care services utilization in Nigeria. Pan Afr Med J. 2015;21:321.
35. Tesfahun F, Worku W, Mazengiya F, Kifle M. Knowledge, perception and utilization of postnatal Care of Mothers in Gondar Zuria District, Ethiopia: a cross-sectional study. Matern Child Health J. 2014;18(10):2341–51.
36. Neupane S, Doku DT. Determinants of time of start of prenatal care and number of prenatal care visits during pregnancy among Nepalese women. J Community Health. 2012;37(4):865–73.
37. Rwabufigiri NB, Mukamurigo J, Thomson RD, Hedt-Gautier LB, Semasaka SJP. Factors associated with postnatal care utilisation in Rwanda: a secondary analysis of 2010 demographic and health survey data. BMC Pregnancy Childbirth. 2016;16:122.
38. Sakeah E, McCloskey L, Bernstein J, Yeboah-Antwi K, Mills S, Doctor HV. Can community health officer-midwives effectively integrate skilled birth attendance in the community-based health planning and services program in rural Ghana? Reprod Health. 2014;11(1):90.
39. Lloyd CB, Gage-Brandon AJ. Women's role in maintaining households: family welfare and sexual inequality in Ghana. Popul Stud. 1993;47(1):115–31.
40. Adongo PB, Phillips JF, Kajihara B, Fayorsey C, Debpuur C, Binka FN. Cultural factors constraining the introduction of family planning among the Kassena-Nankana of northern Ghana. Soc Sci med 1982. 1997;45(12):1789–804.
41. Ganle JK, Obeng B, Segbefia AY, Mwinyuri V, Yeboah JY, Baatiema L. How intra-familial decision-making affects women's access to, and use of maternal healthcare services in Ghana: a qualitative study. BMC Pregnancy Childbirth. 2015;15:173.

42. Somé DT, Sombié I, Meda N. How decision for seeking maternal care is made—a qualitative study in two rural medical districts of Burkina Faso. Reprod Health. 2013;10:8.

43. Furuta M, Salway S. Women's position within the household as a determinant of maternal health care use in Nepal. Int Fam Plan Perspect. 2006;32:17–27.

44. Mullany BC, Becker S, Hindin MJ. The impact of including husbands in antenatal health education services on maternal health practices in urban Nepal: results from a randomised controlled trial. Health Educ Res. 2007;22: 166–76.

3

Prenatal care among rural to urban migrant women in China

Zhanhong Zong[1,2], Jianyuan Huang[1], Xiaoming Sun[2], Jingshu Mao[2], Xingyu Shu[2] and Norman Hearst[3*]

Abstract

Background: There is a very large population of internal migrants in China, and the majority of migrant women are of childbearing age. Little is known about their utilization of prenatal care and factors that influence this. We examined this using data from a large national survey of migrants.

Methods: 5372 married rural to urban migrant women aged 20–34 who were included in the 2014 National Dynamic Monitoring Survey on Migrants and who delivered a baby within the previous two years were studied. We examined demographic and migration experience predictors of prenatal care in the first trimester and of adequate prenatal visits.

Results: 12.6% of migrant women reported no examination in the first trimester and 27.6% had less than 5 prenatal visits during their latest pregnancy. Multivariate analysis indicated that demographic predictors of delayed and inadequate care included lower educational level, lower income and not having childbearing insurance. Migrating before pregnancy, longer time since migration, having migrated a greater distance, and not returning to their home town for delivery were correlated with better prenatal care.

Conclusions: Many internal migrant women in China do not receive adequate prenatal care. While internal migration before pregnancy seems to promote adequate prenatal care, it also creates barriers to receiving care. Strategies to improve prenatal care utilization include expanding access to childbearing insurance and timely education for women before and after they migrate.

Keywords: Prenatal care, Migration, Migrant women, China, Health insurance

Background

In China, the speed of economic development has been rapid since the early 1980s, causing a rapid expansion in migration to industrialized urban areas. Between 1982 and 2015, the number of internal migrants is China is estimated to have increased from 6.5 million to 253 million [1–4]. Most migrants come from relatively poor and underdeveloped rural areas. Under China's longstanding *hukou* (household registration) system, these migrants remain official residents of their communities of origin, a situation that can be an important institutional barrier to equal rights in terms of employment, education, housing, health care and social services, particularly for rural-to-urban migrants [5, 6]. The majority of internal migrants are young workers, and a large percentage of female internal migrants are of childbearing age [7].

Most people migrating from rural to urban areas do so to earn money and have little education, poor healthcare awareness, and limited ability to access health care [8].

Use of prenatal care is associated with reduced maternal mortality [9, 10], may reduce undesirable pregnancy outcomes such as low birthweight and preterm delivery [11], and provides women and their unborn children with access to various screening tests and interventions [12]. The World Health Organization recommends at least four prenatal visits with a detailed list of recommended components of antenatal care for developing and developed countries [13]. In China, prenatal care was regulated under the 1994 Law on Maternal and Infant Health, and these services are covered under the medical insurance system [14]. The recommendation is for at least five antenatal visits, beginning with at least one visit in the first trimester and two visits each in the second and third trimesters, with additional visits as needed [15, 16]. But uptake of healthcare services varies

* Correspondence: norman.hearst@ucsf.edu
[3]Department of Family and Community Medicine, University of California, San Francisco, CA, USA
Full list of author information is available at the end of the article

greatly between maternal populations. Absent or inadequate prenatal care was commonly reported among Chinese women in a study covering the years 1997 to 2015 [17].

Previous studies of migrant women have indicated that their utilization of prenatal care is lower than in the general population [18]. Compared to local residents, migrant women were substantially less likely to have prenatal examinations in one study (43.5% vs. 84.2% in Guangzhou [19]; 84.4% vs. 91.7% in Jiangsu province [20]). Another study in Shanghai showed that while 90.1% of migrant women had at least one prenatal care visit, only 49.7% had the five or more antenatal care visits recommended and only 19.7% visited an antenatal care center during the first trimester [16]. Other studies among migrant women of reproductive age showed that proportions receiving 5 or more prenatal examinations ranged from 37.6% in Beijing [21], 43.3% in Nanjing [22], and 72.3% in Wuhan to 75.5% in Jilin [23]. But such studies have been limited to specific samples in a few urban areas.

A few of these studies have also examined predictors of receiving inadequate prenatal care. Migrant women with younger age, lower educational level, and lower household income were less likely to have 5 or more prenatal examinations [16, 24]. Factors associated with higher likelihood of receiving adequate prenatal care include longer residency in the receiving community, first pregnancy, having medical insurance, husbands with higher educational level, and staying in the receiving community during pregnancy (as opposed to returning to their home town) [4, 20, 25, 26].

These previous studies of prenatal care among migrant women in China provide important insights, but they have limitations. Local studies may not necessarily be representative of China as a whole. Hospital-based studies of women delivering in urban areas exclude the large proportion of women who return to their home towns for pregnancy and delivery. Also, most studies have not measured important aspects of women's migration experience, such as how long ago they migrated and from how far away. We therefore analyzed data from a large national survey of internal migrants in China conducted in 2014 to further examine these issues.

Methods
Setting
China has a longstanding household registration system under which official place of residence is based on place of birth and can only be permanently changed under certain limited circumstances with official permission. Internal migrants thus retain their official resident registration in their sending communities even after moving across administrative boundaries within or between municipal jurisdictions or between provinces. After leaving their homes for a month, they are officially considered migrants or "floaters." No matter how long ago they moved, most internal migrants are not eligible for many public services, including government-provided health care, in their receiving communities since they don't have official resident registration at the destination [27]. An important exception is family planning services, for which all married women of reproductive age are eligible, wherever they live. Health care is also readily available in urban areas from private or public providers, but this must be paid out of pocket without the medical insurance that local urban residents usually have.

Migrant women are eligible for rural health insurance in their sending communities (which requires them to actively enroll and pay nominal premiums). But rural health insurance does not directly cover services outside their home towns. In some circumstances, they can pay out-of-pocket for health care in their receiving communities and submit bills for reimbursement, but the process is cumbersome and reimbursement rates are incomplete and variable. They are not eligible for the urban health insurance that is available to people born in their receiving communities. The Chinese government has for many years had a stated goal of combining the rural and urban health insurance systems, but this has economic and administrative obstacles and there is no specific timeline for implementation.

Migrant women with full time official employment with a labor contract are eligible for separate childbearing insurance included in employee health insurance that covers both maternal medical care and salary for a three to four-month maternity leave and which is mostly paid by the employer, but this does not apply to the majority of female migrant workers who often have part time or temporary jobs or work in the informal sector [28]. Many migrant women stop working and return to their home towns when they are pregnant, typically from the second trimester through delivery [29].

Data source
This study examined a subsample of the 2014 National Dynamic Monitoring Survey on Migrants. This large national survey has been conducted every year since 2009 by the China Population and Development Research Center of the National Health and Family Planning Commission (CPDRC). The Investigators applied for and were granted access to the data in 2014. This study could be considered a secondary data analysis in that none of the investigators were directly involved in data collection. The data that we received did not include any personal identifiers. All data were stored in password-protected form.

The Health and Family Planning Commissions of each province undertook the field work for this survey. This included providing basic data for CPDRC to compile the sampling frame, investigator training in the sampled cites, organizing field surveys, data input, data auditing and quality checks. The sampling frame was first initially compiled according to annual reports of internal migrants from each province in 2013 and then refined with new information provided by each province in April 2014. Overall coordination of the survey, including compiling the final sampling frame, sampling, questionnaire design, training of supervisory personnel, field supervision, quality control, data upload, and data management, was directed at the national level.

The total sample was chosen with a stratified, multistage and Probability Proportional to Size (PPS) sampling method. Survey information was collected by structured face-to-face interview. Domains included demographic characteristics, employment and family income and expenditure, public health and medical service utilization, childbearing, and family planning service utilization among internal immigrants, both men and women, aged 15–59 throughout China in May 2014. Each of 31 provinces and 1 provincial management unit (XPCC), were regarded as strata. The sample had three stages (sub-district/town, neighborhood or village committee, and individual) and was proportional to the size of the migrant population in each. The sample size by province was also roughly proportional to the size of the migrant population: 14000 interviewees in Zhejiang province, 12,000 in Jiangsu and Guangdong, 10,000 in Heilongjiang, 8000 in Beijing and Shanghai, 7000 in Fujian and Hunan, 6000 in 9 provinces including Tianjin and Shandong, 5000 in 9 provinces including Hebei and Shanxi, and 4000 in Jilin, Guizhou, Tibet, Ningxia, Xinjiang and XPCC. According to the survey plan, 201,000 interviewees were to be interviewed; the final sample size was 200,937.

Supervisors in charge of quality control and training at the provincial level were trained at the national level. Uniform survey manuals and investigator handbooks were printed and distributed to each province by CPDRC. In the field, investigators visited the sampled migrants and interviewed them for the survey. Each interview took about 20–30 min. Potential participants received a printed information sheet explaining the study and informing them that participation is voluntary. They then either declined or gave verbal consent to participate. Refusals were rare (as is common for such surveys in China) and were not tabulated; sampled individuals who did not participate were replaced. Completed questionnaires were checked for quality by supervisors. Each province scheduled and finished the survey in May 2014. Further details of the overall survey methodology are available in the "2015 Report on China's Migrant Population Development." [30]

This study was conducted on a subset of the survey described above. Criteria included a rural *Hukou* (household

registration), female, married, aged 20–34, and having delivered a baby since January of 2012. This subset thus included women giving birth at ages as young as 17 years 8 months and accounted for 93.6% of all women in the larger survey from rural *Hukous* who gave birth in the previous two years. The resulting sample size was 5372. Prenatal care utilization data were considered for the youngest child if a respondent had more than one delivery since 2012.

Dependent variables

Regarding prenatal care utilization, there were 2 dependent variables considered. The first was a yes or no question as to whether a respondent received an examination in the first trimester of this pregnancy with an answer of not remembering being considered as a missing value. The second was whether or not the woman had at least 5 prenatal visits. Respondents were asked how many total visits for prenatal examinations they had during this pregnancy, and we dichotomized this as 5 or more (the minimum standard for adequate prenatal care in China) or less than 5.

Independent variables

Two main groups of independent variables were analyzed: those related to demographic characteristics and those related to migration characteristics. For the demographic characteristics, age was divided into 3 categories: 20–24 years, 25–29 years, and 30–34 years; educational level was asked with 7 options (illiterate, elementary, middle school, high school, junior college, undergraduate, graduate) and was recoded into 4 categories: elementary school, middle school, high school, or college; area of origin was recoded into 3 categories: east, central, and west (these are recognized regions of China with substantial differences in development); birth order of this child was coded 1st, 2nd, and 3rd or more (only 17 migrant women had 4 children and one woman had 5); having medical insurance was recoded into 4 categories: rural medical insurance, childbearing insurance, both insurances, and no insurance; household monthly income per capita (CNY) was divided into 4 categories: < 1000, 1000–2000, 2000–3000, and > =3000. For migration characteristics, migration before this pregnancy was coded yes or no (some women did not first migrate until after their recent pregnancy); geographic spread of migration was recoded into 3 categories: between provinces (from a province of origin to another province), between municipal jurisdictions within province (from a city of origin to another city in a province), and within municipal jurisdiction (municipal jurisdictions in China often include large surrounding rural areas.) Staying at one's rural hometown during pregnancy was coded yes or no. Time since first migration (in years) was a numerical variable calculated with

2 time variables: time of first migration and time of the survey.

Data analysis

Data were analyzed with SPSS 20.0. The bivariate associations between prenatal examinations and demographic and migration characteristics were examined using the chi-square test and the F test for the continuous variable of time since migration. We assessed independent predictors of dependent variables with forward stepwise logistic regression that retained predictors with $p < 0.05$ in the final multivariate model. Women who had not yet migrated at the time of their pregnancy were excluded from analyses that included variables that did not apply to them at the time they were pregnant: geographic spread of migration, whether they stayed at their home town during pregnancy, and time since migration.

Results

Sample composition

The sample consisted of 5372 married rural-to-urban migrant women, 48.6% of whom were aged 25–29 years, 92.6% had at least a middle school education, 75.8% migrated from central or west China, 72.7% had only rural medical insurance, 78.8% had migrated before this latest pregnancy, and 50.2% had monthly household per capita income of 1000–2000 CNY (Table 1). Among these migrant women, 37.5% had older children, of whom 93.1% had one child previously and 63.8% had a girl. Regarding specific migration characteristics, nearly half of migrant women (48%) moved from one province to another, and 23.7% went back and stayed at their rural home town during pregnancy. The average time since first migration was 5 years (standard deviation (SD) = 4), with a maximum of 26.

Prenatal care utilization in the first trimester

Regarding initiation of prenatal care, 12.6% of migrant women reported they had no examination in the first trimester of pregnancy, and 3% could not remember this information clearly. Among 5213 respondents with complete data, bivariate predictors of not initiating prenatal care in the first trimester included age, although differences by age group were small (as presented in Table 2.) Stronger predictors of delayed initiation of prenatal care included lower educational level, central and west region of origin, lower monthly per capita household income, lack of insurance, and higher birth order. In the multivariate logistic model, only 4 variables were independent predictors of late initiation of prenatal care. These included lower educational level (elementary school, odds ratio [OR] = 1.98, confidence interval [CI] = 1.31 to 3.01; middle school, OR = 1.50, CI = 1.08 to 2.10; high school, OR = 1.18, CI = 0.82 to 1.70; index category,

Table 1 Sample Characteristics ($N = 5372$)

Characteristics	n(%)
Age group	
20–24	1554(28.9)
25–29	2608(48.6)
30–34	1210(22.5)
Educational level	
Elementary	395(7.4)
Middle school	3025(56.3)
High school	1228(22.9)
College	724(13.5)
Area of origin	
East	1311(24.4)
Central	2171(40.4)
West	1890(35.2)
Monthly household income per capita(CNY)[a]	
< 1000	995(18.5)
1000–2000	2697(50.2)
2000–3000	923(17.2)
≥ 3000	757(14.1)
Medical insurance	
Rural insurance	3908(72.7)
Childbearing insurance	487(9.1)
Both	131(2.4)
None	846(15.7)
Birth order of this child	
1st	3358(62.5)
2nd	1874(34.9)
3rd	140(2.6)
Migrated before this pregnancy	
Yes	4233(78.8)
No	1139(21.2)
Geographic spread of migration	
Between provinces	2565(47.7)
Between municipal jurisdictions within province	1728(32.2)
Within municipal jurisdiction (rural to urban)	1079(20.1)
Stayed at home town during pregnancy	
Yes	1274(23.7)
No	4098(76.3)
Time since first migration (years)	
mean ± SD	5 ± 4

[a] 1 US dollar is approximately 6.5 CNY

college), region of origin (east region, OR = 0.68, CI = 0.53 to 0.86; central region, OR = 1.10, CI = 0.92 to 1.34; index category, west region), birth order (the third child, OR = 3.17, CI = 2.13 to 4.74; the second child,

Table 2 Bivariate predictors of low prenatal care utilization

Characteristics	None in 1st trimester, N = 5213 n(%)	Less than 5 visits, N = 5372 n(%)
Age group	p = 0.04	p = 0.70
20–24	189(12.5)	434(27.9)
25–29	295(11.6)	705(27.0)
30–34	171(14.6)	341(28.2)
Educational level	p = 0.000	p = 0.000
Elementary	78(20.5)	182(46.1)
Middle school	415(14.2)	888(29.4)
High school	116(9.7)	291(23.7)
College	46(6.5)	119(16.4)
Area of origin	p = 0.000	p = 0.000
East	106(8.2)	233(17.8)
Central	302(14.3)	644(29.7)
West	247(13.6)	603(31.9)
Household income per capita(CNY)	p = 0.001	p = 0.000
< 1000	148(15.4)	363(36.5)
1000–2000	342(13.1)	738(27.4)
2000–3000	85(9.5)	226(24.5)
≥3000	80(10.8)	153(20.2)
Medical insurance	p = 0.000	P = 0.000
Rural insurance	517(13.7)	1173(30.0)
Childbearing insurance insurance	27(5.6)	63(12.9)
Both	9(7.0)	22(16.8)
None	102(12.3)	222(26.2)
Birth order pregnancy	p = 0.000	P = 0.000
1st	303(9.3)	820(24.4)
2nd	313(17.2)	584(31.2)
3rd	39(28.7)	76(54.3)
Migrated before his pregnancy	p = 0.91	p = 0.000
Yes	517(12.5)	1076(25.4)
No	138(12.7)	404(35.5)
Geographic spread of migration[a]	P = 0.002	p = 0.000
Between provinces	277(14.0)	509(25.1)
Between municipal jurisdictions within province	136(10.0)	317(22.9)
Within municipal jurisdiction (rural to urban)	104(13.2)	250(30.5)
Stayed at home town during pregnancy[a]	P = 0.06	p = 0.003
Yes	78(15.2)	165(30.6)
No	439(12.2)	911(24.7)

Table 2 Bivariate predictors of low prenatal care utilization (Continued)

Characteristics	None in 1st trimester, N = 5213 n(%)	Less than 5 visits, N = 5372 n(%)
Time since first migration(years)[a]	P = 0.26	p = 0.09
Eta correlation	0.01	0.1

[a]Includes only women who migrated before pregnancy (N = 4233)

OR = 1.78, CI = 1.49 to 2.12; index category, the first child), and medical insurance (childbearing insurance, OR = 0.61, CI = 0.39 to 0.97; rural medical insurance, OR = 1.11, CI = 0.88 to 1.39; both, OR = 0.67, CI = 0.33 to 1.38; index category, no insurance.) Variables not significantly associated with late initiation of prenatal care in the multivariate model included age group, household income, and migration before pregnancy.

Adequate number of prenatal examinations

Among all respondents, the number of prenatal examinations ranged from 1 to 28 with a mean of 7 and standard deviation [SD] of 3. 72.4% of migrant women had 5 or more examinations during pregnancy, 42.9% had 8 or more, and 10.4% had at least 12. But 27.6% of migrant women had less than the 5 examinations considered to be the minimum standard in China, and 12.3% had 3 or fewer examinations.

Bivariate predictors of an inadequate number of prenatal examinations included educational level, area of origin, monthly household income, medical insurance, birth order and migration before pregnancy (Table 2.) The average number of prenatal examinations among those migrating before pregnancy was 7 compared to 6 among those migrating after. Table 3 shows significant independent predictors of an inadequate number of prenatal examinations. These included lower educational level, origin in central and west China, higher birth order, not having childbearing insurance, and lower per capita household income. Women who had not yet migrated at the time of their pregnancy were more likely to have an inadequate number of prenatal examinations.

Several variables related to migration experience were significant predictors of an inadequate number of prenatal visits in the multivariate models (Table 3). In model I (including all women), those who migrated after pregnancy were more likely to have an inadequate number of prenatal visits. In model 2 (excluding women who had not yet migrated at the time of pregnancy), women migrating from less distant areas, women who migrated more recently, and women who returned to their home towns during pregnancy were more likely to have an inadequate number of prenatal visits.

Table 3 Multivariate predicators of low prenatal care utilization

Characteristics	Model I		Model II[a]	
	Less than 5 visits, N = 5372		Less than 5 visits, N = 4233	
	OR(95% c.i.)	p	OR(95% c.i.)	p
Educational level		< 0.001		< 0.001
Elementary	2.38(1.76,3.22)	< 0.001	3.00(2.14,4.21)	< 0.001
Middle school	1.39(1.10,1.74)	0.005	1.39(1.08,1.79)	0.012
High school	1.22(0.95,1.55)	0.12	1.18(0.90,1.56)	0.23
College	index			
Area of origin		< 0.001		< 0.001
East	0.58(0.48,0.69)	< 0.001	0.54(0.44,0.67)	< 0.001
Central	0.99(0.86,1.13)	0.83	1.00(0.85,1.17)	0.98
West	index			
Birth order		< 0.001		< 0.001
3rd	1.18(1.03,1.35)	0.015	1.42(1.21,1.66)	< 0.001
2nd	2.80(1.96,3.99)	< 0.001	3.50(2.32,5.26)	< 0.001
1st	index			
Medical insurance		< 0.001		0.002
Rural insurance	1.18(0.99,1.40)	0.062	1.12(0.91,1.36)	0.29
Childbearing insurance	0.62(0.45,0.86)	0.004	0.60(0.42,0.85)	0.005
Both	0.74(0.45,1.21)	0.23	0.86(0.51,1.47)	0.63
None	index			
Household income		0.004		
1000-	1.52(1.21,1.52)	< 0.001		
1000–2000	1.23(1.01,1.51)	0.044		
2000–3000	1.23(0.97,1.56)	0.086		
3000+	index			
Migrated before this pregnancy		< 0.001		
No	1.52(1.31,1.75)			
Yes	index			
Geographic spread of migration				0.005
Between provinces			0.73(0.61,0.89)	0.001
Between municipal jurisdictions within province			0.78(0.63,0.95)	0.016
Within municipal jurisdiction (rural to urban)			index	
Stayed at home town during pregnancy				0.008
Yes			1.32(1.08,1.62)	
No			index	
Time since first migration(years)			0.98(0.96,0.99)	0.005

[a]Includes only women who migrated before pregnancy (N = 4233)

Discussion

These results regarding prenatal care from a large national survey of migrant women show that a substantial minority of migrant women in China receive delayed or inadequate prenatal care and suggest that utilization of prenatal care is influenced by a combination of demand and access factors. The strongest predictors seem to be related to demand, and this seems mainly related to assimilation in their new urban environment. Women who migrated before they became pregnant, who migrated longer ago, and who did not return to their home towns during pregnancy were more likely to begin prenatal care in the first trimester and/or to have an adequate number of prenatal visits. This was observed despite the fact that the great majority of these women did not have adequate insurance coverage for prenatal care in their new urban homes.

Nevertheless, access and insurance also appear to be important, as indicated by the higher rate of early initiation of prenatal care and higher number or prenatal visits for the minority of women with childbearing insurance. It is interesting that having rural insurance tended to *decrease* utilization of prenatal care. While this insurance has promoted health care access for rural people and might improve their economic access [31], it may also be a marker for closer ties to rural culture and less assimilation into migrants' new urban homes. On the other hand, having childbearing insurance (with or without rural insurance) was associated with better utilization of prenatal care, probably because it both improved economic access and also may have been a marker for assimilation in the urban environment.

This study using data from a national survey of internal migrants found that a substantial minority of pregnant migrant women aged 20–34 in China receive either delayed prenatal care or less than the minimum recommended number of examinations: 12.6 and 27.6% respectively. Whether these percentages are "high" or "low" depends on the comparison group. Other studies indicate that these percentages are lower than for rural women in sending communities, but higher than for natives of the cities where these women now live [20, 26, 32]. Our results indicate that women who were migrants when they became pregnant were more likely to receive timely and adequate prenatal care than similar women who migrated after their pregnancy. These findings are consistent with the substantial regional differences in most health and development indicators that currently exist in China.

Migration is usually driven by economic factors initially, and it creates challenges in accessing medical care due to lack of official local residence and medical insurance. On the other hand, it also appears to bring advantages. Migrant women appear to move toward the prenatal care utilization pattern of native women in their new homes, and this becomes more the case the longer they stay and the more assimilated they become (for example, not returning to their home town for delivery and not maintaining rural health insurance in their communities of origin.) This influence appears stronger than the negative effect of barriers to care that migrants face.

Nevertheless, economic factors remain important, as demonstrated by the much higher rates of early and adequate prenatal care among women with childbearing insurance. Findings from other studies about demographic predictors of inadequate prenatal care are consistent with the results of this study regarding lower educational level, lower household income, and the latter birth order of the child [16, 19]. Adequate prenatal care is important for

realizing China's health goals for maternal and child health adopted in 2016. These include reducing maternal mortality rate from 20.1/100,000 in 2015 to 18/100,000 in 2020 and reducing infant mortality from 8.1/1000 in 2015 to 7.5/1000 in 2020 and 5.0/1000 in 2030 [33]. In 2010, maternal mortality rates in the mainly rural central and western regions of China (29.1 and 45.1 per 100,000 respectively) were higher than that in the eastern region (17.8 per 100,000) [34]. High maternal mortality rates have also been found among rural-to-urban migrant women in some cities [35]. Maternal health has become one of the three major health priorities for migrants, the other two being infectious diseases and occupational diseases and injuries [7].

International studies in both developing countries and developed countries also concluded that migrant women were more likely to have inadequate prenatal care, with some of the same socioeconomic predictors as found in this study, including lower education, lower income and lack of insurance [13, 36]. One study in Malaysia found that while few migrant women never received any prenatal care during their pregnancy, they tended to initiate prenatal care as late as 7 months compared to local citizens starting prenatal care early in the first trimester [37]. Another study of migrant women in India indicated that only 37% of rural to urban migrants had adequate prenatal care and that recent migrants had prenatal visits significantly less than those who were more settled (35% VS. 39%) [38].

This study has many limitations. It did not include a comparison group of non migrant women for direct comparison. Cross-sectional surveys only measure association and cannot prove cause and effect. There may have been recall bias when respondents reported their prenatal care experience; indeed, 3% of women said that they could not remember if they had care in their first trimester. Although this study was based on a national survey, it is possible that participants were not fully representative of all migrant women in China. The questionnaire may not have captured all aspects of the migration experience and other important confounding variables.

Conclusion

Many young rural-to-urban migrant women report no prenatal care in the first trimester of pregnancy and an inadequate number of prenatal visits during pregnancy. Internal migration before pregnancy seems to promote adequate prenatal care compared to women who remain in rural areas, but it also creates barriers to access of care, and migrant women receive less care than native women in their new cities. Migrant women who are less educated, who have lower income, who do not have childbearing insurance, and who migrate from more nearby rural areas are more likely to have inadequate prenatal care suggesting strategies for targeting services.

Our results suggest several strategies that might increase prenatal care for migrant women. These include increasing access for migrant women to childbearing insurance and/or other medical insurance to cover prenatal care in their new homes. Efforts to coordinate services for the large number of women who return to their home towns for delivery might encourage these women to initiate care earlier (before returning home) and to receive more care overall. Education about the importance of prenatal care is also key. Ideally, this should take place in rural areas before these women migrate and by middle school at the latest. Such efforts would benefit not only women who migrate but also those who remain in rural areas.

Abbreviation
CPDRC: China Population and Development Research Center of the National Health and Family Planning Commission

Acknowledgements
We acknowledge the China Population and Development Research Center and the Department of Services and Management for Migrant Population of the National Health and Family Planning Commission for providing the data of the 2014 National Dynamic Monitoring Survey on Migrants.

Authors' contributions
ZZ was the principal investigator of this analysis and obtained access to the data, conducted the statistical analyses, and drafted the manuscript. JH assisted with data analysis and preparing the manuscript. XS contributed to designing the study and preparing the manuscript. JM contributed to data analysis and preparing the manuscript. XS contributed to data analysis and preparing the manuscript. NH contributed to the data analysis and interpretation and preparing the manuscript. All authors read and approved the final manuscript.

Consent for publication
Not applicable

Competing interests
The authors declare that they have no competing interests.

Author details
[1]School of Public Administration, Hohai University, Nanjing, China. [2]School of Sociology and Population Sciences, Nanjing University of Posts and Telecommunications, Nanjing, China. [3]Department of Family and Community Medicine, University of California, San Francisco, CA, USA.

References
1. Shen J, Huang YF. The working and living spaces of the floating population in China. Asia Pacific Viewpoint. 2003;44(1):51–62.
2. Zai L, Ma Z. China's floating population: new evidence of from the 2000 census. Popul Dev Rev. 2001;30:467–88.
3. Zou X. Analysis of population movement and distribution based on sixth census. Popul Econ. 2011;189(6):23–8.
4. Gong SY, Wang H, Liu DM. Analysis on prenatal care utilization among married migrant women Maternal and Child Health Care of China. 2017,32(10):2187–2189.
5. Solinger D. Contesting citizenship in urban China: peasant migrants, the state, and the logic of the market. Oakland: University of California Press; 1999.
6. Wu X, Treiman DJ. The household registration system and social stratification in China:1955-1996. Demography. 2004;41(2):363–84.
7. Cheung NF, Pan A. Childbirth experience of migrants in China: a systematic review. Nurs Health Sci. 2012;14:362–71.
8. Zhou JF, Mantell J, Ru XM. Reproductive and sexual health of Chinese migrants. J Reprod Contracept. 2009;20:169–82.
9. Zhang J, Zhang X, Qiu L, Zhang R, et al. Maternal deaths among rural-urban migrants in China: a case-control study. BMC Public Health. 2014;14:512.
10. Fan X, Zhou Z, Dang S, et al. Exploring status and determinants of prenatal and postnatal visits in western China: in the background of the new health system reform. BMC Public Health. 2017;18(1):39.
11. Schillaci MA, Waitzkin H, Carson EA, Romain SJ. Prenatal care utilization for mothers from low-income areas of New Mexico, 1989–1999. PLoS One. 2010;5(9):e12809. https://doi.org/10.1371/journal.pone.0012809.
12. Rowe RE, Magee H, Quigley MA, Heron P, Askham J, Brocklehurst P. Socialand ethnic differences in attendance for antenatal care in England. Public Health. 2008;122(12):1363–72.
13. Simkhada B, Teijlingen ER, Porter M, Simkhada P. Factors affecting the utilization of antenatal care in developing countries: systematic review of the literature. J Adv Nurs. 2008;61(3):244–60.
14. National Health and Family Planning Commission of the People's Republic of China(NHFPC). Notification of Implementing National Basic Public Health Services in 2013. (Available from: http://www.nhfpc.gov.cn/jws/s3577/201306/b035feee67f9444188e5123baef7d7bf.shtml) [22 Mar 2016].
15. National Health and Family Planning Commission of the People's Republic of China(NHFPC). Notification of releasing the Maternal Health Care Regulation and the Maternal Health Care Specification (Available from: https://wenku.baidu.com/view/e4d04f18c281e53a5802ff82.html). Accessed 23 Mar 2012.
16. Zhao Q, Huang Z, Yang S, et al. The utilization of antenatal care among rural-to-urban migrant women in shanghai: a hospital-based cross-sectional study. BMC Public Health. 2012;12:1012.
17. Gao Y, Zhou H, Singh NS, et al. Progress and challenges in maternal health in western China: a countdown to 2015 national case study. Lancet Glob Health. 2017;5(5):523–36.
18. Boerleider AW, Wiegers TA, Manniën J, Francke AL, Devillé WL. Factors affecting the use of prenatal care by non-western women in industrialized western countries: a systematic review. BMC Pregnancy Childbirth. 2013;13:81.
19. Chen Q, Zeng FL, Ping W. Analysis on maternal care and factors among migrant women in Guangzhou. Guangzhou Medical Journal. 2004;35(5):59–61.
20. Hai G, Hua Y, Weiqing N. Internal migration and maternal health service utilisation in Jiangsu, China. Tropical Med Int Health. 2017;22(2):124–32.
21. An L, GAO Y, GUO C, et al. Study on health care status of Women's and child migrants in Beijing. Chinese Primary Health Care. 2007;21(1):47–50.
22. Li J, Mo BQ. Analysis on maternal health care among migrant women at childbearing age in Xiagua district, Nanjing. Maternal & child Health Care of China. 2008;23(32):4545–6.
23. Wen YL, Chen HH, Li L. Analysis of the utilization and its influencing factors of antenatal examination among migrating women in a hospital, Wuhan. Med Soc. 2013;26(2):26–8.
24. Liu YT, Chen G, Lv J, et al. Analysis of factors influencing the pregnant and maternal Care of the Migrant Women. Chinese J Practice. 2006;9(7):546–8.
25. Ye MF, Huang HY, Liang HP. Influencing factors and measures on prenatal examination in migrating population. J Hainan Med Coll. 2008;14(4):347–9.
26. Han RF. Analysis on factors for prenatal examinations. Maternal & child Health Care of China. 2011;26:4344–5.
27. Hu X, Cook S, Salazar MA. Internal migration and health in China. Lancet. 2008;372(9651):1717–9.
28. Liang JJ, Liu FC. Analysis on bottlenecks and countermeasures of fertility insurance policy among female migrants in China. Maternal & child Health Care of China. 2014;29(1):5–8.
29. Lou CH, Zhao SL, Gao ES. Status and needs of reproductive health among female migrant workers in cities. Population Research. 2001;25(3):61–4.
30. Department of Services and Management for Migrant Population of NHFPC(DSMMP). 2015 Report on China's migrant population development. Beijing: China Population Publishing House; 2015.
31. Liang Y, Lu PY. Medical insurance policy organized by Chinese government and the health inequity of the elderly: longitudinal comparison based on effect of new cooperative medical scheme on health of rural elderly in 22 provinces and cities. Int J Equity Health. 2014;13:37–51.

32. Bao HH, Liu MT, Xu XJ, et al. Study on maternal care utilization among married migrant women in Jilin Province. Maternal & child Health Care of China. 2015;30(22):3767–70.

33. The State Council of the People's Republic of China(SCPRC). Program outline on health China 2030. http://www.gov.cn/zhengce/2016-10/25/content_5124174.htm. Accessed 25 Oct 2016.

34. Zhou YY, Zhu J, Wang YP. Etc. trend on maternal mortality rate of 1996-2010 in China. Chinese J Preventive Med. 2011;45(10):934–9.

35. Tang S, Meng Q, Chen L, Bekedam H, Evans T, Whitehead M. Tackling the challenges to health equity in China. Lancet. 2008;372:1493–501.

36. Heaman M, Bayrampour H, Kingston D. Etc. migrant women's utilization of prenatal care: a systematic review. Matern Child Health J. 2013;17(5):816–36.

37. Siti NZ, Khin MU, Khairuddin Y, Wong YL. Maternal and child health in urban Sabah, Malaysia: a comparison of citizens and migrants. Asia Pac J Public Health. 1994;7(3):151–8.

38. Yadlapalli SK, Rita K, Sonia K. Migration and access to maternal healthcare: determinants of adequate antenatal care and institutional delivery among socio-economically disadvantaged migrants in Delhi, India. Tropical Med Int Health. 2013;18(10):1202–10.

4

Course of depression symptoms between 3 and 8 months after delivery using two screening tools (EPDS and HSCL-10) on a sample of Sudanese women in Khartoum state

Dina Sami Khalifa[1,2]*, Kari Glavin[3], Espen Bjertness[1] and Lars Lien[4,5]

Abstract

Background: Effects of depression on parenting and on cognitive development of newborns are augmented when symptoms continue throughout the first postnatal year. Current classification systems recognize maternal depression as postnatal if symptoms commence within four to six weeks. Traditional cultural rituals in Sudan offer new mothers adequate family support in the first 6–8 weeks postpartum. The course of postnatal depression symptoms beyond that period is not explored in such settings. We therefore aim to investigate the change in screening status and in severity of depression and distress symptoms between three and eight months postpartum among a sample of Sudanese women using the Edinburgh Postnatal Depression Scale (EPDS) and a locally used tool: the 10-items Hopkins Symptoms Checklist (HSCL-10).

Methods: Three hundred pregnant women in their 2nd or 3rd trimester were recruited from two clinics in Khartoum state. They were followed up and screened for depression symptoms eight months after delivery by EPDS at ≥12, and by HSCL-10 at ≥1.85. The same sample was previously screened for depression at three months after birth.

Results: Prevalence of postnatal depression symptoms by EPDS was lower at eight months compared to three months after birth (3.6% at eight months (8/223) compared to 9.2% at three months (22/238), $p < 0.001$). Eight Mothers exhibited depression symptoms eight months after birth. Depressed mothers at three months had a 56% reduction in EPDS mean scores by eight months and 96.4% of participants either remained in the same EPDS category, or improved eight months after birth. Four participants with major depression symptoms at eight months were also depressed three months after birth and four participants had new onset depression symptoms. The HSCL-10 measured higher distress than EPDS across the two screening points (19.3% at three months, 9.1% at eight months postpartum, $p < 0.001$). Nonetheless, the two tests correlated positively at both points.

Conclusions: Repeated screenings by EPDS (depression surveillance) is recommended during the first postnatal year because a subset of mothers can have symptoms beyond the early postnatal period. Existing depression screening instruments can be assessed for their validity to detect PND.

Keywords: Postnatal depression, Course of depression, Maternal distress, Screening, EPDS, HSCL-10

* Correspondence: dinasami5071@hotmail.com; d.m.sami@studmed.uio.no
[1]Department of Community Medicine, Institute of Health and Society, Faculty of Medicine, University of Oslo, Postboks 1130 Blindern, 0318 Oslo, Norway
[2]Faculty of Health Sciences, Ahfad University for Women, Khartoum, Sudan
Full list of author information is available at the end of the article

Background

Depression is classified as postnatal depression (PND) by the 10th revision of the International Statistical Classification of Diseases and Related Health Problems (ICD-10) if symptoms occur within the first six weeks after birth, and by the Diagnostic and Statistical manual for Mental Disorders (DSM) if symptoms occur within the first four weeks after birth [1, 2]. Postnatal depression affects a mother's capacity to form and maintain attachment with her newborn increasing the risk of attachment disorders during infancy and childhood [3]. Compared to a previous report by the World Health Organization (WHO) on PND in low and lower middle income countries (LLMIC) [4], recent reviews on prevalence of postnatal depression show higher estimates. Norhayati et al. [5] reported from LLMIC, based on screening results by the Edinburgh Postnatal Depression Scale (EPDS), prevalence estimates ranging from 12.9 to 50.7% at less than four weeks screening, 4.9–50.8% at four to eight weeks, 8.2–38.2% at six months after birth and 21.0–33.2% in the first postnatal year.

Prolonged postnatal depression is linked to maternal morbidity and to poor childhood cognitive and behavioral development [6]. Minkovitz et al. [7] followed children in the US up to age three and reported that mothers diagnosed with postnatal depression accessed well-baby and immunization visits at a lesser rate than mothers without depression, and they utilized emergency services for their infants at a higher rate. A 16 months US follow-up study on infant and maternal health-related quality of life by Darcy et al. [8] reported that maternal depressive symptoms at four months after birth predicted poorer infant health at 8, 12 and 16 months assessments. O'Brian et al. [9] examined two years old children in the UK and reported that those with faltering growth are more likely to have depressed mothers than children who are gaining weight appropriately. These findings elucidate the risk of continuing or "chronic depression" on health of children due to longer periods of maternal negative affects. The well-documented evidence on impact of PND on the quality of life of both mother and child makes it logical to identify and treat it. Wickramaratne et al. [10] reported that early remission of maternal depression leads to improvement in all child outcomes.

Many health systems worldwide advocate for universal screening for postnatal depression to increase detection rate, but the optimum time for screening or the frequency of screening needed during the postnatal period is still unclear. This issue has been raised by few scholars [11–13]. The DSM 4 and 5, as well as the ICD-10, do not classify late onset postnatal depression [2, 14]. For that reason, exploration of the course of depressive symptoms after birth has become paramount.

A number of systematic reviews and longitudinal studies illustrated the course of depression symptoms after birth. Halbreich and Karkun [15] reviewed studies from high and low income countries. They showed that higher estimates of depression prevalence are commonly noticed during periods closer to birth than periods further away when brief instruments are used for screening, mostly EPDS [15]. Goodman's [16] study reviewed PND beyond the early postnatal period (from 6 months up to 2 1/2 years after delivery) in high-income countries and reported that a significant proportion of mothers continue with depressive symptoms for months and years after giving birth. Vliegen et al. [17] reported on seven longitudinal studies that followed mothers up to three years after birth in high-income countries. The review showed a general reduction in severity of depression symptoms throughout pregnancy and the postnatal period, but not all reductions were statistically significant [17]. They also reported prevalence estimates from 20 longitudinal studies on community-based and clinical samples. They concluded that 30% of depressed mothers from community samples and 50% of depressed mothers from clinical samples remain depressed throughout and beyond the first postnatal year [17].

Studies from the US also reported continued symptoms of depression one and two years after birth [18, 19]. A study from Pakistan recruited 701 mothers during their third trimester of pregnancy and assessed them for depression at 3, 6 and 12 months after birth [20]. Fifty-six percent of mothers that completed follow-up exhibited depression symptoms at all points of assessment [20].

We have previously reported on the three months prevalence of PND symptoms using the EPDS [21]. We have little knowledge on how postnatal depressive symptoms evolve in a North African context: how many cases have a more prolonged course and will new cases appear after the three months period? In addition, will those new cases be "normal" depressive episodes or late postnatal depression? There is also a need to find out if other screening instruments for depressive symptoms used locally are useful in the detection of symptoms in the postnatal period.

The objective of this article is to investigate the course of depressive symptoms up to eight months after birth in a Sudanese sample using the Edinburgh Postnatal Depression Scale (EPDS). In addition, we want to explore correlations between the EPDS and a locally used tool for screening for depression outside pregnancy: the 10-items Hopkins Symptoms Checklist (HSCL-10) points.

Methods

Study design

This is a follow-up study of 300 women recruited during pregnancy. Women attending two antenatal clinics

(ANC) in two major public tertiary hospitals consented to participate in the study. They were screened for symptoms of postnatal depression at three and eight months by EPDS and HSCL-10. The clinics provide routine antenatal care services for pregnant women living within or outside the hospitals' catchment population. The hospitals were Omdurman Maternity Teaching Hospital and Ibrahim Malik Teaching Hospital. Compared to other states in Sudan, Khartoum state has the highest level of utilization of ANC services and the highest level of institutional deliveries as well [22]. Antenatal care attendance in Khartoum state is 88% [22]. This is the proportion of women that attend "at least one" ANC visit provided by a skilled provider. Women from all localities of Khartoum state can access services in Omdurman Maternity Hospital irrespective of their residence [23]. The sample size was calculated using the prevalence of PND in Nigeria, an African country with a similar social context to Sudan [24]. Inclusion criteria were women of Sudanese nationality, in their 2nd or 3rd trimester, of any parity and with full contact information (at least two working telephone numbers). Availability of two working phone numbers was imperative to improve follow-up rates through house visits, as the address system in that context was unclear. Illiteracy was not an exclusion criterion as data collection was via interviews. The study protocol was approved in Sudan by the Sudan Ministry of Health and in Norway by REK (Regional

Committees for Medical and Health Research Ethics, reference no. 2013/353/REK).

Study procedure

Recruitment was intermittent during the period of April 2013 until April 2014. More than 5000 women attended the clinics during that period; the principle investigator approached approximately 700 women. The attending physician screened attendants for the required gestational age and introduced the investigator to each prospective participant at the end of her ANC visit. Random sampling from a list of ANC attendees was not possible in that setting. Approximately four hundred women were not included: almost two hundred women refused to be part of a research study and the remaining were excluded due to none eligibility because they had no telephone number. No information was available of those who refused participation. Recruitment continued during that period until 300 women consented to participate in the study. They were interviewed at recruitment (T0), and screened at three months (T1) and eight months postpartum (T2). Figure 1 illustrates the follow-up process.

First interview (T0, n = 300)

Full contact information was obtained at recruitment to optimize follow-up and screening rate for PND after delivery. Median age of women at recruitment was 28 years

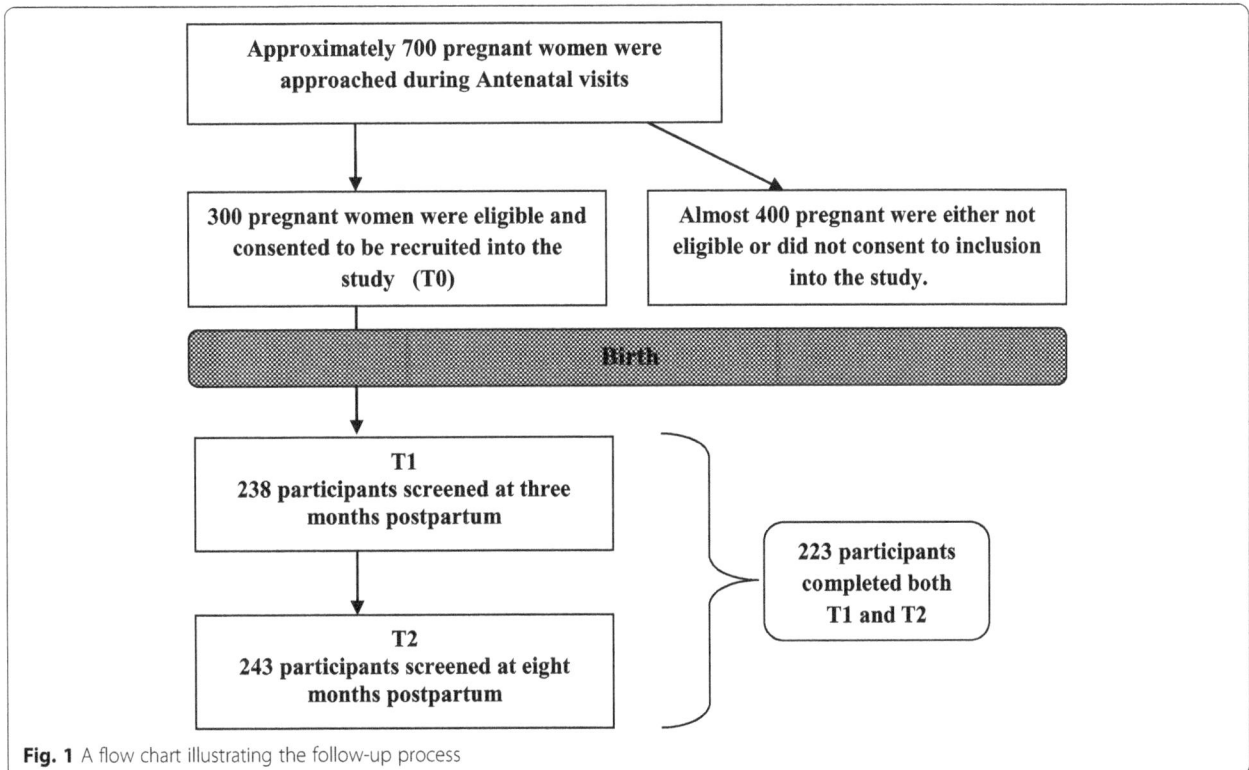

Fig. 1 A flow chart illustrating the follow-up process

(range 15 to 43); 41% were between the ages of 15–25. Twelve percent held an occupation. The majority (215 women) had no previous employment (72%), 10% (31 women) had an occupation before marriage or childbirth, and 6% (17 women) were students. [21]

Second interview (first screening) (T1, n = 238)

At three months postpartum, participants were interviewed regarding circumstances of the index pregnancy. The interview was either face-to-face (at home or ANC clinic), or through phone. Phone interviews were conducted to minimize loss of follow-up only when women were away from Khartoum state or refused home interviews. The first EPDS and HSCL-10 screening was conducted at that time. A single interviewer conducted the interviews. As reported from a previous analysis in the same study [21], the response rate at T1 was 79.3% (62 participants were lost to follow-up). The loss to follow-up was due to personal refusal (14 participants), husband's refusal (13 participants), and contact failure (35 participants). Participants lost to follow-up were not significantly different from participants who completed the follow-up in age (the median age was 27 years old for both groups), in parity (the median parity was 1.9 children and 1.8 children, respectively) or in educational level (Pearson chi-square p-value = 0.70) [21].

Third interview (second screening) (T2, n = 243)

At eight months postpartum, 243 women were screened for PND with EPDS and HSCL-10 resulting in a follow-up rate of 81%. Fifty-seven women were lost in the second screening due to contact failure (27 participants), personal refusal (15 participants), and husband refusal (15 participants).

Measurement tools
EPDS

The Edinburgh Postnatal Depression Scale (EPDS) is a self-reporting tool specifically developed for screening for symptoms of postnatal depression at primary healthcare level [25]. It has been translated and validated into 57 languages including Arabic [26–28]. We have validated the Arabic EPDS in this sample and we have described its validity indices against a diagnostic tool [21]. The EPDS screens for PND through ten inventory questions investigating new feelings felt by the mother within the previous seven days. Each question has four possible answers rated from 0 to 3 and the scale has a total score of 30. In this study, EPDS was administered through personal interviews and a test is "positive" for major depression if the woman scores 12 or more out of 30 as set by Cox et al. [25]. A cut-off point of ≥10 is optimum for screening for minor and major depression combined [25]. Combined subscale analysis of EPDS confirms that

there is an anxiety scale embedded within the tool and that the whole 10 item tool measures both depression and anxiety [29].

Although it is a self-administered tool, studies have shown that administering EPDS through directed interviews is an equivalent screening technique [30]. According to Ghubash et al. [27], the Arabic EPDS has good internal consistency and reliability with a Cronbach's coefficient of 0.84. In the current study, the Cronbach's coefficient was 0.83.

Prevalence of PND symptoms at T1 with the EPDS at ≥12 was 9.2% [21]. Validity indices of the EPDS were 89% sensitivity, 82% specificity, 98.7% NPV and 33% PPV [21].

Only a subsample of participants was clinically interviewed for assessment of their depression symptoms (the EPDS "test positives" at T1 and their matched controls). Clinically depressed participants were referred to the outpatient mental health clinic in Khartoum for further management.

HSCL-10

Originally the Hopkins Symptoms Checklist was a 58-item self-reporting inventory symptom checklist developed in the mid-1970s for psychological distress [31]. A ten items version as well as 35, 25 and five items versions were also developed and validated against the extended version and were found of equal performance [32, 33]. The first four items in the 10-item tool evaluate "anxiety" and the remaining six items "depression". Each item has a 4-point scale ranging from "not at all" to "extremely". The symptoms screened were in the seven days prior to screening. HSCL-10 final score is the average of the total score. The cut-off score for "distress" used in this study is ≥1.85 [32]. It has been translated to Arabic and validated on Arab speaking populations [34]. HSCL-10 is brief and simple. It has well-documented reliability and validity and is an easily administered instrument. In this analysis, it has an acceptable internal consistency of 0.77.

Statistical analysis

Prevalence of major depression symptoms at eight months postpartum (T2) was calculated based on EPDS at a cut-off point ≥12/30. The prevalence of depression symptoms at T1 and T2 with EPDS at a cut-off score ≥ 10/30 was also explored (reflecting prevalence of major and minor depression combined).

Prevalence of psychological distress with HSCL-10 at three months (T1) and eight months (T2) postpartum was calculated at a cut-off point ≥1.85. Correlation coefficients among scores of the two tests were computed. Numbers of new and continuous depression symptoms between the two screening points, based on EPDS, were calculated. The change in EPDS test status between T1 to T2 was analysed for its statistical significance (i.e. if individual scores and mean scores fell below cut-off score) and for its clinical reliability using the Reliability Change Index method (RCI) as described by Jacobson and Truax [35]. This analysis is on data of participants that completed follow-up at T1 *and* T2 (i.e. participants with complete follow-up).

Results

Participants lost to follow-up at the eight months' screening were not significantly different from women that were screened in terms of median age; 27 years old and 28 years old respectively, in parity (2 children and 1.8 children, respectively, p-value = 0.48) or in educational level (Pearson chi square p-value = 0.78).

Participants with complete follow-up at T1 and T2 were 223 (74.3% of sample) and 77 participants did not complete screening either at T1 or at T2 (see Fig. 1). Mean scores of EPDS at T1 and T2 for the entire sample were compared with mean scores for the 223 participants. Differences in mean scores (between 0 and 0.06 points on a 30-point scale) were insignificant between participants that had complete follow-up and participants that were lost at either T1 or T2. Table 1 illustrates the characteristics of women that completed follow-up.

Course of postnatal depression symptoms among women with "complete follow up"

Twenty participants at three months and eight participants at eight months tested "positive" by EPDS at a cut-off score of ≥12 (correlation coefficient = 0.57; $p < 0.001$). To reflect minor and major depression combined, 26 participants at three months and 10 participants at eight months scored ≥10 cut-off score. A paired-samples t-test was conducted on EPDS scores across T1 and T2. There was a significant reduction of EPDS mean scores between T1 and T2 (Table 2). A mixed between-within subjects ANOVA was conducted to assess the effect of time on depression status. Figure 2 illustrates the change in mean scores over time for EPDS test "positives" and "negatives" from T1 until T2. There was a significant interaction between time and depression status (Wilks' Lambda = 0.69, F (1,221) =98.9, $p < .0005$, partial eta squared = 0.31) meaning that the change of scores across time was different between depressed and non-depressed mothers. Mothers with depression symptoms at three months were more likely to recover by eight months. Their mean EPDS score was 15.3 (SD = 3.2) at T1 and 6.7 (SD = 5.7) at T2. There was 56% reduction in mean scores to below the cut-off score of <12. Non-depressed mothers at three months showed stable symptomology up to eight months after birth.

The next set of analysis was about EPDS "test positives" at T1 (20 women) (see Fig. 3). Sixteen out of those

Table 1 Characteristics of women with complete follow-up (n = 223)

Variable	No. (%)
Educational level	
University and Postgraduate	89 (39.9%)
Secondary	64 (28.7%)
Primary	65 (29.1%)
No education	5 (2.2%)
Parity	
Primigravida	56 (25.1%)
Multigravida(1–4)	147 (65.9%)
Grandmultipara (= > 5)	20 (9%)
Polygamy	
Yes	17 (7.6%)
No	206 (92.4%)
Place of delivery	
Health Facility	206 (92.4%)
Home	17 (7.6%)
Mode of delivery	
Vaginal (incl. abortion)	139 (62.3%)
C/section	84 (37.7%)
History of psychological condition	
Yes	18 (8.1%)
No	205 (91.9%)
Family history of a psychological condition	
Yes	37(16.6%)
No	186(83.4%)

20 women scored below 12 at T2. The Reliable Change Index Score for each of the 16 was more than 1.96 (two standard deviations) indicating reliable change. They constitute the remission group. The remaining four participants experienced "continuing depression" The Reliable Change Index Score for each was below 1.96 indicating unreliable change (i.e. we are 95% confident that change in EPDS scores was not real and most likely due to measurement error). All four "continuing depression" participants were clinically diagnosed with depression at T1 by a diagnostic interview and all had corresponding scores above ≥1.85 by HSCL-10 at both screening points. Their ages were 23, 26, 27 and 30 years, Two had a history of domestic violence, one had a perceived history of depression before pregnancy. One participant suffered from anemia during pregnancy and all had term pregnancies. With regard to newborn illness: one participant had a newborn suffering from a congenital anomaly. Three participants had primary level education and one was a university student.

In addition, four other participants developed *new* major depressive symptoms at eight months after

Table 2 Prevalence of depression and distress symptoms at 3 months (T1) and 8 months (T2) postpartum with EPDS and HSCL-10 (n = 223)

	Prevalence	Mean of scores(SD)	Difference of means	SD	95% CI	P value
EPDS T1[a]	9.2%	4.37(4.5)	1.83	3.8	1.33–2.33	< 0.001
EPDS T2	3.6%	2.54(3.3)				
HSCL-10T1[b]	13.5%	1.44(0.38)	0.13	0.32	0.08–0.16	< 0.001
HSCL-10 T2	5.8%	1.31(0.28)				

[a]Cut-off score ≥ 12/30
[b]Cut-off score ≥ 1.85/4

delivery (EPDS score was ≥12 at T2). They constitute the "incident" depression group. Their ages were 28 (2 women), 32 and 37 years. None of them had a history of domestic violence or of a perceived past psychological condition. One suffered a stillbirth. Otherwise, their medical and obstetrical history was unremarkable. Mothers with new onset symptoms at 8 months seem to have higher parity compared to mothers with continuing depression symptoms (the former had two, four, and six children compared to no children, one and two children). Figure 3 illustrates the results of the EPDS across the two screening points.

The majority of the respondents (89.2%) remained in the same EPDS category across the two time points (always scoring <12 in EPDS). In fact, 96.4% of participants either remained in the same EPDS category, or improved eight months after birth.

Only three participants diagnosed with clinical depression by a clinical interview at T1 responded to our referral to the local psychiatric outpatient clinic and received

appropriate management. One of them was lost to follow-up at 8 months and the other two participants scored below 12 at 8 months.

Prevalence of maternal distress by HSCL-10 at the two screening points

At a cut-off point of ≥1.85, HSCL-10 measured higher distress among participants than EPDS. At three months after birth, 30 participants (13.5%) had high distress symptoms. At eight months screening (T2) 13 participants (5.8%) had high distress (Table 2). A paired-samples t-test was performed on HSCL-10 scores on T1 and T2. Mean scores of HSCL-10 significantly decreased by 8.3% at T2 for all 223 participants (Table 2).

There were strong and positive correlations between depression and distress at the two screening points (Table 3). Correlations between EPDS total scores and the two anxiety and depression subscales of HSCL-10 were similarly positive and significant but stronger at T1 than T2. Higher scores of HSCL-10 are strongly

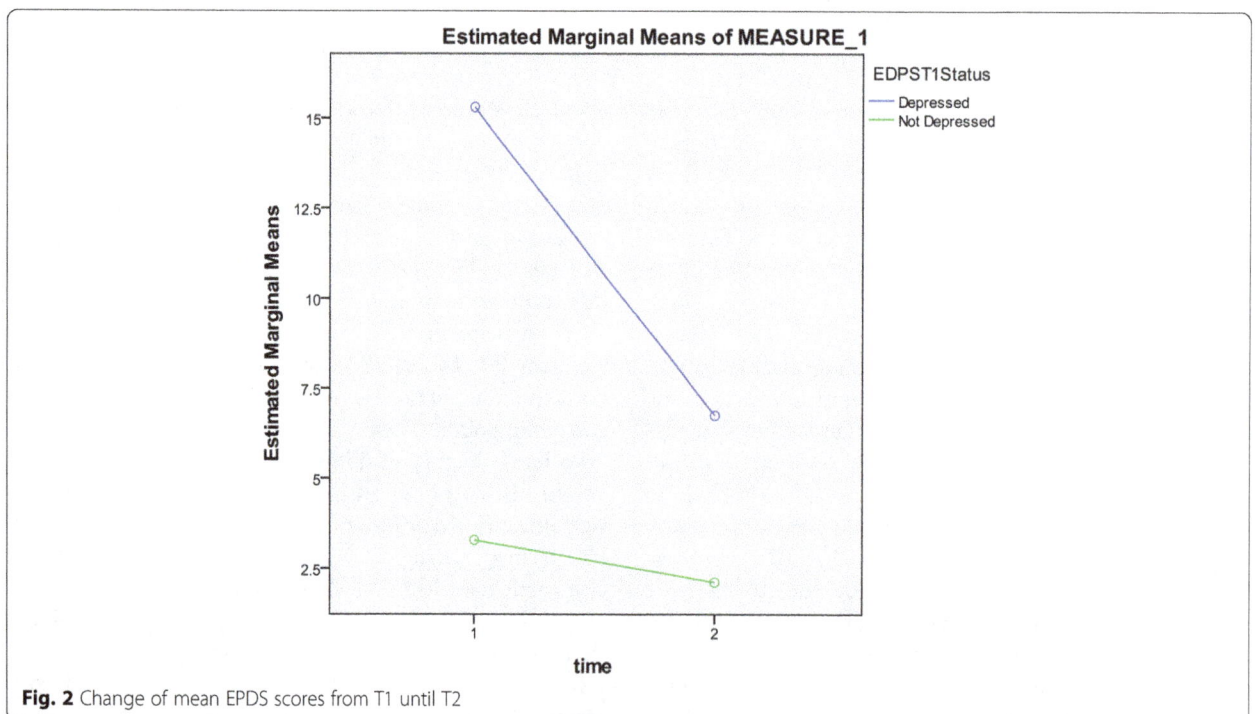

Fig. 2 Change of mean EPDS scores from T1 until T2

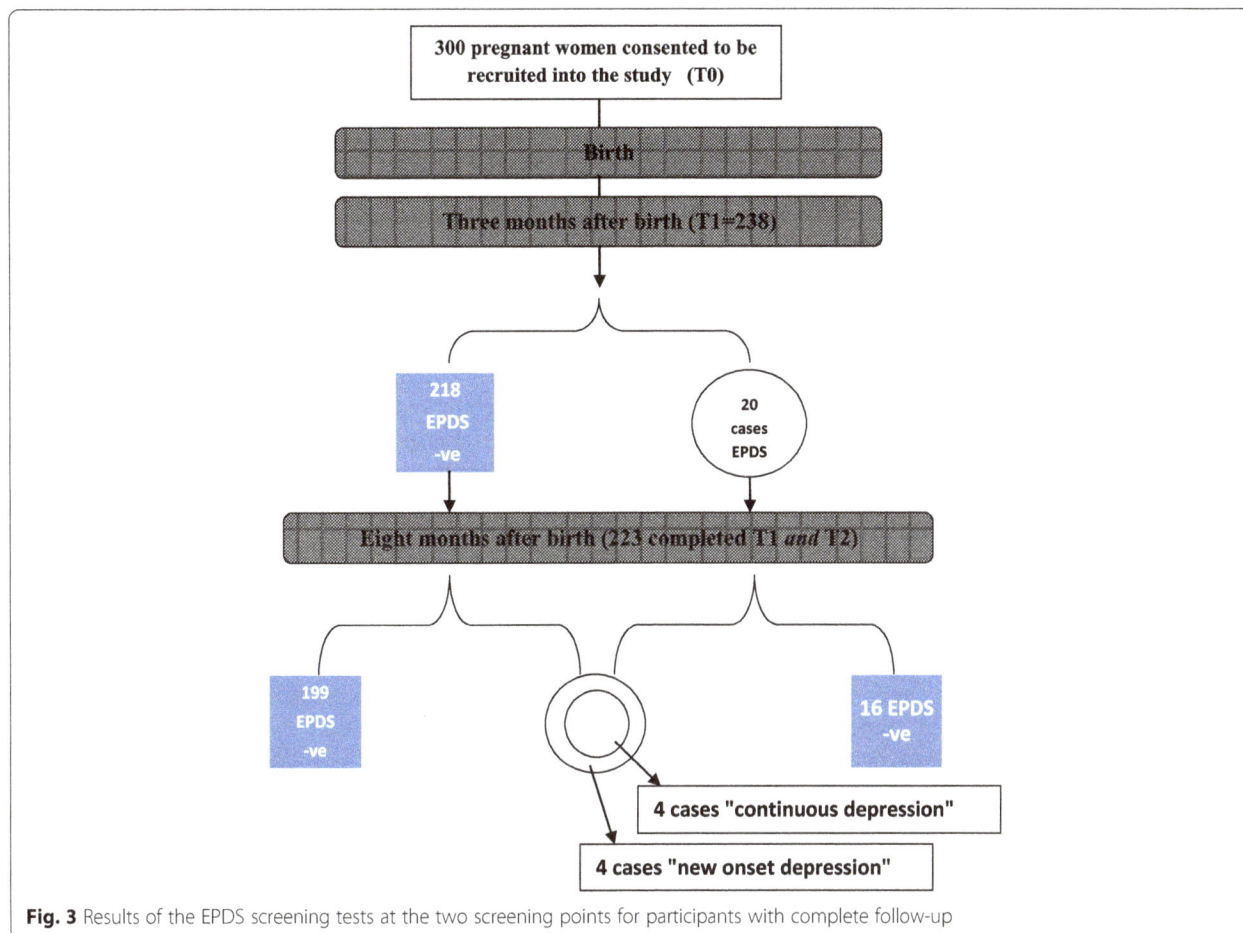

Fig. 3 Results of the EPDS screening tests at the two screening points for participants with complete follow-up

associated with higher scores of EPDS, and HSCL-10 explained almost 60% of the depression symptoms detected by the EPDS in the sample.

Discussion

The study illustrates that depression symptoms can exist well beyond the early postnatal period on a subset of women. The study also showed a general reduction of severity of symptoms for most mothers

Table 3 Correlations between EPDS & HSCL-10 at 3 and 8 months postpartum

	Correlation with EPDS	P value[a]
At T1 (3 months postpartum)		
Total HSCL-10 score	0.77	<.001
Depression subscale	0.69	
Anxiety subscale	0.67	
At T2 (8 months postpartum)		
Total HSCL-10	0.78	<.001
Depression subscale	0.59	
Anxiety subscale	0.59	

[a]P value is for Pearson correlation coefficient

further away from birth. The decrease in the level of depression symptoms was probably not due to active treatment of clinically diagnosed cases, as very few proactively sought our referral services. We also showed that depression at three months constitutes higher risk and could predict depression later on in the first postnatal year. These findings were paralleled by both screening tests: all mothers reporting high depressive symptoms also showed a similar pattern of heightened distress Heron et al. [36] assessed the pattern of symptoms in a large community sample in England ($n = 8323$) during pregnancy up to 8 months after birth by self-reporting tools [37]. They reported a mean decrease in depression and anxiety across the period. McMahon et al. followed 100 postnatal mothers in Australia and measured depression symptoms by self-reporting tools one year after delivery [37]. They reported that 30% of all mothers and 60% of those depressed at 4 months continued to report significant depression at one year [37]. They also reported on factors predicting the persistence of depressive symptoms. Horowitz et al. [38] followed mothers that had high depression symptoms when screened 2 to 4 weeks after birth. Two years after birth, 30% of these mothers continued with depressive symptoms [38]. Women with a chronic course of depression were more likely to have suffered from previous depression, have high parental distress and limited current partner support [38]. Depression symptoms with atypical time of onset or course have raised the argument whether symptoms are in fact PND or an undiagnosed bipolar disorder that was triggered by the birth experience. Recent studies have explored the possibility of PND being an indicator for underlying bipolar depression. Liu et al. [39] conducted a Danish register-based cohort study and reported that the risk of bipolar depression among women with postnatal depression symptoms was higher than in women with depression outside the first year after birth. Sharma et al. [40] reported that 21.4–54% of women with PND in different studies have a diagnosis of bipolar depression. Having a mood disorder during such sensitive periods has tremendous impact on the mother, child, partner, and family. A chronic course of depression will involve more impairment and role limitations for depressed mothers. The period during and after pregnancy in low resource settings is a time of highest contact between mothers and healthcare services and it is a missed opportunity to detect and manage depression symptoms, whether it is unipolar or bipolar.

This article adds to existing research from North Africa by taking a prospective approach, measuring, and monitoring the course of depression and distress symptoms after the customary period for postnatal screening. This analysis highlights to healthcare personnel that they should not rule out PND if symptoms occur after the early postnatal period [41]. Women may not recognize the symptoms and may not seek help in the immediate weeks following birth. There are still limits in existing classifications of postnatal depression by the Diagnostic and Statistical Manual for Mental disorders (DSM 4 and 5) and in ICD-10 in spite of clear evidence from studies on late postnatal onset of depression [41–43]. Nonetheless, a depression screening strategy should take into account potential relapse or chronic course of depression symptoms. Women with relevant risk factors are more likely to have a consistent level of depression symptoms throughout the first postnatal year [44]. Hence, it will be cost-effective, in low resource settings, to redirect repeated screening and follow-up care to women at higher risk of depression, as the number of women may be small. Low risk mothers will be reached through health promotion and awareness raising, even if they are not targeted for repeated screening for depression. That way they are equipped with knowledge if they do suffer from symptoms during pregnancy or after birth. To prevent a chronic course of postnatal depression, it may be

necessary to identify symptoms and risk factors as well [44]. As our study showed, a negative early screening test may predict a continued negative test later on and this reduces the need for repeated screening for all women.

The study suggests that existing screening tools used to screen for depression can correlate with tools developed to detect women at risk for PND, especially in low resource settings where the possibility of adopting new tools is difficult. Further studies to compare performance of HSCL-10 against a diagnostic tool are needed to optimize cut-off points suitable for the perinatal period. We also recommend further qualitative studies on why women are reluctant to respond to referrals to mental health services.

Our study had several limitations. We relied on self-reporting instruments, not on clinical interviews, to measure severity and course of symptoms. In addition, the study did not investigate onset of depression symptoms during pregnancy. We missed the opportunity to assess if antenatal depression predicted the prevalence and course of postnatal depression. Due to this limitation, we illustrated our results as new onset late postnatal depression. Also, repeated screening by the investigator may have provided participants with some supportive talk therapy that could have biased (underestimated) our eight months screening results. Studies have shown that the most desired method of treatment by women feeling depressed is talking about their feelings with a sympathetic listener who understands the nature and extent of their feelings [45]. On the other hand, the concept of repeated screening may have raised feelings of stigma or intrusion among our respondents. This may have increased the number of participants who ignored or refused our second screening, although this risk was investigated statistically and was proved minimal. In addition, we do not consider our estimates generalizable to all women in Sudan. Our estimates may underestimate the magnitude of PND among mothers, for example, in the Eastern and Southern regions of Sudan, which are states suffering from political unrest and other psychosocial risk factors.

Conclusion
The ICD-10 and DSM-5 PND onset classification does not reflect consistent evidence brought about from longitudinal studies. Hence, postnatal depression will remain underdiagnosed with consequent policy implications. Screening strategies should advocate repeated screening during the first postnatal year as symptoms could persist or relapse beyond the early postnatal period. In low resource settings, repeated screening could be directed to mothers with relevant risk factors for depression.

Abbreviations

ANC: Antenatal care; CI: Confidence interval; DSM: The Diagnostic and Statistical Manual for Mental disorders; EPDS: Edinburg Postnatal Depression Scale; HSCL: Hopkins Symptoms Checklist; ICD: International Statistical Classification of Diseases and Related Health Problems; LLMIC: Low and lower middle income countries; NPV: Negative protective value; PND: Postnatal depression; PPV: Positive predictive value; REK: Regional Committees for Medical and Health Research Ethics; WHO: World Health Organization

Acknowledgments

The authors are grateful to Ms. Rania Adam and the clinical psychologist Ms. Fatma Fazaa for their support and help during the follow-up phase in the data collection and clinical interview.

Funding

This research received no specific grant from a funding agency in the public, commercial, or not-for profit sectors. Author "A" received a State Educational Loan Fund in support of an educational program.

Authors' contributions

DSK was responsible for designing the original study protocol, recruiting and informed consent, follow-up of study participants, data entry and analysis, and preparation of the initial draft of this article. LL, KG and EB provided constructive criticism on the design of the study, data interpretation and on each draft of this article until the final version was ready for submission. All authors read and approved the final manuscript.

Competing interests

The authors declare that they have no competing interests.

Author details

[1]Department of Community Medicine, Institute of Health and Society, Faculty of Medicine, University of Oslo, Postboks 1130 Blindern, 0318 Oslo, Norway. [2]Faculty of Health Sciences, Ahfad University for Women, Khartoum, Sudan. [3]VID Specialized University, Oslo, Norway. [4]National Advisory Board on Dual Diagnosis, Innlandet Hospital Trust, Hamar, Norway. [5]Department of Public Health, Hedmark University College, Elverum, Norway.

References

1. World Health Organization. The ICD-10 classification of mental and behavioral disorders. Diagnostic criteria for research. Geneva: World Health Organization; 1993.
2. Association D-AP. Diagnostic and statistical manual of mental disorders. Arlington: American Psychiatric Publishing; 2013.
3. Henshaw C, Cox J, Barton J. Modern management of perinatal psychiatric disorders. London: RCPsych Publications; 2017. http://rcpsych.ac.uk/usefulresources/publications/books/rcpp/9781909726772.aspx.
4. Fisher J, Cabral de Mello M, Patel V, Rahman A, Tran T, Holtona S, Holmesf W. Prevalence and determinants of common perinatal mental disorders in women in low- and lower-middle-income countries: a systematic review. Bull World Health Organ. 2012;90:139–149G.
5. Norhayati M, Hazlina NN, Asrenee A, Emilin WW. Magnitude and risk factors for postpartum symptoms: a literature review. J Affect Disord. 2015;175:34–52.
6. Wachs TD, Black MM, Engle PL. Maternal depression: a global threat to children's health, development, and behavior and to human rights. Child Dev Perspect. 2009;3(1):51–9.
7. Minkovitz CS, Strobino D, Scharfstein D, Hou W, Miller T, Mistry KB, Swartz K. Maternal depressive symptoms and children's receipt of health care in the first 3 years of life. Pediatrics. 2005;115(2):306–14.
8. Darcy JM, Grzywacz JG, Stephens RL, Leng I, Clinch CR, Arcury TA. Maternal depressive symptomatology: 16-month follow-up of infant and maternal health-related quality of life. J Am Board Fam Med. 2011;24(3):249–57.
9. O'Brian LM, Heycock EG, Hanna M, Jones PW, Cox JL. Postnatal depression and faltering growth: a community study. Pediatrics. 2004;113(5):1242–7.
10. Wickramaratne P, Gameroff MJ, Pilowsky DJ, Hughes CW, Garber J, Malloy E, King C, Cerda G, Sood AB, Alpert JE. Children of depressed mothers 1 year after remission of maternal depression: findings from the STAR* D-child study. Am J Psychiatr. 2011;168(6):593–602.
11. Knights JE, Salvatore ML, Simpkins G, Hunter K, Khandelwal M. In search of best practice for postpartum depression screening: is once enough? Eur J Obstet Gynecol Reprod Biol. 2016;206:99–104.
12. Kabir K, Sheeder J, Stafford B, Stevens-Simon C. Screening for postpartum depression at well-child visits: is once enough during the first six months of life? J Pediatr Adolesc Gynecol. 2008;21(2):62–3.
13. Dennis C-L. Can we identify mothers at risk for postpartum depression in the immediate postpartum period using the Edinburgh postnatal depression scale? J Affect Disord. 2004;78(2):163–9.
14. Association AP. Diagnostic and statistical manual of mental disorders, revised, vol. 943. Washington DC: American Psychiatric Association; 2000. p. 2000.
15. Halbreich U, Karkun S. Cross-cultural and social diversity of prevalence of postpartum depression and depressive symptoms. J Affect Disord. 2006;91: 97–111.
16. Goodman JH. Postpartum depression beyond the early postpartum period. J Obstet Gynecol Neonatal Nurs. 2004;33(4):410–20.
17. Vliegen N, Casalin S, Luyten P. The course of postpartum depression: a review of longitudinal studies. Harv Rev Psychiatry. 2014;22(1):1–22.
18. Mayberry LJ, Horowitz JA, Declercq E. Depression symptom prevalence and demographic risk factors among US women during the first 2 years postpartum. J Obstet Gynecol Neonatal Nurs. 2007;36(6):542–9.
19. Beeghly M, Weinberg MK, Olson KL, Kernan H, Riley J, Tronick EZ. Stability and change in level of maternal depressive symptomatology during the first postpartum year. J Affect Disord. 2002;71(1):169–80.
20. Rahman A, Creed F. Outcome of prenatal depression and risk factors associated with persistence in the first postnatal year: prospective study from Rawalpindi, Pakistan. J Affect Disord. 2007;100(1):115–21.
21. Khalifa DS, Glavin K, Bjertness E, Lien L. Postnatal depression among sudanese women: prevalence and validation of the Edinburgh postnatal depression scale at 3 months postpartum. Int J Women's Health. 2015;7:677.
22. Federal Ministry of Health and Central Bureau of Statistics, Sudan Household and Health Survey -2. National report. Khartoum: Federal Ministry of Health and Central Bureau of Statistics; 2012.
23. Ibnouf AH, Borne HW, Maarse JA. Utilization of antenatal care services by Sudanese women in their reproductive age. Saudi Med J. 2007;28(5):737–43.
24. Abiodun OA. Postnatal depression in primary care populations in Nigeria. Gen Hosp Psychiatry. 2006;28:133–6.
25. Cox J, Holden J, Sagovsky R. Detection of postnatal depression: development of the 10-item Edinburgh Postnatal Depression Scale. Br J Psychiatry. 1987;150:782–6.
26. Cox J, Holden J, Henshaw C. Perinatal mental health. The Edinburg postnatal depression scale (EDPS) manual, 2nd ed. London: RCPsych Publications; 2014.
27. Ghubash R, Abou-Saleh MT, Daradkeh TK. The validity of the Arabic Edinburgh Postnatal Depression Scale. Soc Psychiatry Psychiatr Epidemiol. 1997;32:474–6.
28. Abou-Saleh MT, Ghubash R. The prevalence of early postpartum psychiatric morbidity in Dubai: a transcultural perspective. Acta Psychiatr Scand. 1997; 95(5):428–32.
29. Brouwers EP, van Baar AL, Pop VJ. Does the Edinburgh postnatal depression scale measure anxiety? J Psychosom Res. 2001;51(5):659–63.
30. Kaminsky LM, Carlo J, Muench MV, Nath C, Harrigan JT, Canterino J. Screening for postpartum depression with the Edinburgh postnatal depression scale in an indigent population: does a directed interview improve detection rates compared with the standard self-completed questionnaire? J Matern Fetal Neonatal Med. 2008;21(5):321–5.
31. Derogatis LR, Lipman RS, Rickels K, Uhlenhuth EH, Covi L. The Hopkins symptom checklist (HSCL): a self-report symptom inventory. Behav Sci. 1974; 19(1):1–15.
32. Müller JM, Postert C, Beyer T, Furniss T, Achtergarde S. Comparison of eleven short versions of the symptom checklist 90-revised (SCL-90-R) for use in the assessment of general psychopathology. J Psychopathol Behav Assess. 2010;32:246–54.
33. Rosen C, Drescher KD, Moos R, Finney JW, Murphy R, Gusman F. Six and ten item indices of psychological distress based on the Symptom Checklist-90. Assessment. 2000;7(2):103–11.
34. Kobeissi L, Peters TJ, Araya R, Ghantous Z, Khoury B. The Arabic validation of the Hopkins Symptoms Checklist-25 against MINI in a disadvantaged

suburb of Beirut, Lebanon Ziyad Mahfoud Weill Cornell Medical College, Doha-Qatar. Int J. 2013;13:1.

35. Jacobson NS, Truax P. Clinical significance: a statistical approach to defining meaningful change in psychotherapy research. J Consult Clin Psychol. 1991; 59(1):12.

36. Heron J, O'Connor TG, Evans J, Golding J, Glover V. Team AS: The course of anxiety and depression through pregnancy and the postpartum in a community sample. J Affect Disord. 2004;80(1):65–73.

37. McMahon C, Barnett B, Kowalenko N, Tennant C. Psychological factors associated with persistent postnatal depression: past and current relationships, defence styles and the mediating role of insecure attachment style. J Affect Disord. 2005;84(1):15–24.

38. Horowitz JA, Goodman J. A longitudinal study of maternal postpartum depression symptoms. Res Theory Nurs Pract. 2004;18(2–3):149–63.

39. Liu X, Agerbo E, Li J, Meltzer-Brody S, Bergink V, Munk-Olsen T. Depression and anxiety in the postpartum period and risk of bipolar disorder: a Danish nationwide register-based cohort study. J Clin Psychiatry. 2017;78(5):e469.

40. Sharma V, Doobay M, Baczynski C. Bipolar postpartum depression: An update and recommendations. J Affect Disord. 2017;219:105-11.

41. Stowe ZN, Hostetter AL, Newport DJ. The onset of postpartum depression: implications for clinical screening in obstetrical and primary care. Am J Obstet Gynecol. 2005;192(2):522–6.

42. Seguin L, Potvin L, St-Denis M, Loiselle J. Depressive symptoms in the late postpartum among low socioeconomic status women. Birth. 1999;26(3): 157–63.

43. Stuart S, Couser G, Schilder K, O'hara MW, Gorman L. Postpartum anxiety and depression: onset and comorbidity in a community sample. J Nerv Ment Dis. 1998;186(7):420–4.

44. Klier CM, Rosenblum KL, Zeller M, Steinhardt K, Bergemann N, Muzik M. A multirisk approach to predicting chronicity of postpartum depression symptoms. Depress Anxiety. 2008;25(8):718–24.

45. Dennis CL, Chung-Lee L. Postpartum depression help-seeking barriers and maternal treatment preferences: a qualitative systematic review. Birth. 2006; 33(4):323–31.

5

Husbands' involvement in antenatal care and its association with women's utilization of skilled birth attendants in Sidama zone, Ethiopia

Wondwosen Teklesilasie[1,2*] and Wakgari Deressa[3]

Abstract

Background: There is limited evidence about husbands' roles on women's utilization of skilled maternity care in Ethiopia, a country with low utilization coverage of skilled birth attendants and high maternal mortality. This study examined the association between husbands' involvement in antenatal care and women's use of skilled birth attendants in Sidama zone, Southern Ethiopia.

Methods: Using a cohort study design, we followed a random sample of 709 antenatal women until delivery from June 01 to November 30, 2015. Main exposure variable was husband's involvement in at least one antenatal care visit, and outcome variable was women's use of skilled attendants during birth. Data were analysed using SPSS software-version20. We computed univariate and bivariate analyses to describe characteristics of the study subjects. A chi-square test with p-value < 0.05 level of significance and logistic regression analyses with odds ratio and 95% confidence interval were computed to test homogeneity of the two groups' baseline characteristics and examine the association between husbands' involvement in antenatal care and women's use of skilled attendants during birth. Model assessment of the regression equation was checked using a likelihood ratio test, score test, and Hosmer-Lemeshow goodness-of-fit test.

Results: Women who reported at least one antenatal care visit in which their husbands accompanied them were 6. 27 times (95% Confidence interval: 4.2, 9.3) more likely to use skilled birth attendants compared to women attended antenatal care alone.

Conclusion: There was a strong statistically significant association between husbands' involvement during antenatal care and women's use of skilled attendants during birth. This implies that woman's utilization of skilled attendants during birth can be improved by involving their husbands in at least one antenatal care visit.

Keywords: Husband, Male involvement, Antenatal care, Skilled birth attendant, Ethiopia

* Correspondence: wondeti@yahoo.com
[1]School of Public and Environmental Health, College of Medicine and Health Sciences, Hawassa University, Hawassa, Ethiopia
[2]Department of Reproductive Health and Health Service Management, School of Public Health, College of Health Sciences, Addis Ababa University, Addis Ababa, Ethiopia
Full list of author information is available at the end of the article

Background

Globally, in 2015, approximately eight hundred and thirty women were dying every day due to pregnancy and childbirth complications. Almost all these deaths (99%) occurred in low-resource settings, and more than half occur in sub-Saharan Africa [1–3]. The probability that a 15 year-old girl in sub-Saharan Africa eventually dying from a maternal cause was as high as 1 in 36 compared to 1 in 4900 in developed Region [1, 4].

Ethiopia is one of the six countries that account for 50% of maternal deaths globally [3]. Trends in maternal mortality ratios (MMRs) in Ethiopia, however, showed a significant reduction of maternal deaths from 897 per 100,000 live births in 2000 to 353 per 100,000 live births in 2015 [1]. There is no doubt that the country will need to make huge reductions in MMRs to meet the target of MDG5 and Sustainable Development Goals (SDG3), a transformative new agenda for maternal health towards ending preventable maternal mortality [1]. This will require a great commitment from the government and its partners [5] with community effort.

The challenges of maternal mortality and morbidity in Ethiopia are aggravated by the underutilization of skilled delivery services [6]. The proportion of births with skilled attendants is still very low in Ethiopia [5, 7]. Unskilled persons assist the majority of births at home and only 16% of births are at health facilities in 2014, in Ethiopia [7]. Even though the percentage of facility births continues to be low in Ethiopia, it increased from 5% in 2000 to 16% in 2014 in the last 15 years. In Southern region, 11.7% of the women delivered by SBAs, which is lower than other similar regions in Ethiopia [7].

Ethiopian Federal Ministry of Health (EFMOH), as part of reproductive health (RH) strategies to reduce MMR, had planned to raise the number of deliveries attended by SBAs from 16% in 2006 to 60% by 2015 [5]. This RH strategy did not consider the roles of men in maternal health services. However, the majority of studies in Ethiopia indicates men's roles as head of the households and key decision-makers of all issues including women's need for health care services. Moreover, common reasons cited by many studies in Ethiopia for the low utilization of SBAs are focused on the socio-demographic and maternal characteristics, and little has been done to involve male partners in maternal health care services [6, 8, 9].

Evidence from an interventional study in African countries suggest that the three exposure indexes consistently and significantly associated with women's use of SBAs are husband's involvement in decision-making, couple's discussion and planning within the household, and having received counselling on birth preparedness during ANC [8]. Despite that fact, research about the association between husbands' involvement in ANC visits and women's utilization of SBAs is limited. Therefore, identifying such association would be important for policy and program planning for maternal health care, specifically to improve women's utilization of skilled birth attendants. Using a cohort study design, our study sought to determine whether husbands' involvement in ANC visits is associated with women's utilization of SBAs.

Methods

Design, aim, and setting of the study

This study employed a prospective cohort design to examine the relationship between husbands' involvement in ANC visits and women's utilization of SBAs during birth, in Sidama zone, Southern Nations, Nationalities, and People's Region (SNNPR) of Ethiopia, from June 1, 2015 to November 30, 2015. SNNPR is one of the regions in Ethiopia, with 14 administrative zones and 13 special weredas. One of the most populous zones in the region is Sidama zone. The capital of Sidama zone as well as the region is Hawassa town, which is situated 275 km south of Addis Ababa. The total population size of the zone was 2,966,652; of which 49.5% was females and 5.5% are urban inhabitants [10, 11]. The population density in the zone was 452/km^2 with an average household size of 4.9 persons. Women of reproductive age (15–49 years) and children under-one-year of age were estimated to be 23 and 3% of the total population, respectively [10]. According to the zonal health department's report, there are seven primary (district) hospitals, one general hospital (a comprehensive and specialized university hospital), one-hundred and twenty-seven health centres, and five-hundred and twenty-four health posts in the zone. According to 2011 EDHS report, the total fertility rate of the region (SNNPR) was 4.9 children per woman, which was almost similar to the national fertility level of 4.8 children per woman in three years preceding the survey [12]. Skilled ANC, delivery care, and postnatal care (PNC) services (within two days after birth) utilization coverage of the region in the five years preceding the survey were 39, 11.7, and 11.1%, respectively [7].

Study population and sampling technique

The study was conducted on a random sample of 709 antenatal women who were eligible to be included in this study. The sample-size was estimated by using 'Power and Sample-Size' software Program' (PS version 3.1.2) [13]. The computation was made with 95% confidence level, 5% alpha (α), 80% power (β), and with 1:1 ratio of independent exposed and unexposed groups. We used 90 and 82% of the women attended by SBAs (outcome variable) among women who attended ANC education with their husbands (intervention group) and those who did not attend the services (control group) respectively, from a study in Nepal [14]. The calculated sample-size indicated an appropriate sample size of 638 women. Assumed loss to follow-up was 10%. Hence, total sample of 702 pregnant women were needed to test the hypothesis that women whose husbands were involved during ANC visit are more likely to utilize SBAs during birth compared to women whose husbands were not involved during ANC visit. Then, we applied a random sampling technique to select the study sample. First, we randomly selected eight out of twenty-one weredas in Sidama Zone using a lottery method. Lists of all pregnant women between 24th and 36th weeks of gestational age from June 01 to November 30, 2015 (i.e. 712 women) were prepared using household survey, health institutional records reviews, and by linking them at follow-up schemes with collaborations of the health extension workers (HEWs). Women on the lists were sent invitation letters to participate in the study. Finally, 709 pregnant women were included.

Inclusion and exclusion criteria

Women with a gestational age (G.A.) between 24th weeks to 36th weeks, living with their husbands for at least a year in the study area and those who initiated ANC service in the selected health institutions before or during the study period were asked to participate. Mothers were excluded if they had complications of pregnancy (high-risk pregnancy confirmed during ANC check-up), being unmarried, and those who were sick and unable to undergo an interview during the study period.

Definition of exposure and outcome variables

In this study, *husbands' involvement in antenatal care* (ANC) is the exposure variable- defined as- women who were accompanied by their husbands at least once for ANC visits, and women who attended ANC visits without their husbands were considered as 'non-exposed'. *Women's use of skilled birth attendants* (SBAs) was an outcome indicator to evaluate the effect of husbands' involvement in ANC visits. Women used SBAs - means women were assisted by SBAs during births in health institutions or at home. *Skilled Birth Attendants* (SBAs) – are doctors, nurses, and midwives who have a special training on childbirth practices [8].

Data collection

Data were collected using a semi-structured follow-up questionnaire, which was prepared for a progressive evaluation of maternal conditions (Additional file 1). Twenty-eight nurses who were working in maternity units and five supervisors collected data after they were trained for three days. Both data collectors and supervisors had a bachelor degree in nursing and a master degree in public health, and had at least one experience in quantitative data collection. The interviews were conducted using the local language (Sidamigna and Amharic) after the questionnaire was pretested for cultural appropriateness and clarity. Data collectors were fluent speakers of both the local and Amharic languages. The questionnaire included three major components: background information of study subjects, past and current obstetric conditions, utilization status of ANC services, husband's involvement status during ANC visits, and women's utilization status of SBAs during births.

Data collections were conducted *at three time points.* At the beginning, data collectors approached each potential subject to inquire about their eligibility and interest in volunteering for this study. This inquiry included a description of the study, its importance for maternal health care, responsibilities for participating, and potential benefits of participating.

The questions to confirm eligibility included

Information on maternal characteristics such as month of pregnancy, pregnancy intention, initiation of ANC visit, marital status, number of U5 children currently alive, 'Are you living with your husband or not?', and 'Did your husband accompany you for at least one ANC visit in this recent pregnancy?', and information on women's background characteristics. All mothers who met the study criteria were asked to participate and give informed consent. Study aids included a client information booklet, writing pad with pen and pencil to calculate expected date of delivery (E.D.D), 'fundal height' measurement guide for abdominal palpation were given to data collectors; and telephone numbers of the study team to all HEWs for advice in case of complications or questions regarding follow up visits. During initial assessment, data collectors and supervisors estimated each woman's date of last ANC check-up (or at 9 months of pregnancy) for next contact.

The *first interviews* with the women were conducted at their last ANC check-up according to the estimated schedule for each woman (or at 9 months of pregnancy). It was to ascertain information on women's utilization status of ANC services (the number of ANC visits) and the status of their husbands' involvement in ANC visits (did your husband accompany you for at least one ANC visit? [yes/no]). These included a baseline evaluation and planned visits according to the schedule given for every woman. The *second interviews* were conducted on date of delivery (or within a week after birth) to collect data on women's place of birth and utilization status of SBAs during birth. If place of births were at health facility, data collectors checked the information available in the delivery care 'logbook'. Each specific date of interview for every woman was estimated beforehand, based on gestational age by data collectors and supervisors as well as principal investigator. In addition, HEWs at each kebele were assigned to assist data collectors during home visits according to the given schedule. The HEWs in the selected weredas used telephone reminders for upcoming study visits, which was no less frequently than once every month or when there was unscheduled or unexpected childbirth.

Data processing and analysis

After appropriate coding, data were entered from the completed questionnaires to computer software (SPSS version20) for analysis. Data entry was validated (logic checks including range checks and missing value checks) by visual inspection. Monitoring of the interviews occurred regularly through site visits by supervisors and principal investigator. This included ensuring all questionnaires were completed, few questionnaires were matched randomly with the source of information, and all scheduled and unscheduled visits were documented. Inconsistencies were resolved by contacting the study participants.

We hypothesized that SBA would be higher in the exposed group than in the control group. Study participants were coded as lost to follow-up if the questionnaire on delivery care was not completed. Descriptive statistics were presented mainly as frequency listings and percentages because most of the variables were categorical. For continuous variables, we computed means and standard deviations. We used a chi-square ($\chi 2$) goodness-of-fit test with p-values < 0.05 for level of significance to test the comparability (homogeneity) of women's baseline variables (their proportions) in our sample population.

Bivariate logistic regression analyses were computed to examine the association between exposure and outcome variables. Then, we computed multivariate logistic regression analyses to evaluate the independent effects of each predictor variable on the outcome variable by controlling for confounding factors. Odds ratios with 95% confidence intervals (C.I.) were used to evaluate the direction and strength of associations. We checked presence of interaction effects between independent variables, performed an overall model evaluation, statistical test of individual predictors, and goodness-of-fit statistics of the model using SPSS software *version20* (Additional file 2). As women's demographic and maternal characteristics were a priori expected to have moderation or interaction effects on the relationship between husbands' involvement and women's use of SBAs, stratified odds ratios of the exposure and outcome variables were estimated for each independent factor, but are only reported when found to be statistically significant.

Results

Of 709 study participants, 54% (n_1 = 385) reported at least one ANC visit, in which they were accompanied by their husband whereas 46% (n_2 = 324) reported that they were never accompanied by their husbands. On the first interview dates, women were asked about the total number of ANC visits and whether their husbands' were involved in at least one or not. This helped to cross-check their first and second responses, and we took the similar (agreed) responses as a true response to ascertain exposure status. Moreover, 41% (n = 143) of the women from the exposed group were observed with their husbands at health facilities for at least one ANC visit during the initial assessment. Fortunately, we did not find variations between the two responses with respect to their husbands' involvement. During *the second interview sessions*, 664 women (100% of the exposed and 86% of the non-exposed groups) completed their follow-up, yielding a 93.6% response rate. Incomplete follow-up for 45 (6.3%) women from the non-exposed group was due to those who changed their residence with unknown reason even though repeat visits took place.

Characteristics of study subjects

One hundred and seventy-five (26.4%) respondents were 15 to 24 years of age and 110 (16.6%) were 35 to 49 years of age when their last children were born. (Table 1) Mean age was 28.2 (SD ± 5.43 years). Among these women, 141 (21.2%) had no formal education, 248 (37.3%) had attended primary education, and 176 (26.5%) of the women had attained secondary education. A higher proportion (77.3%, n = 513) of the women were 'housewives'; and the majority (67.6%, n = 449) were Protestants while others belonged to Muslim, Orthodox and Catholic religion. (Table 1) The proportion of births at health facility (329; 49.5%) and at home (335; 50.5%) was nearly equal. Similarly, the women's responses on use of skilled birth attendants (SBAs) and health facility delivery (HFDs) were equal. The two groups of women had nearly even distributions by place of residence, age, level of education, and number of under five children at recent pregnancy (Table 1).

A higher proportion of the exposed group used SBAs compared to the non-exposed group (67.5%, n = 260 versus 24.7%, n = 69)). (Table 2) *Variance inflation factors* (VIFs) for each covariate were between '1.06 to 1.278', indicating *no multicollinearity;* since the values are < 5.0 (Additional file 3) [15]. However, the results of stratified analyses showed instability of ORs for 'initiation of ANC visits during the recent pregnancy', which has both confounding and modification effect on the relationship between the number of ANC visits and the outcome variable. Due to this reason, the variable 'initiation of ANC visit' dropped from the final model.

Bivariate and multivariate logistic regression analyses

Bivariate analysis showed that husbands' involvement during ANC visit was statistically significantly associated with women's use of SBAs during births [COR 6.33, 95% C.I.: 4.5, 8.9]. (Table 2) Regarding women's background

Table 1 Baseline characteristics of women in the two groups, in Sidama zone, Southern Ethiopia, 2015

| Characteristics | Was your husband involved at least in one ANC visit? | | | |
	Yes, (%) (n = 385)	No, (%) (n = 279)	Total (N = 664)	X², (p-value)
Residence				
Urban	194 (60.1)	129 (39.9)	323	1.117 (=0.291)
Rural	191 (56.0)	150 (44.0)	341	
Age in year				
15–24	103 (58.9)	72 (41.1)	175	0.090 (=0.956)
25–34	218 (57.5)	161 (42.5)	379	
35–49	64 (58.2)	46 (41.8)	110	
Education level				
Tertiary	62 (62.6)	37 (37.4)	99	3.010 (=0.390)
Secondary	103 (58.5)	73 (41.5)	176	
Primary	134 (54.0)	114 (46.0)	248	
None	86 (61.0)	55 (39.0)	141	
Occupation type				
Government employee	64 (69.6)	28 (30.4)	92	6.159 (=0.046)*
Businesswomen	35 (59.3)	24 (40.7)	59	
Housewife	286 (55.8)	227 (44.2)	513	
Religion				
Protestant	251 (55.9)	198 (44.1)	449	8.908 (=0.031)*
Orthodox	45 (63.4)	26 (36.6)	71	
Catholic	47 (73.4)	17 (26.6)	64	
Muslim	42 (52.5)	38 (47.5)	80	
Initiation of ANC visit				
1st trimester	41 (71.9)	16 (28.1)	57	9.764 (=0.008)**
2nd trimester	231 (60.0)	154 (40.0)	385	
3rd trimester	113 (50.9)	109 (49.1)	222	
Number of ANC visits				
4+	64 (76.2)	20 (23.8)	84	13.087 (< 0.001)***
1 to 3	321 (55.3)	259 (44.7)	580	
Number of under 5 children				
< 1	127 (62.0)	78 (38.0)	205	1.918 (=0.166)
> 1	258 (56.2)	201 (43.8)	459	
Is the pregnancy planned?				
Yes	280 (64.2)	156 (35.8)	436	20.282 (< 0.001)***
No	105 (46.1)	123 (53.9)	228	

***P-value < 0.001, **p-value < 0.01, and *P-value < 0.05, indicate the significance differences of the two groups (women with husbands' involvement and without involvement by indicated variables)

and maternal factors, nine variables were significantly associated with women's use of SBAs during births, though there was a weak association with women's age. All independent variables, which had a p-value < 0.25 in the bivariate analysis were included in a multivariate regression analysis to ascertain their independent effects on women's utilization of SBAs during deliveries. (Table 2) On a multivariate analysis, husbands' involvement during ANC visits and women's use of SBAs during birth showed a strong significant association [AOR 6.27, 95% C.I.: 4.2, 9.3] (Table 2).

There was no homogeneity of the odds ratios for the relationship between 'husbands' involvement during ANC visit' and 'women's use of SBA' across categories of place of residence and women's age (as layer variables). (Table 3) However, across categories of women's education (as layer

Table 2 Logistic regression analysis of skilled birth attendant utilization by selected characteristics, Sidama Zone, Ethiopia, 2015

Characteristics		Have you received SBAs' service?			
		Yes, n (%)	No, n (%)	COR (95%C.I.)	AOR (95%C.I.)
Husband involved in ANC	Yes	260 (67.5)	125 (32.5)	6.33 (4.5, 8.9)*	6.27 (4.2, 9.3)*
	No	69 (24.7)	210 (75.3)	1.00	1.00
Place of residence	Urban	193 (59.8)	130 (40.2)	2.2 (1.6, 3.0)*	1.7 (1.14, 2.5)*
	Rural	136 (39.9)	205 (60.1)	1.00	1.00
Age in year	15–24	100 (57.1)	75 (42.9)	1.9 (1.2, 3.1)*	–
	25–34	184 (48.5)	195 (51.5)	1.4 (0.9, 2.1)	–
	35–49	45 (40.9)	65 (59.1)	1.00	–
Education level	Tertiary	61 (61.6)	38 (38.4)	1.9 (1.14, 3.3)*	1.6 (0.8, 2.9)
	Secondary	102 (58.0)	74 (42.0)	1.7 (1.06, 2.6)*	1.3 (0.7, 2.2)
	Primary	102 (41.1)	146 (58.9)	0.8 (0.5, 1.3)	0.6 (0.4, 1.1)
	None	64 (45.4)	77 (54.6)	1.00	1.00
Occupation type	Government employee	56 (60.9)	36 (39.1)	1.8 (1.2, 2.8)*	–
	Businesswomen	36 (61.0)	23 (39.0)	1.8 (1.05, 3.2)*	–
	Housewife	237 (46.2)	276 (53.8)	1.00	–
Religions	Protestant	207 (46.1)	242 (53.9)	1.5 (0.9–2.5)	1.7 (0.9, 3.1)
	Orthodox	49 (69.0)	22 (31.0)	3.9 (1.9–7.8)*	3.8 (1.7, 8.6)*
	Catholic	44 (68.8)	20 (31.2)	3.8 (1.9–7.8)*	3.4 (1.5, 7.8)*
	Muslim	29 (36.2)	51 (63.8)	1.00	1.00
Planned pregnancy	Yes	262 (60.1)	174 (39.9)	3.6 (2.6–5.1)*	2.5 (1.7, 3.7)*
	No	67 (29.4)	161 (70.6)	1.00	1.00
Number of U5 year children	≤ 1	135 (65.9)	70 (34.1)	2.6 (1.9–3.7)*	2.5 (1.6, 3.8)*
	> 1	194 (42.3)	265 (57.7)	1.00	1.00
Initiation of ANC visit	1st trimester	37 (64.9)	20 (35.1)	3.2 (1.7, 5.8)*	–
	2nd trimester	210 (54.5)	175 (45.5)	2.0 (1.5, 2.9)*	–
	3rd trimester	82 (36.9)	140 (63.1)	1.00	–
Number of ANC visits	4+	66 (78.6)	18 (21.4)	4.4 (2.6–7.6)*	3.3 (1.7, 6.5)*
	1 to 3	263 (45.3)	317 (54.7)	1.00	1.00

COR Crude Odds Ratio, AOR Adjusted Odds Ratio
*Where 95% C.I. does not include 'one', it shows a significant association between the outcome and the factor
The sign"------"indicates the variable was not included in the multivariate analysis

variable), a significance value of homogeneity test was greater than 0.10, indicating homogeneous odds ratios among categories. (Table 3).

Among women's background and maternal factors, place of residence, religion, number of under five children, and number of ANC visits attended by women during the recent pregnancy were found to be significant predictors for women's use of SBAs during births, after controlling for confounding variables. Women with one or no U5 children during the recent pregnancy were 2.5 times more

Table 3 Homogeneity tests for Odds Ratio of factors (layer variable), in Sidama zone, Southern Ethiopia, 2015

Layer variable (by categories)		Chi-Squared	df	Asymp. Sig. (2-sided)
Place of residence (2 categories.)	Breslow-Day	9.808	1	0.002
	Tarone's	9.806	1	0.002
Women's age (3 categories)	Breslow-Day	21.613	2	0.000
	Tarone's	21.455	2	0.000
Women's education level (4 categories)	Breslow-Day	4.114	3	0.249*
	Tarone's	4.112	3	0.250*

*p-value > 0.10, indicating homogeneity of the odds ratios among categories of a particular variable

likely to use SBAs during births compared to women with more than one U5 children during the recent births [AOR 2.5, 95%C.I.: 1.6, 3.8]. Similarly, urban women were 1.7 times more likely to use SBAs during births compared to rural women [AOR 1.7, 95% C.I.: 1.14, 2.5]. (Table 2) Women who belong to Orthodox [AOR 3.8, 95% C.I.: 1.7, 8.6] and Catholic [AOR 3.4, 95% C.I.: 1.5, 7.8] religions were 3.8 and 3.4 times more likely to use SBAs during births compared to Muslim women. (Table 2).

The odds of using SBAs during birth for women with planned pregnancies were 2.5 more times as likely as women with unplanned pregnancies [AOR 2.5, 95%C.I.: 1.7, 3.7]. Women who attended four or more ANC visits during recent pregnancies were 3.3 times more likely to use SBAs during birth compared to women who attended less than or equal to three ANC visits [AOR 3.3, 95% C.I.: 1.7, 6.5]. In addition, there was a positive relationship between number of ANC visits and odds of using SBAs during births. (Table 2).

Discussion

A higher proportion of women from the exposed group attended skilled assistance during birth compared to the non-exposed group. Husbands' involvement in their wives' ANC visits was an important predictor found to be strongly and significantly associated with women's use of SBAs during birth. This is consistent with other studies in Africa including Ethiopia, and Asia [16–20]. This could be due to a man involved in ANC who is more likely to discuss and jointly decide on his wife's place of birth than an uninvolved man. This is supported by studies in Ethiopia and Uganda [16, 21]. Male partners' concern and the presence of open discussion between partners may help a woman to use SBAs during birth. Similarly, our finding reinforces studies in Uganda [18] and Bangladesh [19] showing that women were more likely to have better outcomes when their husbands were directly involved in maternal health care by attending ANC visits and by supporting them during pregnancy. This implies that the influences from other people (especially, partners) are important determinants of women's delivery place [8, 17, 20].

There were variations in the influence of husbands' involvement during ANC visits on women's use of SBAs across categories of residence and women's age, although it did not differ with respect of categories of women's education levels. This implies that women's odds of using SBAs during births may be increased by targeting husbands of both rural women and young women (age 15–25 years old) to be involved in their wives' ANC visits. Women who reside in urban places were more likely to use SBAs during births compared to rural women. This is consistent with other studies in Ethiopia and other African countries [6, 9, 22]. A likely explanation for this relationship is that urban women are more accessible for health information through either mass media or other sources. Moreover, as in most sub-Saharan African countries, urban women in Ethiopia tend to benefit from relatively easy access to maternal health services [22]. However, currently, the Ethiopian government has tried to reach rural communities with health information through HEWs as well as some electronic media like television and mobile phones.

Women who belong to Orthodox and Catholic religions were more likely to use SBAs during birth than women belong to Muslim religion. This is consistent with other studies in Ethiopia, Asia, and Kenya [6, 22–29]. A previous study in Ethiopia, however, did not find a significant association between religion and SBAs utilization [9]. This difference might be due to the difference in study context, study design and sample size. Further studies are needed to ascertain the discrepancies with respect to religion.

The relationship between level of education and women's use of SBAs during birth did not attain statistical significance. It is similar with another study in Ethiopia that showed women's education is a weak predictor of the use of skilled assistance at birth [6]. Other studies in Ethiopia [9, 11, 22, 28], however, documented that women's education is a major factor influencing maternal health care utilization, but these addressed maternity care services in general and utilization of SBAs not as a separate issue. It is commonly believed that education serves as proxy for information and knowledge of available health care services [30]. Moreover, education enhances level of women's autonomy and increases decision-making power that results in improved freedom to make decisions including the use of maternal health care [31]. A study in Tanzania reported that educated women were more likely to make decisions to use assistance from medical personnel at birth themselves compared to their uneducated counterparts [32]. Similarly, studies in Bangladesh [33] and Turkey [34] found that women's education was a strong determinant of the use of skilled assistance at birth. Possible explanations for the differences may be, first, due to differences in study designs and sample sizes; second, it could be due to an effect modification between women's education levels and our main exposure variable in the association with the outcome variable. So, how women's education levels influence SBAs utilization with and without the influence of husbands require further study.

The association of women's use of SBAs during birth with the number of ANC visits, the number of under five children, and the pregnancy intention are consistent with three studies in Ethiopia [6, 35, 36], studies in Kenya [17, 37], Tanzania [38] and Nepal [39]. It is, however, not only the quantity but also the quality of ANC that influences care seeking during birth [8]. Although this study did not address quality of ANC services, a study in Africa showed that women with the highest focused ANC Index scores (care involved both quantity and quality) were three times more likely to deliver in health facilities than women with the lowest scores. This illustrates that even in an area where women have a strong preference to use traditional birth attendants for delivery, quality and quantity of ANC can have a major impact on care-seeking [8]. Women who had one or no under-five children were more likely to use SBAs during birth than those with more than one. Similarly, women whose pregnancy was planned were more likely to use SBAs during birth compared to women with unplanned pregnancy. This is consistent with studies in South and South-East Ethiopia [6, 35] and Kenya [17, 37]. Women with two or more under five children may prefer to deliver at home because of experiences from previous birth. Parents with fewer children lack experience and thus may seek more easily professional care [9, 28]. In addition, the first deliveries tend to be more difficult and that may motivate women for institutional delivery [6, 28].

Study limitation

Loss of follow up was a limitation in this cohort study. Respondents often changed their place of residence during follow-up time. To manage this, we tried repeated visits during data collection periods. To examine the effect of the lost follow-up cases, we computed an intent-to-treat analysis and there was no significant difference on the outcomes. The other potential biases in this study may be social desirability bias in favour of their husbands' involvement in ANC service. To reduce this, we tried to interview each woman in a separate room by explaining the benefits of their honest responses for improvement of maternal health services, and we used repeated interviews (before and after delivery) to ensure the response was genuine. Further limitation of this study is data on service quality were not included. Also data on household income were incomplete, since most respondents did not volunteer to respond to such questions due to unknown reasons. This may have influenced both husbands' involvement and women's use of skilled services.

Strengths of the study

The strengths of this study were, first, a cohort design and an adequate sample size. Secondly, the observations of up to 41% of women being accompanied by their husbands lend credence to the findings from the interviews. Moreover, it is the first study in the region to determine the relationship between husbands' involvement in ANC services and women's utilization of skilled birth attendants during delivery.

Conclusions and recommendations

The strong relationship between husband's involvement during ANC visits and women's use of SBAs during birth implies that raising awareness about husbands' involvement during ANC visits through mass media, religious leaders and community elders should be given due attention, especially in regions and areas with contextual similarities. Besides that, there is a need to promote husbands' involvement in their wives' ANC visits by targeting large proportions of rural and young women. Further, it is necessary to provide information and advice on the frequency of ANC visits, at least four visits per pregnancy through contextual based couple's ANC counselling sessions. Therefore, there is a need for planners of maternal health programs to develop contextual-based approaches that promote husbands' involvement in maternal health care at Wereda, Zone and Regional levels. Our findings also strongly recommend a policy to mainstream male involvement in routine maternal health care. Such policies should address husbands' roles and constraints, as well as an educational component to sensitize husbands to the benefits of their involvement in pregnancy care and outcomes. Based on our findings, we also strongly recommend health institutions to start well-organized ANC couples' counselling sessions at least once after the first ANC visit of every pregnant woman based on the women's consent. Antenatal care couple-counselling sessions should address the benefits of skilled maternal health care in general; and the benefits of repeated ANC visits and postpartum services in particular. For men, such efforts could help to deflate the assumption that maternal health care is an exclusively women's concern.

Additional files

Additional file 1: Participants' Information Sheet & Consent-form.

Additional file 2: SPSS Output-logistic regression table. The data described the output of a multivariate analysis of selected predictors for women's utilization of skilled birth attendants; and it is the best-fitted model selected from six models constructed by forward log-likelihood methods in SPSS.

Additional file 3: Multicollinearity statistics output table. The data described the multicollinearity statistics output- i.e. the tolerance and Variance Inflation Factor- of selected independent variables.

Additional file 4: English version Interview Questionnaire.

Abbreviations

ANC: Antenatal Care; AOR: Adjusted Odds Ratio; CI: Confidence Interval; COR: Crude Odds Ratio; E.D.D.: Expected Date of Delivery;; EDHS: Ethiopia Demographic and Health Survey; EFMOH: Ethiopia Federal Ministry Of Health; G.A.: Gestational Age; HEW: Health Extension Worker; MMR: Maternal Mortality Rate/Ratio; OR: Odds Ratio; PNC: Postnatal Care; RH: Reproductive Health; SBA: Skilled Birth Attendant; SDG: Sustainable Development Goals; SNNPR: Southern Nation Nationality and People's Region; SPSS: Statistical Software Package for Social Science; VIF: Variance Inflation Factor

Acknowledgements
We are grateful to Addis Ababa University School of Public Health for supporting this study. We would like to extend our appreciation to the entire Wereda Health Team of Regional and Sidama Zone Health Bureaus and Wereda Health Offices for their co-operation. Finally, our special thanks go to data collectors and study participants who took part in this study.

Authors' contributions
WT and WD contributed equally during the process of proposal development. WT participated in data collection, data analysis and in preparing the draft manuscript. WT and WD made significant contributions in revising the manuscript. Finally, both authors read and approved the final version of the manuscript.

Ethics approval and consent to participate
Before the commencement of the study, ethical approval letter was obtained from the Institutional Review Board of the College of Health Sciences, Addis Ababa University in Ethiopia (Protocol No. 067/13/SPH and Approval Meeting No.054/13). Then we obtained permission letters from South Region and Sidama Zone Health Bureaus, as well as from Weredas Health Offices and health institutions (Additional file 4). Before started data collection, written informed consent was obtained from respondents. With regard to participants under the age of 18 years, the parent provided written informed consent on behalf of them. They were informed to interrupt the interview at any time that they desire if they are not willing to continue with the interview. To ensure confidentiality, codes instead of names were used during data entry and in depicting the results of the study. In addition, the questionnaires and other collected information were kept locked and only the P.I had access. Participants found sick were referred to the nearby health centre for medical care.

Competing interests
The authors declare that they have no competing interests.

Author details
[1]School of Public and Environmental Health, College of Medicine and Health Sciences, Hawassa University, Hawassa, Ethiopia. [2]Department of Reproductive Health and Health Service Management, School of Public Health, College of Health Sciences, Addis Ababa University, Addis Ababa, Ethiopia. [3]Department of Preventive Medicine, School of Public Health, College of Health Sciences, Addis Ababa University, Addis Ababa, Ethiopia.

References
1. World Health Organization (WHO). Trends in maternal mortality: 1990 to 2015. Estimates by WHO, UNICEF, UNFPA, the World Bank and the United Nations population division. Geneva: WHO. p. 2015. http://apps.who.int/iris/bitstream/10665/194254/1/9789241565141_eng.pdf?ua=1. Accessed 1 Aug 2018.
2. World Health Organization (WHO). Trends in Maternal Mortality: 1990 to 2010. Geneva Switzerland: WHO; 2014. http://apps.who.int/iris/bitstream/handle/10665/44874/9789241503631_eng.pdf?sequence=1. Accessed 1 Aug 2018.
3. Hogan MC, Foreman KJ, Naghavi M, Ahn SY, Wang M, Makela SM, et al. Maternal mortality for 181 countries, 1980-2008: a systematic analysis of progress towards millennium development goal 5. Lancet. 2010;375(9726):1609–23.
4. World Health Organization. Global Health Observatory (GHO) Data, 2015. http://apps.who.int/iris/bitstream/handle/10665/170250/9789240694439_eng.pdf?sequence=1. Accessed 1 Aug 2018.
5. UNDP- Ethiopia. Analyzing Performance and Regional Disparities in Health Outcomes in Ethiopia; 2012; No.2/2012. http://www.undp.org/content/dam/ethiopia/docs/Analyzing%20Regional%20Performance%20and%20Disparities%20in%20Health%20outcome%20in%20Ethiopia.pdf. Accessed 1 Aug 2018.
6. Fekadu M, Regassa N. Skilled delivery care service utilization in Ethiopia: analysis of rural-urban differentials based on national demographic and health survey (DHS) data. Afr Health Sci. 2014;14(4) https://doi.org/10.4314/ahs.v14i4.29.
7. Ethiopia Mini Demographic and Health Survey 2014. Central statistical agency; Addis Ababa, Ethiopia 2016.
8. Family Care International (FCI'S Skilled Care Initiatives). Testing Approaches for Increasing Skilled Care during Childbirth: Key Findings. Technical Brief, October 2007. http://www.familycareintl.org/UserFiles/File/SCI%20Kenya%20Report%20March%202008.pdf. Accessed 1 Aug 2018.
9. Mekonnen Y., Mekonnen A. Utilization of maternal health Care Services in Ethiopia Calverton, Maryland, USA: ORC macro: 2002.
10. FDRE. Central statistics authority (CSA): summary and statistical report of the 2007 population and housing census results of Ethiopia. Addis Ababa: UNFPA, Population Census Commission; 2008.
11. Regassa N. Antenatal and postnatal care service utilization in southern Ethiopia: a population-based study. Afr Health Sci. 2011;11(3):390–7.
12. Central Statistical Agency (CSA) [Ethiopia] and ICF Macro. Ethiopia Demographic and Health Survey 2011. Addis Ababa, Ethiopia, and Calverton, Maryland, USA: Central Statistical Agency and ICF Macro. 2012.
13. Dupont WD, Plummer WD. Power and sample size calculations for studies involving linear regression. Control Clin Trials. 1998;19:589–601. http://biostat.mc.vanderbilt.edu/wiki/Main/PowerSampleSize. Accessed 1 Aug 2018.
14. Mullany BC, Becker S, Hindin MJ. The impact of including husbands in antenatal health education services on maternal health practices in urban Nepal: results from a randomized controlled trial. Health Educ Res. 2007;22(2):166–76.
15. Robert M. O'brien. A Caution Regarding Rules of Thumb for Variance Inflation Factors. Quality and Quantity. 2007;41:673–690. USA; Springer, 2007.
16. Lingerh W, Ababeye B, Ali I, Nigatu T, et al. Magnitude and factors that affect males' involvement in deciding partners' place of delivery in Tiyo District of Oromia region. Ethiopia Ethiop J Health Dev. 2014:6–13.
17. Judith NM, Ann M, Samwel M, Vincent M. Male involvement in maternal health care as a determinant of utilization of skilled birth attendants in Kenya. ICF Maryland, USA: United States Agency for International Development.DHS working papers; 2013. No. 93
18. Kabakyenga JK, Östergren PO, Turyakira E, Pettersson KO. Influence of birth preparedness, decision-making on location of birth and assistance by skilled birth attendants among women in south-western Uganda. PLoS One. 2012;7(4):e35747.
19. Story TW, Burgard SS, Lori RJ, Taleb F, Ali AN, Hoque ED. Husbands' involvement in delivery care utilization in rural Bangladesh: a qualitative study. BMC Pregnancy Childbirth. 2012;12:28.
20. Rahman MM, Haque SE, Zahan MS. Factors affecting the utilization of postpartum care among young mothers in Bangladesh. Health Soc Care Community. 2011;19(2):138–47.
21. Kabakyenga JK, Ostergren PO, Turyakira E, Pettersson KO. Influence of birth preparedness, decision-making on location of birth and assistance by skilled birth attendants among women in southwestern Uganda. PLoS one. 2012;7(4):e35747. https://doi.org/10.1371/journal.pone.0035747.
22. Abera M, Belachew T. Predictors of safe delivery service utilization in Arsi zone, south-East Ethiopia. Ethiop J Health Sci. 2012;21(3):101–13.
23. Baral YR, Lyons K, Skinner J, van Teijlingen ER. Determinants of skilled birth attendants for delivery in Nepal. Kathmandu University Med J. 2010;8(3):325–32.
24. Singh A, Kumar A, Pranjali P. Utilization of maternal healthcare among adolescent mothers in urban India: evidence from DLHS-3. PeerJ. 2014;2:e592. https://doi.org/10.7717/peerj.592.
25. Shah N, Rohra DK, Shams H, Khan NH. Home Deliveries: Reasons and Adverse Outcomes in Women Presenting to a Tertiary Care Hospital. J Pak Med Assoc. 2010;60(7):555.
26. Wabuge E.M. Obstetric Care in the Home Delivery among women in Lugari District, Western Province, Kenya. JKUAT Abstracts of Post Graduate Thesis. 2010. Available at http://www.researchkenya.or.ke/api/content/abstract/Lugari+District. Accessed 1 Aug 2018.
27. Wanjira C, M. Mwangi, E. Mathenge, G. Mbugua. Delivery Practices and Associated Factors among Mothers Seeking Child Welfare Services in Selected Health Facilities in Nyandarua South District, Kenya. BMC Public Health. 2011; 11(1): 360.
28. Paavilainen Miia and Matti Salo. Men's socio-demographic background and maternal health care utilization in Ethiopia. International health. August 2013.
29. Mehari, A. Levels and determinants of use of institutional delivery care services among women of childbearing age in Ethiopia: analysis of EDHS 2000 and 2005 data. ICF International Calverton, Maryland, USA, 2013.
30. Babalola S, Fatusi A. Determinants of use of maternal health services in Nigeria-- looking beyond individual and household factors. BMC Pregnancy Childbirth. 2009;9:43. https://doi.org/10.1186/1471-2393-9-43.

31. Acharya DR, Bell JS, Simkhada P, Van Teijlingen ER, Regmi PR. Women's autonomy in household decision-making: a demographic study in Nepal. Reprod Health. 2010; https://doi.org/10.1186/1742-4755-7-15.
32. Mrisho, M., Schellenberg, J.A., Mushi,A.K, Obrist,B., Mshinda, H., Tanner,M., Schellenberg, D. Factors affecting home delivery in rural Tanzania, Tropical Medicine & International Health. 2007;volume 12, Issue 7 pages 862–872.
33. Chakraborty N, Islam MA, Chowdhury RI, Wasimul Bari W, Akhter HH. Determinants of the use of maternal health services in rural Bangladesh. Health Promot Int. 2003;18(4):327–37.
34. Celik Y, Hotchkiss DR. The socio-economic determinants of maternal health care utilization in Turkey. Soc Sci Med. 2000;50(12):1797–806.
35. Amano A, Gebeyehu A, Birhanu Z. Institutional delivery service utilization in Munisa Woreda, south East Ethiopia: a community based cross-sectional study. BMC; Pregnancy and Childbirth. 2012;12:105.
36. Teferra AS, Alemu FM, Woldeyohannes SM. Institutional delivery service utilization, and associated factors among mothers who gave birth in the last 12 months in Sekela District, North West of Ethiopia: A community-based cross sectional study. BMC, Pregnancy Childbirth. 2012;12:74. https://www.ncbi.nlm.nih.gov/pmc/articles/PMC3449175/pdf/1471-2393-12-74.pdf. Accessed 1 Aug 2018.
37. Van Eijk A, Bles H, Odhiambo F, Ayisi J, Blokland I, et al. Use of antenatal services and delivery care among women in rural western Kenya: a community based survey. J Reprod Health. 2006;3(2):1–9.
38. Lwelamira J, Safari J. Choice of place for childbirth: prevalence and determinants of health facility delivery among women in Bahi District, Central Tanzania. Asian J Med Sci. 2012;4(3):105–12. ISSN: 2040-8773
39. Karkee R, Binns CW, Lee AH. Determinants of facility delivery after implementation of safer mother programme in Nepal: a prospective cohort study. BMC Pregnancy and Childbirth. 2013;13:193.

6

Mother–infant interaction quality and sense of parenting competence at six months postpartum for first-time mothers in Taiwan: a multiple time series design

Fen-Fang Chung[1,2], Gwo-Hwa Wan[3,4,5*], Su-Chen Kuo[6], Kuan-Chia Lin[7] and Hsueh-Erh Liu[1,8,9*]

Abstract

Background: For first-time mothers, not knowing how to interact with newborn infants increases anxiety and decreases the quality of the parent–infant interactions. A substantial lack of interactional knowledge can ultimately limit the adjustments necessary for a stable transition into motherhood. This study investigated how postpartum parenting education influenced first-time mothers' mother–infant interaction quality and parenting sense of competence.

Methods: Eighty-one healthy first-time-mother and infant dyads were recruited. The control group ($n = 40$) received postpartum care based on the medical and cultural norms practiced in Taiwan, while the experimental group ($n = 41$) received, on top of typical care, education by way of a 40-min videotape on infant states, behaviors, and communication cues, as well as a handout on play practices. Data were collected at five points: within the first week, and during follow-ups in the first, second, third, and sixth months after birth. We administered the Chinese versions of the Parenting Sense of Competence Scale and Edinburgh Perinatal Depression Scale, and used the Nursing Child Assessment Teaching Scale to score videotaped mother–infant interactions.

Results: We observed an increase in the quality of mother–infant interaction within the experimental group only. Furthermore, at the five assessment points, we observed no significant changes in perceived parenting competence. Among all subjects, there were correlations between postpartum depression scores, parenting competency, and quality of mother–infant interaction.

Conclusions: Our results indicate that first-time mothers in Taiwan who are provided with extra education on infants' abilities and how to effectively play with infants are likely to exhibit improvements in quality of interaction.

Keywords: Parenting education, First-time mothers, Parent–infant interaction quality, Parenting sense of competence

Background

The mother–infant interaction is the first and most important intrapersonal interaction that deeply affected a trust-building relationship in life [1]. It has substantial influences on infants' language development, [2] emotional regulation, [3] and cognitive development [4, 5], while children whose mothers regularly engage in quality interaction with them tend to exhibit a high mental development index at 2 years old [6]. If the parents' behavior shows strong intent for interaction, it attracts the attention of infants and initiates mutual exchange, response, and participation [7, 8]. In such cases, the infants actively contribute to social engagements and learn from these to anticipate social responses from caregivers [7]. Parent–child interaction is a shared, reciprocal experience within the dyads, whereby the experience of each has an impact on

* Correspondence: ghwan@mail.cgu.edu.tw; sarah@mail.cgu.edu.tw
[3]Department of Respiratory Therapy, College of Medicine, Chang Gung University, 259, Wen-Hwa 1st Road, Kwei-Shan, Taoyuan 333, Taiwan, Republic of China
[1]Department of Nursing, College of Nursing, Chang Gung University of Science and Technology, Taoyuan, Taiwan
Full list of author information is available at the end of the article

the experience of the other [7]. Effective parent–child interaction requires that both the infant and parent (or caregiver) send clear cues and respond to each other, thus facilitating the development of an interactive environment that continues the interaction [9, 10]. The parent and infant learn to adapt, modify, and change their behaviors in response to the other in every interaction process [11].

Researchers have determined that educational programs can be helpful means of improving first-time mothers' abilities to interact with their infants [12–17]. Dickie and Gerber indicate that providing information on infant development, temperament, and cues in 4- to 12-month-old infants to their parents during a 16-h class was helpful in understanding the demands of newborns, providing appropriate contingent responses for parents, and producing feedback and increasing behavior predictability for infants [18]. A randomized controlled trial, based on Brazelton's Neonatal Behavior Assessment Scale (NBAS) intervention, showed that a one-hour video and discussion on the behaviors and status of newborns for first-time mothers, delivered within 1 month postpartum, can increase the quality of mother–infant interactions. The results of this trial are based on the effect of information presented, about the newborn's competence to interact, on a mother's sensitive responsiveness toward her infant, thus promoting affectionate handling of the infant and motivating the mothers to become more involved and interact with their infants [15]. Similarly, another study similarly showed that a 45-min educational video on newborn behaviors for first-time pregnant women at 38 weeks' gestation enhanced the quality of mother–infant interaction during the 24 h following birth. More specifically, the scores for newborns' sensitivity to cues and socioemotional growth were found to be higher in the experimental group than in the control group that did not watch the video [12].

Furthermore, postpartum women must not only recover physically, but also, via mother–infant interaction, learn the skills necessary for caring for and identifying with their newborns, consequently developing their maternal role and behavior [19, 20]. The lack of understanding of newborns can increase mothers' anxiety, thereby influencing mother–infant interaction [12, 21–23], maternal confidence [22, 24–26], and even mothers' adaption to the maternal role [27]. Clark and Affonso report that it is exceedingly important for first-time mothers, in the first month after delivery, to deal with the gap in expectations and reality of maternal life, improve their own parenting skills, and establish a good relationship with the newborn [28].

Parenting sense of competence (PSOC) refers to the subjective feeling of a mothers' ability to take care of their infants and understand their infants' needs [29]. For first-time mothers, the most confusing period is 1–2 weeks after discharge from the hospital, after which their self-confidence

in motherhood tends to increase [30–33]. Maternal confidence and ability tends to increase with time after birth, with the highest confidence and ability appearing at 4 months postpartum [34]. Improving mothers' parenting skills can facilitate and enhance their sense of competence and satisfaction with the maternal role, and can prevent postnatal depression that fostering positive neonates' psychosocial development [29]. However, PSOC is not related to mothers' actual parenting abilities [35–37].

At 6 months postpartum, the postpartum depression symptoms can interfere with perceived parenting knowledge [38]. Women with postpartum depression showed a lower sense of mother role competence and satisfaction [29]. A Japanese study showed that mothers with higher postpartum depression score were more likely to engage in neglectful or aggressive parenting behaviors [39]. The depressed mothers were likely to show more negative and less positive behavior toward their infants than did the nondepressed mothers [40]. A negative correlation was found between the postpartum depression scores and PSOC [41–43] and parent–infant interaction quality [40, 44–46].

In Taiwan, women giving birth in the hospital are usually discharged three or 5 days after birth, depending on normal spontaneous delivery (NSD) or cesarean section (C/S). General postpartum care provided by hospitals concentrates on mothers' physical care, observation of urine and stool, instructed uterine massage, normal change in lochia, perineal douche, postnatal exercises, episiotomy or C/S wound care, neonatal bathing, and treatment of physical problems. In Taiwan, few hospitals provided postpartum care, but even so, postpartum home visits focused on lactation consultation for promoting the breastfeeding behavior. It rarely provided parents the information about how to be sensitive to child's signals, interpret them, and respond with emotional attunement. Previous studies have primarily focused on parenting stress and maternal confidence in Taiwanese postpartum women [30, 32]. Furthermore, Chinese typically express their emotions in more subtle forms than Western people. Chinese parents rarely praise their children verbally, because their culture encourages modesty and humility. Thus, human cultural factors influence beliefs and expressive behaviors in interaction [5, 47, 48]. Therefore, this study evaluated how mother-infant interactions and parenting competence are affected by a parenting competence education and how they change as the infant matures up to 6 months postpartum in Taiwan.

Methods
Study design and population
This study used a single-blind multiple time series design. In Taiwan, when visiting the doctor, pregnant

women who come for prenatal examination and postpartum women who come for postnatal 6 weeks examination sit in the same waiting area. The pregnant and postpartum women could share and discuss the information of this study with each other. To avoid affecting the authenticity of the data, we approached the potential participants for the experimental group after the last postpartum woman in the control group had finished her postnatal 6 weeks examination. In other words, after the last participant in the control group had completed her postnatal examination, the experimental group recruitment began.

Study subjects were recruited from a 260-bed medical center in northern Taiwan between August 1, 2010 and February 2, 2012. The inclusion criteria were (1) primiparas; (2) 20–34 years old; (3) normal term and singleton birth; (4) no diagnosed complications of gestational diabetes mellitus, pregnancy-induced hypertension, preterm birth, placental abruption, postpartum hemorrhage, postpartum thrombophlebitis, or perinatal depression; (5) understood and spoke Mandarin or Taiwanese; (6) lived in northern Taiwan; and (7) signed an informed consent form. The necessary sample size was calculated by considering mother–infant interaction score as the primary outcome (Cohen's d = 0.50) [8], while incorporating a 10% attrition rate. Given a 90% power and 5% type 1 error, the sample size was 82 dyads. This study received institutional review board (IRB) approval (no. 99-0243B).

Materials

This study provided self-compiled CDs and manuals of "Tips on caring for your baby" to the postpartum women in the experimental group. The 40-min content of the CD was modified from the self-instructional video series entitled "Keys to caregiving" on infant, behaviors, communication cues, and state modulation [49]. Then, we translated the sub-titles of the film to Chinese. The content of the manuals mainly introduced the sensory development of newborns aged 0–6 months and summarized the CD's content.

Instruments

We conducted the study using two instruments: the Nursing Child Assessment Teaching Scale (NCATS) and the Chinese version of the Parenting Sense of Competence (C-PSOC) Scale. In addition, we collected data from Additional file 1 (Questionnaires A. demographic and background information) and Additional file 2 (Questionnaires B. breastfeeding and baby care practices), and at the same time used the Chinese version of the Edinburgh Perinatal Depression Scale (C-EPDS) to monitor postpartum depression.

The NCATS is a standardized tool for assessing interactions between caregivers and infants aged between 0 to 36 months [11, 16]. The NCATS was widely used in research and clinical practice for families and young children [2, 12, 17, 43, 50]. The NCATS consists of 73 binary items, divided into six subcategories: the caregiver's sensitivity to cues, response to distress, social-emotional growth-fostering behaviors, and cognitive growth-fostering behaviors; the child's clarity of cues and responsiveness to caregiver. In addition, the tool captures contingency items, such as the behavior of one member of the dyad affects the response from the other. The scale showed good internal consistency (0.76–0.87) and 4-week test-retest reliability (0.55–0.85) [11]. The Cronbach's α of caregiver's and child's subscales in this study were 0.84 and 0.76, respectively.

The PSOC Scale was developed in 1978 [51] and the C-PSOC Scale. The latter had been validated with 0.85 internal consistency and 0.87 4-week test-retest reliability in a sample of Hong Kong Chinese mothers. Significant correlations with measures of self-esteem ($r = 0.60$, $p < 0.01$) and depression ($r = - 0.48$, $p < 0.01$) demonstrated good construct validity [52]. The Cronbach's α of the PSOC Scale in this study was 0.90.

The questionnaires B were developed by the researcher for this study. The questionnaires B was collected from the postpartum mothers who self-reported that they were primary caregivers or not, and recalled how much time they spent to care for and handle with their babies in a week. The content validity was done by five obstetrics experts, who were asked to rate each item based on relevance, clarity, simplicity, and ambiguity on the 5-point Likert scale. The Content Validity Index (CVI) was 0.86–0.94.

The C-EPDS, which was developed by Cox, Holden, and Sagovsky in 1987 [53], has been validated in a sample of Taiwanese mothers [54]. The Cronbach's α of C-EPDS in this study was 0.79. The 12/13 cutoff point was used to monitor postpartum depression [55] in our study. If necessary, the subjects were referred to the psychiatrist for further diagnosis, and if they were diagnosed with postpartum depression, the data collection was stopped and the subjects were excluded.

Experimental procedure and data collection

One researcher identified women from the prenatal and delivery records who met the inclusion criteria and approached them in the postnatal ward at least 3 days after delivery (before they were discharged). Potential participants were first given written and verbal information about the study and then written informed consent was obtained. The mothers who agreed to participate in the study were asked to provide their addresses and phone numbers to contact them for their first visit after discharge. Their contact information was kept confidential for the purpose of the study.

The participants were visited five times – within the first week, the 1st month, the 2nd month, the 3rd month, and the 6th month after delivery – in postpartum nursing centers and/or their homes. Most Taiwanese conduct the ritual 'Do the months' (30-day period) after delivery [56], a form of support for postpartum women that originated in the Chinese culture [57]. Either the woman's mother or mother-in-law assists her by taking care of her personal needs, helping her care for the newborn baby, taking care of any other children, and doing the housework [58]. Nowadays, around half of the new mothers choose to stay in postpartum nursing centers in northern Taiwan. It is a professional home-like health care facility operated by registered nurses. They provide postpartum services (for about a month) to facilitate the recovery of a postpartum woman and take care of her newborn baby, thus, conducting the 'Doing the month' ritual.

Each visit concluded with the administration of the above mentioned self-report questionnaires. The data collection procedure is presented in Fig. 1. When the baby was ready (in quiet alert state), the researcher (first author) introduced the task by giving a toy (rattle, block, or squeak toy) to the mother to play with her baby. We provided a new toy in each visit for hygiene considerations. To assess mother–infant interactions, we videotaped first-time mothers when they introduced new toys to their children and completed the task and when they needed to soothe their children. We videotaped for as long as the mothers interacted with their infants, which ranged from 2 to 16 min, depending on the actual interaction time until the mothers claimed they had done with teaching their infants [11]. The scoring was done by first researcher, certified in the use of NCATS tools (achieved an inter-rater reliability score of 90%). In this study, all toys, missions, and administration were taken and followed from the "Caregiving/Parent–Child Interaction Teaching Manual" as per NCATS protocol [11].

After videotaping, both the groups were given general postpartum guidance: (1) demo bathing of the baby and umbilical cord care skills, manually expressing breastmilk skills; (2) discussing breastfeeding problems and selection of breastfeeding pumps, to relieve baby gas/red spot on baby's face; (3) providing the information on adding food to the baby's diet; (4) listening and providing emotion support. However, there was no discussion of mother–infant interaction or parenting competence in the control group. The data collection procedure was conducted by a specific researcher to reduce the data collection bias and ensure the privacy and safety of videotaped information.

Statistical analysis

All statistical analyses were conducted using SPSS Statistics 21.0 (IBM Corp., Armonk, NY, USA). The significance level for all tests was 0.05. The independent two-sample t test was used to identify the group differences in normally distributed continuous variables, while the chi-square test was used to determine group differences in categorical variables. The generalized estimating equation (GEE) analysis is a very useful technique when subject attrition threatens the power of longitudinal studies [59, 60]. In this study, we examined the trends in dependent variables, mother–infant interaction (NCATS) and PSOC using the GEE model, and set up "within-subject variable" = time; "covariance matrix" = robust estimator; "working correlation matrix" = exchangeable; "predictors factor" = group, time, and group time; "model" = group, time, group time and propensity scores. The propensity scores were calculated for parents' age, education, and work status; mothers' body mass index (BMI) before pregnancy, weight gain during pregnancy, and abortion history; whether the pregnancy was planned; mothers' parenting knowledge; delivery method; and child's gender and birth weight.

Results

Participants

Eighty-one primiparous mothers (40 in control group and 41 in experimental group) and their newborn infants were recruited for the study. One subject withdrew after 1 month because her mother-in-law held traditional views of parenting, such as newborns do not need much interaction or play. The dropout rate was 1.2%. No mother was referred to the psychiatrist in our study.

In the control group, around 30% of first-time mothers held no religious beliefs and only three mothers had ever had a smoking habit. In the experimental group, 17.3% held no religious beliefs, and two participants previously had smoking and drinking habits, while one still had a smoking habit (about 10 cigarettes per day). The BMI before pregnancy and the weight gain during pregnancy were in the normal range for both the groups. Approximately 93% of the subjects had obtained parenting information during their pregnancy, but none of this education had covered the topics taught in this study. Although infants' body weight was significantly heavier in the control group than in the experimental group, the other basic characteristics and pregnancy/delivery data did not differ significantly (see Table 1).

Infant care pattern in six months postpartum

Sixty percent of the control group and 65.9% of the experimental group chose a postpartum nursing center or a babysitter to assist in infant care during the first month postpartum. All first-time mothers self-reported that they spent a considerable amount of time on infant care during that first month. The exclusive breastfeeding rate was 58% in control group and 59% in experimental group. After 6 months, the infant care time and exclusive breastfeeding

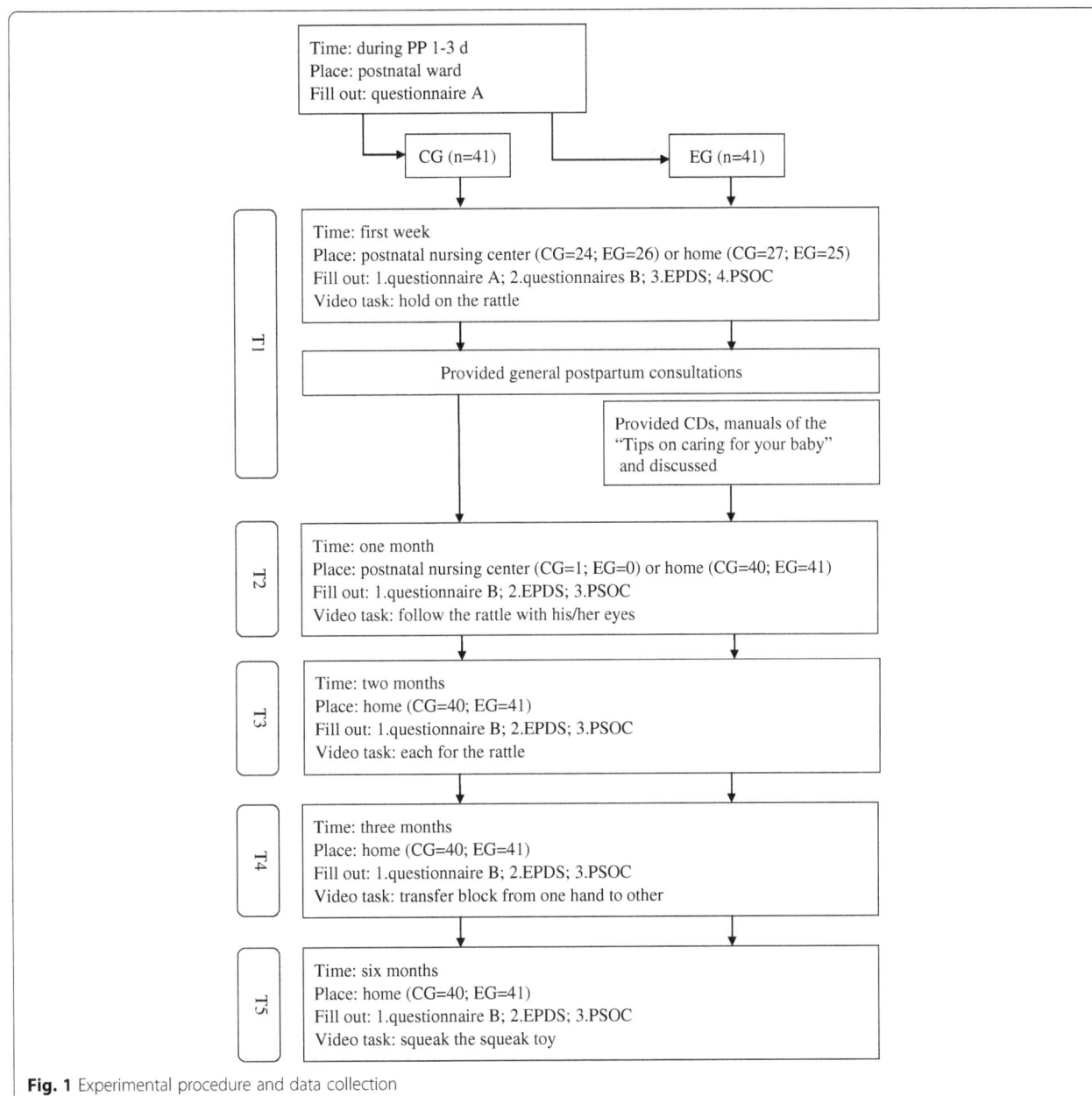

Fig. 1 Experimental procedure and data collection

rates had reduced in both groups. There was no difference in infants' time schedules, caregiving patterns, milk-feeding types, or mothers' perceived resting frequency across any of the points in time or between groups (see Table 2).

Most Chinese postpartum women undergo food therapy, that is, eating yang foods and avoiding yin foods, and engage in plenty of good rest in order to recover physically in the first month postpartum [58]. Common yang foods include chicken, egg, pig kidney, chicken or fish soup, ginger, and brown sugar. Common yin foods include most fresh fruits and vegetables, ice, and salt [61]. This diet is followed to compensate for the blood loss during childbirth [57].

Trends in mother–infant interaction quality

Figure 2 shows the results of the NCATS for caregivers and infants (caregivers: (sensitivity to cues, response to distress, social-emotional growth fostering, and cognitive growth fostering; infants: clarity of cues and responsiveness to caregiver). The sensitivity to cues score for caregivers showed a slight decreasing trend in the second (T3) and sixth (T5) months compared to the first week postpartum. Furthermore, the score of social-emotional growth fostering, cognitive growth fostering, and responsiveness to caregiver showed a decrease at 6 months. All the other scores for mother–infant interaction increased over time. Overall, the results indicated that the caregiver scores (Fig. 3a), child

Table 1 Personal characteristics and pregnancy/delivery information

	CG ($n = 40$)	EG ($n = 41$)	t / χ^2 value	p value
Mother's age, yrs	32.35 ± 2.80	33.49 ± 3.38	2.720	0.103
BMI, kg/m^2	20.46 ± 2.17	20.49 ± 3.03	0.002	0.962
BW increase during pregnancy, kg	14.51 ± 3.90	15.29 ± 6.56	0.430	0.514
Father's age, yrs	34.68 ± 3.94	36.15 ± 4.39	2.517	0.117
Infant BW, kg	3278.38 ± 377.06	3096.34 ± 371.54	4.789	0.032
Mother's education			2.483	0.283
High school	1 (2.5)	4 (9.8)		
Junior college	26 (65.0)	21 (51.2)		
College or above	13 (32.5)	16 (39.0)		
Mother's work status			2.614	0.282
Housewife	6 (15.0)	10 (24.4)		
Part-time Job	2 (5.0)	0		
Full-time job	32 (80.0)	31 (75.6)		
Father's education			3.952	0.165
High school	0	4 (9.7)		
Junior college	20 (50.0)	17 (41.5)		
College or above	20 (50.0)	21 (48.8)		
Father's work status			1.307	0.513
None	1 (2.5)	0		
Part-time Job	3 (7.5)	2 (4.9)		
Full-time job	36 (90.0)	39 (95.1)		
Abortion history	12 (30.0)	5 (12.2)	3.871	0.049
Pregnancy planned	27 (67.5)	29 (70.7)	0.099	0.753
Received parenting information	37 (92.5)	38 (92.7)	0.001	1.000
Delivery			2.102	0.147
NSD	16 (40.0)	23 (56.1)		
C/S	24 (60.0)	18 (43.9)		
Infant gender			0.307	0.579
Boy	21 (52.5)	19 (46.3)		
Girl	19 (47.5)	22 (53.7)		

CG control group, *EG* experimental group

scores (Fig. 3b), total scores (Fig. 3c), and contingency scores (Fig. 3d) at the 1st to the 6th month were evidently higher in the experimental group than in the control group.

Trends of the sense of parenting competence

We observed no difference in C-PSOC scores between the control group (mean = 67.28, SD = 10.18) and experimental group (mean = 65.46, SD = 12.56) in the first week (Fig. 3e). The C-PSOC scores then showed a decrease (control group: mean = 65.05, SD = 10.06; experimental group: mean = 63.56, SD = 15.15) at the 1st month, before gradually increasing from the 2nd to the 6th month. At no point were the C-PSOC scores significantly different between the two groups.

Effectiveness on PCI and PSOC

This study evaluated the intervention effect on mother–infant interaction quality and PSOC using a GEE model (Table 3). We found no differences in sensitivity to cues, response to distress, social-emotional growth fostering, cognitive growth fostering, clarity of cues, or responsiveness to caregiver in the first week between the two groups. Notably, caregiver scores, child scores, total scores, and contingency scores for infants in the experimental group did not significantly differ from those in the control group. For the experimental group, a significant increasing trend was observed in sensitivity to cues, social-emotional growth fostering, cognitive growth fostering, clarity of cues, and responsiveness to caregiver, as well as overall caregiver scores, child scores, total scores,

Table 2 Infant care pattern during six months postpartum

	1st week	1st month	2nd month	3rd month	6th month
Baby average day wake time, hr./ day					
CG	5.3 ± 2.0	5.5 ± 2.7	5.6 ± 2.1	6.5 ± 2.4	8.8 ± 2.3
EG	4.8 ± 2.0	5.2 ± 2.6	5.9 ± 2.3	7.3 ± 2.1	9.0 ± 2.4
p value	0.281	0.636	0.581	0.124	0.758
Baby primary caregiver, n (%)					
CG					
Mother	18 (50.0)	37 (92.5)	26 (66.7)	13 (32.5)	10 (25.0)
Family	1 (2.8)	2 (5.0)	7 (17.9)	16 (40.0)	17 (42.5)
Others	17 (47.2)	1 (2.5)	6 (15.4)	11 (27.5)	13 (32.5)
EG					
Mother	13 (31.7)	40 (97.6)	31 (75.6)	19 (46.3)	16 (39.0)
Family	0	0	5 (12.2)	14 (34.1)	15 (36.6)
Others	28 (68.3)	1 (2.4)	5 (12.2)	8 (19.5)	10 (24.4)
p value	0.081	0.487	0.666	0.423	0.389
Care baby time per week, hr					
CG	119.6 ± 54.9	153.3 ± 38.7	138.7 ± 43.1	107.0 ± 47.1	100.4 ± 47.8
EG	123.8 ± 50.8	163.9 ± 20.6	148.4 ± 34.4	123.7 ± 47.2	121.1 ± 44.9
p value	0.730	0.127	0.271	0.115	0.048
Exclusive Breastfeeding, n (%)					
CG	19 (52.8)	23 (57.5)	17 (43.6)	18 (45.0)	19 (47.5)
EG	23 (56.1)	24 (58.5)	16 (39.0)	18 (43.9)	18 (43.9)
p value	0.770	0.925	0.678	0.921	0.745
Perceived resting frequency, n (%)					
CG					
Often	21 (58.3)	13 (32.5)	20 (51.3)	33 (82.5)	34 (85.0)
Sometimes	10 (27.8)	16 (40.0)	11 (28.2)	6 (15.0)	4 (10.0)
Seldom	5 (13.9)	11 (27.5)	8 (20.5)	1 (2.5)	2 (5.0)
EG					
Often	17 (41.5)	12 (29.3)	24 (58.5)	35 (85.4)	33 (80.5)
Sometimes	14 (34.1)	16 (39.0)	11 (26.8)	5 (12.2)	8 (19.5)
Seldom	10 (24.4)	13 (31.7)	6 (14.6)	1 (2.4)	0
p value	0.295	0.907	0.741	0.934	0.124

CG control group, EG experimental group

and contingency scores at the 1st month, the 2nd month, the 3rd month, and the 6th month. This indicated that receiving postpartum parenting education led to an increase in mother–infant interaction quality among first-time mothers in the 6 months after delivery, except for the aspect of interaction related to response to distress.

The PSOC at baseline in the experimental group was similar to that in the control group. Furthermore, we observed no change in the PSOC in the experimental group between the 1st month and the 6th month, indicating that while the postpartum parenting education appeared to help improve mother–infant interaction quality, it has no effect on the PSOC of first-time mothers. Among all subjects, clear correlations were found between postpartum depression, parenting competency, and quality of mother–infant interaction (see Table 4).

Discussion

In this study, we evaluated how postpartum parenting education influenced the quality of mother–infant interaction and PSOC in the 6 months after delivery among first-time mothers in Taiwan. The education was evidently helpful in improving overall mother–infant interaction quality during the 6 months after delivery, but it

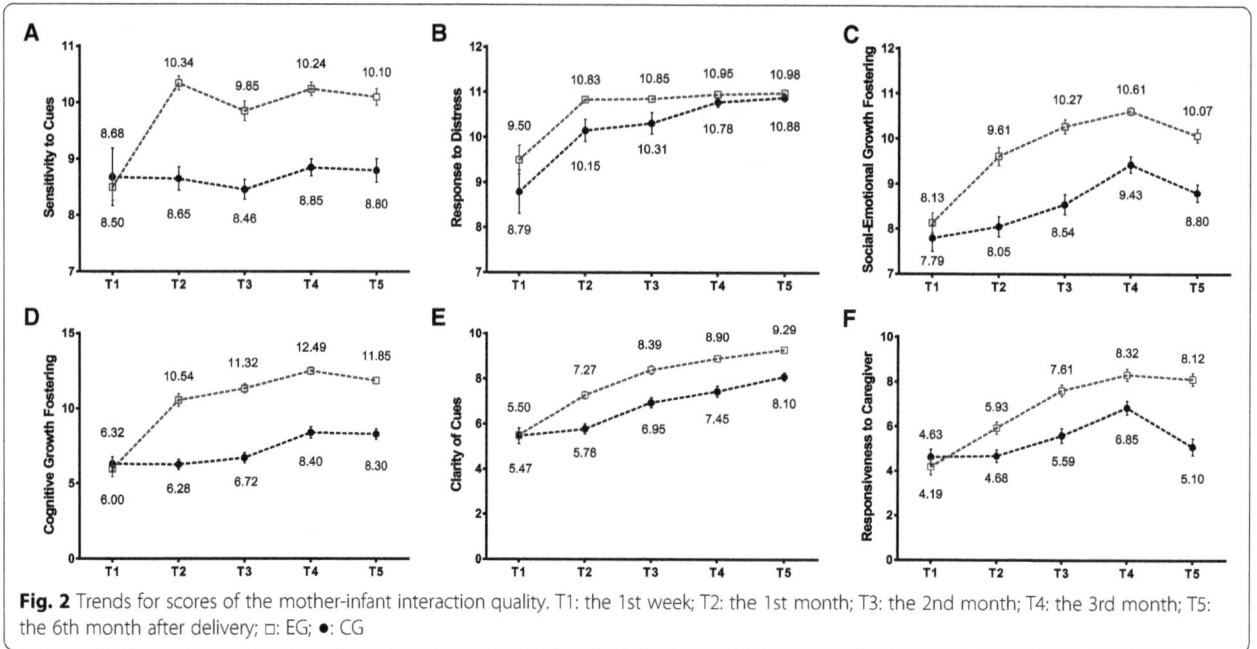

Fig. 2 Trends for scores of the mother-infant interaction quality. T1: the 1st week; T2: the 1st month; T3: the 2nd month; T4: the 3rd month; T5: the 6th month after delivery; □: EG; ●: CG

had no effect on the response to distress aspect of that interaction. This result was in accordance with the findings of previous studies indicating that postpartum parenting education is effective in improving mother–infant interaction quality [12–15, 18, 62, 63]. It should be noted that, while the interaction scores of the mother's response to infant's distress in the first and second month after delivery were higher in the experimental group than in the control group, there was no significant difference in the magnitude of the progress between the two groups. A possible reason for this is that first-time mothers must be able to manage infants' distress, for example, crying, being fussy, or generally upset in everyday life. As such, while the intervention education made the mothers in the experimental group learn these skills sooner, the control group mothers were still accumulating parenting experience during the first month after delivery, including how to respond to infants' distress; thus, their abilities would not differ substantially from that of the experimental group. Previous studies have similarly

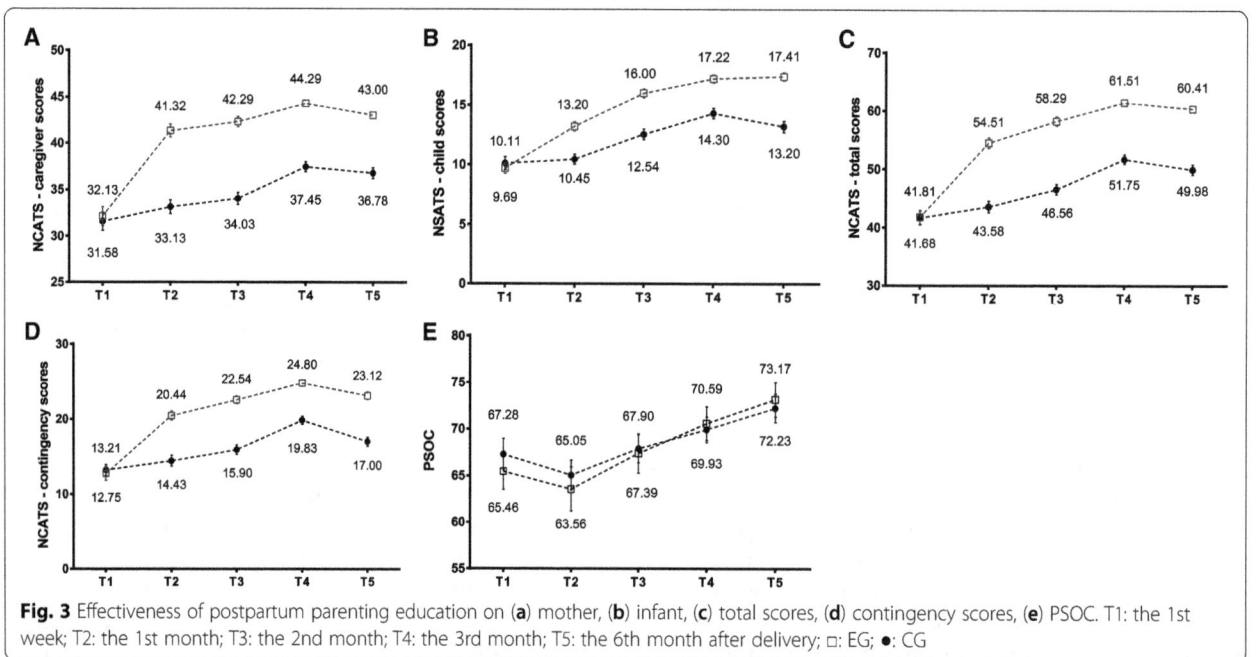

Fig. 3 Effectiveness of postpartum parenting education on (**a**) mother, (**b**) infant, (**c**) total scores, (**d**) contingency scores, (**e**) PSOC. T1: the 1st week; T2: the 1st month; T3: the 2nd month; T4: the 3rd month; T5: the 6th month after delivery; □: EG; ●: CG

Table 3 Effectiveness of postpartum parenting education on the quality of mother-infant interaction and sense changes of parenting competence

| | NCATS | | | | | | | | | | | |
| | Sensitivity to Cues | | | | Response to Distress | | | | Social-Emotional Growth Fostering | | | |
	B	S.E.	Wald χ^2	p value	B	S.E.	Wald χ^2	p value	B	S.E.	Wald χ^2	p value
Intercept	8.68	0.29	924.22**	< 0.001	8.78	0.48	328.50**	< 0.001	7.80	0.29	718.56**	< 0.001
EG[a]	−0.31	0.35	0.77	0.381	0.49	0.54	0.82	0.366	0.26	0.35	0.57	0.452
Time												
1st m vs. 1st wk[b]	−0.10	0.29	0.12	0.728	1.25	0.48	6.69*	0.010	0.18	0.30	0.38	0.539
2nd m vs. 1st wk[b]	−0.29	0.30	0.94	0.334	1.42	0.49	8.32**	0.004	0.66	0.31	4.60*	0.032
3rd m vs. 1st wk[b]	0.10	0.31	0.10	0.751	1.88	0.46	16.92**	< 0.001	1.56	0.31	25.09**	< 0.001
6th m vs. 1st wk[b]	0.05	0.28	0.03	0.866	1.98	0.46	18.83**	< 0.001	0.93	0.34	7.72**	0.005
Interaction												
EG × [1st m vs. 1st wk][c]	1.93	0.36	28.74**	< 0.001	0.08	0.57	0.02	0.890	1.24	0.35	12.60**	< 0.001
EG × [2nd m vs. 1st wk][c]	1.63	0.39	17.53**	< 0.001	−0.06	0.57	0.01	0.913	1.42	0.37	14.60**	< 0.001
EG × [3rd m vs. 1st wk][c]	1.63	0.41	15.75**	< 0.001	−0.42	0.55	0.60	0.438	0.86	0.37	5.34*	0.021
EG × [6th m vs. 1st wk][c]	1.53	0.37	16.85**	< 0.001	−0.50	0.55	0.83	0.364	0.95	0.41	5.48*	0.019
Propensity score	0.21	0.22	0.89	0.347	0.35	0.31	1.28	0.258	0.18	0.28	0.42	0.518

| | NCATS | | | | | | | | | | | |
| | Cognitive Growth Fostering | | | | Clarity of Cues | | | | Responsiveness to Caregiver | | | |
	B	S.E.	Wald χ^2	p value	B	S.E.	Wald χ^2	p value	B	S.E.	Wald χ^2	p value
Intercept	6.67	0.45	222.11**	< 0.001	5.53	0.36	242.18**	< 0.001	4.77	0.36	179.79**	< 0.001
EG[a]	−0.23	0.67	0.15	0.736	0.03	0.38	0.01	0.941	−0.30	0.52	0.33	0.566
Time												
1st m vs. 1st wk[b]	−0.34	0.45	0.55	0.459	0.29	0.39	0.56	0.453	0.03	0.45	0.00	0.957
2nd m vs. 1st wk[b]	0.10	0.45	0.05	0.830	1.47	0.38	14.89**	< 0.001	0.95	0.45	4.53*	0.033
3rd m vs. 1st wk[b]	1.79	0.52	11.62**	0.001	1.97	0.43	21.15**	< 0.001	2.20	0.45	24.24**	< 0.001
6th m vs. 1st wk[b]	1.69	0.54	9.88**	0.002	2.62	0.40	42.71**	< 0.001	0.45	0.54	0.69	0.407
Interaction												
EG × [1st m vs. 1st wk][c]	0.54	0.70	41.62**	< 0.001	1.51	0.45	11.38**	0.001	1.67	0.62	7.32**	0.007
EG × [2nd m vs. 1st wk][c]	4.89	0.69	49.60**	< 0.001	1.45	0.46	9.77**	0.002	2.42	0.61	15.70**	< 0.001
EG × [3rd m vs. 1st wk][c]	4.37	0.75	34.30**	< 0.001	1.47	0.47	9.95**	0.002	1.88	0.63	9.05**	0.003
EG × [6th m vs. 1st wk][c]	3.83	0.72	27.96**	< 0.001	1.21	0.44	7.37**	0.007	3.44	0.74	21.75**	< 0.001
Propensity score	−0.17	0.54	0.10	0.754	−0.13	0.24	0.29	0.590	3.35	0.43	0.67	0.413

| | NCATS | | | | | | | | | | | |
| | Caregiver scores | | | | Child scores | | | | Total scores | | | |
	B	S.E.	Wald χ^2	p value	B	S.E.	Wald χ^2	p value	B	S.E.	Wald χ^2	p value
Intercept	32.01	0.97	1095.92**	< 0.001	10.30	0.56	343.17**	< 0.001	42.30	1.16	1328.29**	< 0.001
EG[a]	0.19	1.30	0.02	0.887	−0.27	0.71	0.15	0.702	−0.11	1.64	0.01	0.946
Time												
1st m vs. 1st wk[b]	0.92	0.92	1.00	0.318	0.31	0.69	0.20	0.652	1.25	1.29	0.93	0.336
2nd m vs. 1st wk[b]	1.81	0.97	3.49	0.062	2.42	0.64	14.45**	< 0.001	4.26	1.31	10.60**	0.001
3rd m vs. 1st wk[b]	5.24	1.03	26.03**	< 0.001	4.16	0.67	38.32**	< 0.001	9.42	1.41	44.64**	< 0.001
6th m vs. 1st wk[b]	4.57	1.00	21.08**	< 0.001	3.06	0.72	18.19**	< 0.001	7.65	1.32	33.57**	< 0.001
Interaction												
EG × [1st m vs. 1st wk][c]	7.82	1.29	36.77**	< 0.001	3.18	0.90	12.43**	< 0.001	11.02	1.77	38.75**	< 0.001

Table 3 Effectiveness of postpartum parenting education on the quality of mother-infant interaction and sense changes of parenting competence *(Continued)*

EG × [2nd m vs. 1st wk]^c	7.91	1.34	35.07**	< 0.001	3.87	0.87	19.98**	< 0.001	11.79	1.79	43.27**	< 0.001
EG × [3rd m vs. 1st wk]^c	6.47	1.44	20.33**	< 0.001	3.35	0.87	14.99**	< 0.001	9.85	1.87	27.73**	< 0.001
EG × [6th m vs. 1st wk]^c	5.85	1.39	17.68**	< 0.001	4.65	0.95	23.68**	< 0.001	10.52	1.82	33.57**	< 0.001
Propensity score	0.57	0.90	0.40	0.528	−0.49	0.55	0.78	0.376	0.84	1.14	0.01	0.941

	NCATS				PSOC			
	Contingency scores							
	B	S.E.	Wald χ^2	p value	B	S.E.	Wald χ^2	p value
Intercept	13.67	0.75	336.23**	< 0.001	66.78	2.30	843.52**	< 0.001
EG^a	−0.36	1.15	0.10	0.751	−2.59	2.94	0.78	0.379
Time								
1st m vs. 1st wk^b	0.91	0.92	0.98	0.323	−2.37	1.27	3.47	0.062
2nd m vs. 1st wk^b	2.40	0.90	7.18**	0.007	0.15	1.13	0.02	0.896
3rd m vs. 1st wk^b	6.31	0.87	52.00**	< 0.001	2.50	1.24	4.09*	0.043
6th m vs. 1st wk^b	3.48	0.78	20.15**	< 0.001	4.80	1.41	11.56**	0.001
Interaction								
EG × [1st m vs. 1st wk]^c	6.53	1.26	26.85**	< 0.001	0.47	1.82	0.07	0.796
EG × [2nd m vs. 1st wk]^c	7.14	1.26	32.05**	< 0.001	1.78	1.74	1.05	0.306
EG × [3rd m vs. 1st wk]^c	5.50	1.31	17.62**	< 0.001	2.62	1.83	2.06	0.151
EG × [6th m vs. 1st wk]^c	6.64	1.29	26.51**	< 0.001	2.91	2.07	1.97	0.161
Propensity score	−0.47	0.82	0.32	0.572	1.92	4.20	0.21	0.647

*: $p < 0.05$, **: $p < 0.01$; df = 1; ^a Reference category: CG; ^b Reference category: 1st week (Baseline); ^c Reference category: CG × 1st week (Baseline)
NCATS nursing child assessment teaching scale, *PSOC* parenting sense of competence, *EG* experimental group, *1st wk* the 1st week, *1st m* the 1st month; *2nd m* the 2nd month, *3rd m* the 3rd month, *6th m* the 6th month

found that first-time mothers apparently show improvements in knowledge of caring for newborns in the two–six weeks after birth [31–33].

However, when observing the influence of time on mother–infant interaction quality, response to distress showed apparent progress at the 1st month, the 2nd month, the 3rd month, and the 6th month, but there was no significant progress in sensitivity to cues over the assessment period. This suggests that mother–infant interaction quality exhibits positive changes through the accumulation of experience between mothers and infants. More specifically, response to distress showed a rather rapid increase, whereas sensitivity to cues might need greater contact time or special instructions. Recognizing that a child is a person

Table 4 Associations between scores of postpartum depression, parenting competency, and quality of mother-infant interaction

Scores		PSOC	NCATS
EPDS	r_s	−0.618**	−0.146**
	p value	< 0.001	0.006
PSOC	r_s	1	0.156**
	p value	–	0.003

PSOC parenting sense of competence, *NCATS* nursing child assessment teaching scale, *EPDS* Edinburgh perinatal depression scale
**: $p < 0.01$

in the environment is considered the basis of personal interaction [9]. Sumner and Spietz report that numerous first-time parents are unable to recognize their newborns' abilities or interact with their infants as people in their environment [11]. First-time parents become familiar with the characteristics and abilities of their newborns through the process of caregiving [19, 20], which makes them more sensitive to newborns' behaviors and demands and engage in more appropriate responses, thus improving interaction quality [10].

Gibaud-Wallston and Wandersman showed that the parenting competence of first-time parents began to increase from about 6 weeks after delivery [51]. Our results showed that postpartum education focusing on infants' states, behaviors, and communication cues using videos and instruction manuals cannot improve PSOC during in the 6 months after delivery. We found that the lowest PSOC scores in both groups were in the first month postpartum, after which they increased until the third month. This is perhaps because, in the first month, first-time mothers spend considerable amount of time taking care of their children rather than recovering. During the first month home visit, we found that the mothers consistently asked questions about infants' crying during the nighttime, bowel movements, and breastfeeding, as well as how to adjust infants' time schedules. Thus, even if first-time mothers might have been thoroughly immersed in the joyful feeling of motherhood, they might have been experiencing feelings of anxiety, frustration, lack of competence, and exhaustion, thus leading to the low PSOC [64].

Past research has shown that newborns' mothers were most stressed in the first month postpartum, after which their stress began decreasing as their understanding of infants, mastery of care skills, and perceived ability to care for the infant increased [34]. This result is similar to that of our own study, wherein PSOC in both the experimental and control groups increased over time, beginning from the second month of delivery. Additionally, mothers' knowledge of newborn care and maternal confidence increased over time. This somewhat consistent with the findings of Wu (2000), who found that providing physical care for newborns, establishing a mother–infant relationship, and instructing first-time mothers on newborns' conditions and behavioral cues during their discharge from the hospital could improve maternal confidence in the second week of postpartum; however, no difference in maternal confidence was found after the first month [31]. Other studies have also demonstrated similar results: Kuo et al. (2000) show that providing instructions on newborns' physical care and behavioral status at postpartum can increase maternal confidence in the second week of postpartum, [32] while Chen (2005) shows that providing instructions on newborns' development and physical care at 32–34 weeks of pregnancy could enhance maternal confidence at 6 weeks' postpartum [33].

Additionally, there was no significant difference between the groups in the magnitude of the change in PSOC between the 1st month and 6th month. Previous studies have emphasized instruction on practical behaviors, such as skills in caring for newborns, as they can facilitate mothers' self-confidence in their parenting skills and ability to understand infants' demands. A possible reason for no significant difference in the magnitude of change was the C-PSOC, which evaluates both self-efficacy and self-satisfaction of mothers' parenting role abilities and is associated more with mothers' personal feelings, but is not representative of their actual abilities [36, 37]. Influenced by modesty and humility in Taiwanese culture [5], mothers underestimate themselves and the maternal role achievement needs more time than maternal skills [19, 20]. Additionally, higher depression scores were correlated with lower parenting competence scores and interaction scores. Also, higher interaction scores were correlated with higher parenting competence scores in this study. These results were similar to the previous studies [38, 39].

In this study, we could not randomly assign the participants to the two groups, and approximately 60% of the participants remained in postpartum nursing facilities for the first month. Thus, we employed the propensity score and GEE model for reducing the selection bias and the influence of missing data. Additionally, further study warrants investigations on the impact of mother–infant interaction quality with the total time of using the CDs/manuals and different child sequence.

We also found that first-time mothers usually focused on completing the task rather than giving new toys to their children for exploration, and seldom praised their children. It was found that 93% of the participants obtained information on raising children from relatives, friends, books, and magazines, other mothers, health care personnel, and the internet. Thus, it would seem necessary to educate Taiwanese first-time mothers on how to play with their infants, as well as how to be sensitive to infants' behaviors. We suggest providing information about newborns' characteristics, their ability to play with parents and grandparents, and postpartum nursing facilities via the internet as well as through service education.

Conclusions

It was helpful in mother–infant interaction quality when the first-time mothers received the parenting educations on infants' abilities and how to play with infants during the 6 months after delivery. An apparent progress on response to distress in mother–infant interaction quality was shown at the 1st, 2nd, 3rd, and 6th months, respectively. The lowest PSOC scores in both groups were found in the first month postpartum, after which they increased until the third month. Significant associations found among postpartum depression, parenting competency, and quality of mother–infant interaction in the two groups.

Abbreviations
BMI: Body mass index; C-EPDS: Chinese version of the Edinburgh Perinatal Depression Scale; C-PSOC: Chinese version of the Parenting Sense of Competence Scale; GEE: Generalized estimating equation; NCATS: Nursing child assessment teaching scale; PSOC: Parenting sense of competence; SD: Standard deviation

Acknowledgments
The authors would like to thank the Chang Gung Memorial Hospital, Taiwan, for financially supporting this research under grants CMRPF1A0031. The funders had no role in study design, data collection and analysis, decision to publish, or preparation of the manuscript. The authors also thank Denise Findlay at University of Washington for her help in the NCATS qualification process and CD production.

Funding
This study was supported by the Chang Gung Memorial Hospital in Taiwan (CMRPF1A0031). The funder had no role in study design, data collection and analysis, decision to publish, or preparation of the manuscript.

Authors' contributions
FFC and HEL supervised the data collection; KCL designed the analysis. FFC analyzed the data under the supervision of SCK, KCL, and HEL. GHW wrote and edited the manuscript. All authors were involved in the design of the study and interpretation of the data; all have approved the final version.

Competing interests

The authors declare that they have no competing interests.

Author details
[1]Department of Nursing, College of Nursing, Chang Gung University of Science and Technology, Taoyuan, Taiwan. [2]Department of Nursing, Linkuo Chang Gung Memorial Hospital, Taoyuan, Taiwan. [3]Department of Respiratory Therapy, College of Medicine, Chang Gung University, 259, Wen-Hwa 1st Road, Kwei-Shan, Taoyuan 333, Taiwan, Republic of China. [4]Department of Obstetrics and Gynecology, Taipei Chang Gung Memorial Hospital, Taipei, Taiwan. [5]Department of Respiratory Care, Chang Gung University of Science and Technology, Chiayi, Taiwan. [6]Department of Midwifery and Women Health Care, National Taipei University of Nursing and Health Sciences, Taipei, Taiwan. [7]Institute of Hospital and Health Care Administration, Community Research Center, National Yang-Ming University, Taipei, Taiwan. [8]School of Nursing, College of Medicine, Chang Gung University, 259, Wen-Hwa 1st Road, Kwei-Shan, Taoyuan 333, Taiwan, Republic of China. [9]Department of Rheumatology, Linkuo Chang Gung Memorial Hospital, Taoyuan, Taiwan.

References
1. Hofer MA. Psychobiological roots of early attachment. Curr Dir Psychol Sci. 2006;15(2):84–8.
2. Magill-Evans J, Harrison MJ. Parent-child interactions and development of toddlers born preterm. West J Nurs Res. 1999;21(3):292–307.
3. MacLean PC, Rynes KN, Aragón C, Caprihan A, Phillips JP, Lowe JR. Mother-infant mutual eye gaze supports emotion regulation in infancy during the still-face paradigm. Infant Behav Dev. 2014;37(4):512–22.
4. Shannon JD, Tamis-LeMonda CS, London K, Cabrera N. Beyond rough and tumble: low-income fathers' interactions and childrens' cognitive development at 24 months. Parenting. 2002;2(2):77–104.
5. Negayama K, Delafield-Butt JT, Momose K, Ishijima K, Kawahara N, Lux EJ, Murphy A, Kaliarntas K. Embodied intersubjective engagement in mother–infant tactile communication: a cross-cultural study of Japanese and Scottish mother–infant behaviors during infant pick-up. Front Psychol. 2015; 6:66. https://doi.org/10.3389/fpsyg.2015.00066.
6. Barnard KE, Eyres SJ. Child health assessment, part 2: the first year of life. Washington, DC: U. S. Government Printing Office; 1979.
7. Trevarthen C, Aitken K. Infant Intersubjectivity: research, theory, and clinical applications. J Child Psychol Psychiatry. 2001;42(1):3–48.
8. Brazelton TB, Koslowski B, Main M. The origins of reciprocity: the early mother-infant interaction. In: Lewis M, Rosenblum LA, editors. The effect of the infant on its caregiver. New York: Wiley; 1974. p. 49–76.
9. White C, Simon M, Bryan A. Using evidence to educate birthing center nursing staff about infant states, cues, and behaviors. MCN Am J Matern Child Nurs. 2002;27(5):294–8.
10. Barnard KE. NCAST: nursing child assessment satellite training: learning resource manual. Seattle: University of Washington; 1978.
11. Sumner G, Spietz A. NCAST caregiver/ parent-child interaction teaching manual. Seattle: NCAST; 1994.
12. Leitch DB. Mother-infant interaction: achieving synchrony. Nurs Res. 1999; 48(1):55–8.
13. Hall LA. Effect of teaching on primiparas' perceptions of their newborn. Nurs Res. 1980;29(5):317–22.
14. Waterston T, Welsh B, Keane B, Cook M, Hammal D, Parker L, McConachie H. Improving early relationships: a randomized, controlled trial of an age-paced parenting newsletter. Pediatrics. 2009;123(1):241–7.
15. Wendland-Carro J, Piccinini CA, Millar WS. The role of an early intervention on enhancing the quality of mother-infant interaction. Child Dev. 1999;70(3):713–21.
16. Letourneau N. Fostering resiliency in infants and young children through parent-infant interaction. Infants Young Children. 1997;9(3):36–45.
17. Letourneau N, Drummond J, Fleming D, Kysela G, McDonald L, Stewart M. Supporting parents: can intervention improve parent-child relationships? J Fam Nurs. 2001;7(2):159–87.
18. Dickie JR, Gerber SC. Training in social competence: the effect on mothers, fathers, and infants. Child Dev. 1980;51:1248–51.
19. Rubin R. Maternal identity and the maternal experience. New York: Springer; 1984.
20. Mercer RT. Nursing support of the process of becoming a mother. J Obstet Gynecol Neonatal Nurs. 2006;35:649–51.
21. Parfitt Y, Pike A, Ayers S. The impact of parents' mental health on parent-baby interaction: a prospective study. Infant Behav Dev. 2013;36(4):599–608.
22. Sumner B, Barnard K. Keys to caregiving. Seattle: NCAST; 1980.
23. Nicol-Harper R, Harvey AG, Stein A. Interactions between mothers and infants: impact of maternal anxiety. Infant Behav Dev. 2007;30(1):161–7.
24. Pridham KF, Chang AS. Transition to being the mother of a new infant in the first 3 months: maternal problem solving and self-appraisals. J Adv Nurs. 1992;17(2):204–16.
25. Ngai FW, Chan SWC. Psychosocial factors and maternal wellbeing: an exploratory path analysis. Int J Nurs Stud. 2011;48(6):725–31.
26. Sayil M, Güre A, Uçanok Z. First time mothers' anxiety and depressive symptoms across the transition to motherhood: associations with maternal and environmental characteristics. Women Health. 2006;44(3):61–77.
27. Guedeney A, Guedeney N, Wendland J, Burtchen N. Treatment-mother-infant relationship psychotherapy. Best Pract Res Clin Obstet Gynaecol. 2014;28(1):135–45.
28. Clark AL, Affonso DD. Childbearing: A nursing perspective. 2nd ed. F. A. Davis Co: Philadephia; 1979.
29. Ngai FW, Chan SWC, Ip WY. Predictors and correlates of maternal role competence and satisfaction. Nurs Res. 2010;59(3):185–93.
30. Hong CH. Postpartum stress and social support of women at different places of their confinement and at different points of time during the puerperium. Public Health Q. 2001;28(3):241–53. (in Chinese)
31. Wu HW. The effects of discharge nursing instruction on primiparas' knowledge and confidence in caring for newborn at home. 2000. http://handle.ncl.edu.tw/11296/ndltd/66938208850651545483. Accessed 2 Feb 2017.
32. Kuo SF, Chen YC, Mao HC, Tsou KI. Effects of individual nursing instruction on infant care knowledge and maternal confidence of primiparas. J Nurs Res. 2000;8(2):152–64. (in Chinese)
33. Chen YS. The effect of a prenatal web-based newborn care education on mother's newborn care knowledge, and maternal confidence. 2005. http://handle.ncl.edu.tw/11296/ndltd/65491529968990327436. Accessed 2 Feb 2017.
34. Liu CC, Chen YC, Yeh YP, Hsieh YS. Effects of maternal confidence and competence on maternal parenting stress in newborn care. J Adv Nurs. 2012;68(4):908–18. https://doi.org/10.1111/j.1365-2648.2011.05796.x. (in Chinese).
35. Gao LL, Xie W, Yang X, Chan SWC. Effects of an interpersonal-psychotherapy-oriented postnatal programme for Chinese first-time mothers: a randomized controlled trial. Int J Nurs Stud. 2015;52(1):22–9.
36. Walker LO, Crain H, Thompson E. Mothering behavior and maternal role attainment during the postpartum period. Nurs Res. 1986;35(6):352–5.
37. Zahr LK. The relationship between maternal confidence and mother-infant behavior in premature infants. Res Nurs Health. 1991;14(4):279–86.
38. Mohammad KI, Gamble J, Creedy DK. Prevalence and factors associated with the development of antenatal and postnatal depression among Jordanian women. Midwifery. 2011; https://doi.org/10.1016/j.midw.2010.10.008.
39. Sagami A, Kayama M, Senoo E. The relationship between postpartum depression and abusive parenting behavior of Japanese mothers: a survey of mothers with a child less than one year old. Bull Menn Clin. 2004;68(2): 174–87.
40. Field T, Healy B, Goldstein S, Guthertz M. Behaviour-state matching and synchrony in mother-infant interactions of nondepressed versus depressed dyads. Dev Psychol. 1990;26(1):7–14.
41. Ngai FW, Chan SWC, Ip WY. The effects of a childbirth psychoeducation program on learned resourcefulness, maternal role competence and perinatal depression: a quasi-experiment. Int J Nurs Stud. 2009;46(10):1298–306.
42. Gao LL, Chan SWC, Sun K. Effects of an interpersonal-psychotherapy- oriented childbirth education programme for Chinese first-time childbearing women at 3-month follow up: randomised controlled trial. Int J Nurs Stud. 2012;49(3):274–81.
43. Chung CC, Liu HE. Mother-infant interaction quality and sense of parenting competence during two months postpartum for first time mothers. J Midwifery. 2015;57:27–38. (in Chinese)
44. Leadbeater BJ, Bishop SJ, Raver CC. Quality of mother-toddler interaction, maternal depressive symptoms, and behaviour problems in preschoolers of adolescent mothers. Dev Psychol. 1996;32(2):280–8.
45. Steadman J, Pawlby S, Mayers A, Bucks RS, Gregoire A, Miele-Norton M, Hogan AM. An exploratory study of the relationship between mother-infant

interaction and maternal cognitive function in mothers with mental illness. J Reprod Infant Psychol. 2007;25(4):255–69.

46. Tronick E, Reck C. Infants of depressed mothers. Harv Rev Psychiatry. 2009; 17(2):147–56.

47. Chao RK. Beyond parental control and authoritarian parenting style: understanding Chinese parenting through the cultural notion of training. Child Dev. 1994;65:1111–9.

48. Liu M, Guo F. Parenting practices and their relevance to child behaviors in Canada and China. Scand J Psychol. 2010;51(2):109–14.

49. NCAST-AVENUW. Keys to caregiving. revised ed. Seattle: NCAST-AVENUW; 2008.

50. Bryan AA. Enhancing parent-child interaction with a prenatal couple intervention. MCN Am J Matern Child Nurs. 2000;25(3):139–44.

51. Gibaud-Wallston J, Wandersman LP. Development and utility of the Parenting Sense of Competence Scale, Paper session presented at the meeting of the American Psychological Association. Canada: Toronto; 1978.

52. Ngai FW, Chan SWC, Holroyd E. Translation and validation of a Chinese version of the parenting sense of competence scale in Chinese mothers. Nurs Res. 2007;56(5):348–54.

53. Cox JL, Holden JM, Sagovsky R. Detection of postnatal depression. Development of the 10-item Edinburgh postnatal depression scale. Br J Psychiatry. 1987;150:782–6.

54. Heh SS. Validation of the Chinese version of the Edinburgh postnatal depression scale: detecting postnatal depression in Taiwanese women. J Nurs Res. 2001;9(2):105–13.

55. Teng HW, Hsu CS, Shih SM, Lu ML, Pan JJ, Shen WW. Screening postpartum depression with the Taiwanese version of the Edinburgh postnatal depression scale. Compr Psychiatry. 2005;46(4):261–5.

56. Liu YQ, Petrini M, Maloni JA. "doing the month": postpartum practices in Chinese women. Nurs Health Sci. 2015;17(1):5–14.

57. Heh SS. "Doing the month" and social support. Fu-Jen. J Med. 2004; 2(2):11–7.

58. Hung CH, Yu CY, Ou CC, Liang WW. Taiwanese maternal health in the postpartum nursing Centre. J Clini Nurs. 2009;19:1094–101.

59. Liang KY, Zeger SL. Longitudinal data analysis using generalized linear models. Biometrika. 1986;73(1):13–22.

60. Zeger SL, Liang KY. Longitudinal data analysis for discrete and continuous outcomes. Biometrics. 1986;42(1):121–30.

61. Ma GN, Bai GJ. Dietary ying yang balance. Clin J Chin Med. 2010; 2(13):77. (in Chinese)

62. Liptak GS, Keller BB, Feldman AW, Chamberlin RW. Enhancing infant development and parent-practitioner interaction with the Brazelton neonatal assessment scale. Pediatrics. 1983;72(1):71–8.

63. Myers BJ. Early intervention using Brazelton training with middle-class mothers and fathers of newborns. Child Dev. 1982;53(2):462–71.

64. Chen MI. A primipara's experience as a new motherhood during the early postpartum period. 1999. http://handle.ncl.edu.tw/11296/4vwtgc. Accessed 2 Feb 2017 (in Chinese).

7

Supporting healthful lifestyles during pregnancy: a health coach intervention pilot study

Michael W. Seward[1], Denise Simon[1], Martha Richardson[2], Emily Oken[1], Matthew W. Gillman[1,3] and Marie-France Hivert[1,4*] (iD)

Abstract

Background: Excessive gestational weight gain (GWG) is associated with adverse health outcomes in both the mother and child. Many previous lifestyle interventions in women with excess weight during pregnancy encouraging appropriate GWG have been unsuccessful, and there remains no consensus about the content, format, or theoretical framework of GWG interventions. We assessed the feasibility and acceptability of a remote health coach intervention to promote healthful lifestyle behaviors and appropriate GWG among overweight pregnant women.

Methods: At one northeastern US clinic, we enrolled 30 overweight (pre-pregnancy BMI $\geq$ 25 kg/m^2) pregnant women at a median gestation of 12.5 weeks (IQR: 11–15) into a one-arm trial. We connected participants with a health coach to provide behavioral support to help participants adopt healthful lifestyles during pregnancy. Health coaches contacted participants by phone every 2–3 weeks to monitor goals, and sent emails and text messages between calls. Participants completed baseline ($N = 30$) and follow-up ($N = 26$) surveys at the end of the intervention (36 weeks gestation), as well as follow-up phone interviews ($N = 18$).

Results: Among 30 participants, median age was 32 years (IQR: 28–33), median self-reported pre-pregnancy BMI was 27. 3 kg/m^2 (IQR: 25.7–31.1), and 17/30 were white, 9/30 African-American, and 3/30 Asian. Three-quarters (22/29) of participants completed at least a college degree. Although 25/30 participants reported in baseline surveys that they worried about being able to lose the weight postpartum that they expected to gain during pregnancy, just 12/26 participants reported the same at follow-up ($P < 0.001$). In follow-up surveys, 21/26 participants reported that health coaches were helpful in keeping them motivated, and 22/26 thought the phone conversations helped them face problems and find solutions. Based on qualitative assessment, several themes emerged in follow-up interviews about the quality of the intervention including accountability and support from health coaches. Participants also expressed desire for more visual resources and integration with standard clinical care to improve the intervention.

Conclusions: We demonstrated feasibility and high participant satisfaction with our remote health coach intervention during pregnancy. We identified areas in which we could refine the intervention for inclusion in a full-scale RCT, such as integration with clinical care and additional visual resources.

Keywords: Gestational weight gain, Goal-setting, Pregnancy, Health coaching

* Correspondence: mhivert@partners.org
[1]Division of Chronic Disease Research Across the Lifecourse, Department of Population Medicine, Harvard Medical School and Harvard Pilgrim Health Care Institute, Boston, MA, USA
[4]Diabetes Unit, Massachusetts General Hospital, Boston, MA, USA
Full list of author information is available at the end of the article

Background

Pregnancy and post-partum are a key period in the life course for the prevention of obesity and cardiovascular disease in both mothers and children. Over 55% of women of reproductive age in the US are overweight or have obesity [1], and these women are two to three times more likely to experience excessive gestational weight gain (GWG) than women of normal weight [2]. The US Center for Diseases Control (CDC) report on GWG from 2012 to 2013 found that 62% of women with overweight had excessive GWG, compared to 37% of normal weight women [3].

Excessive GWG is associated with several health risks for mothers and their children. Excessive GWG increases the risk of gestational diabetes, cesarean delivery, and post-partum weight retention, which may lead to excess weight later in life [4–7]. Children born to mothers who experienced excessive GWG are more likely to have greater adiposity and other cardiovascular risk factors later in life [8–14]. Interventions that promote healthful lifestyles and limit excessive GWG could therefore possibly help reduce obesity and cardiovascular disease risk in two generations.

Although a few previous behavioral interventions during pregnancy have successfully reduced excessive GWG [15–21], several others have not [22–26]. The two largest RCTs that implemented comprehensive behavioral lifestyle interventions during pregnancy had minimal impact on GWG. The LIMIT study, which included over 2000 women with overweight and obesity, did not find that the intervention impacted GWG [27], and the UP-BEAT trial (1500 women with obesity) found only modestly lower GWG (– 0.55 kg) in the intervention group compared to standard care [28]. The reluctance of women to join these trials based on the small proportions of eligible women who decided to participate (19% in UPBEAT, 40% in LIMIT) suggests an additional need to explore the acceptability of behavioral interventions among pregnant women.

Findings from reviews and meta-analyses on the efficacy of GWG interventions are decidedly mixed; even within the few studies that showed some impact of proposed interventions there is no clear consensus about either the content, format, or theoretical framework of GWG interventions [29–33]. Moreover, a review of 5 RCT and 8 qualitative studies before LIMIT and UP-BEAT concluded that women's barriers to behavior change were poorly addressed by existing interventions and that more research is necessary to explore what kinds of interventions are effective. The review found that pregnancy as a period of transition and perceived lack of control emerged as a common theme across the qualitative studies, and suggested that interventions that give women a sense of control may be more effective [30]. This review highlights the need for feasibility studies to ensure proposed interventions are successfully adapted to the needs of pregnant women.

In this mixed methods pilot study, our primary aim was to assess feasibility (recruiting, retention) and acceptability (participant satisfaction) of our intervention. Health coaches used behavioral approaches commonly employed in other behavioral change studies to encourage healthful diets (increase consumption of vegetables and fruits, whole grains, or low mercury fish, decrease fast-food and sugar-sweetened beverage consumption), improve physical activity (increase number of steps/day, increase moderate activity), decrease screen time and optimize sleep duration. We hypothesized that a more flexible delivery of the intervention in terms of the methods of communication with health coaches (e.g. phone call, text, email) would entice recruitment and retention of participants in the study and could promote participant satisfaction with the intervention. We also used surveys and interviews for a secondary goal to explore issues related to weight in pregnancy such as trust in sources of information about weight issues and management, discussions with healthcare providers about weight, and attitudes during pregnancy.

Methods

Recruitment

We recruited between July 2015 and January 2016 at one northeastern US clinic. We included participants if they were less than 16 weeks' gestation at the time of their initial obstetric appointment, overweight or had obesity (pre-pregnancy BMI ≥ 25 kg/m^2), 18 years of age or older, English speaking, and planned to remain at the same obstetric clinic for the duration of their pregnancies. The clinic provided us with monthly lists of appointments for potentially eligible women with pre-pregnancy BMI ≥ 25 kg/m^2 and less than 16 weeks of gestation. Before each scheduled appointment, we notified healthcare providers that their patients could be eligible for the study. At the end of the clinical encounter, healthcare providers asked patients if they would like to meet with research staff to hear about a healthful lifestyle study. Of 37 individuals approached by the healthcare providers, 30 agreed to meet, and all 30 were eligible and gave written informed consent to participate. Two participants later withdrew from the study during the intervention because of concerns about the time commitment (Fig. 1). Our recruitment goal of 30 women was based on recommendations for conducting qualitative in-depth interviews and the need to account for potential loss to follow-up due to pregnancy events or drop-outs. Because our primary aims of this pilot study were to show feasibility and provide qualitative evaluation of the interventions, we did not attempt to show effect on clinical outcomes for which power calculations would be indicated.

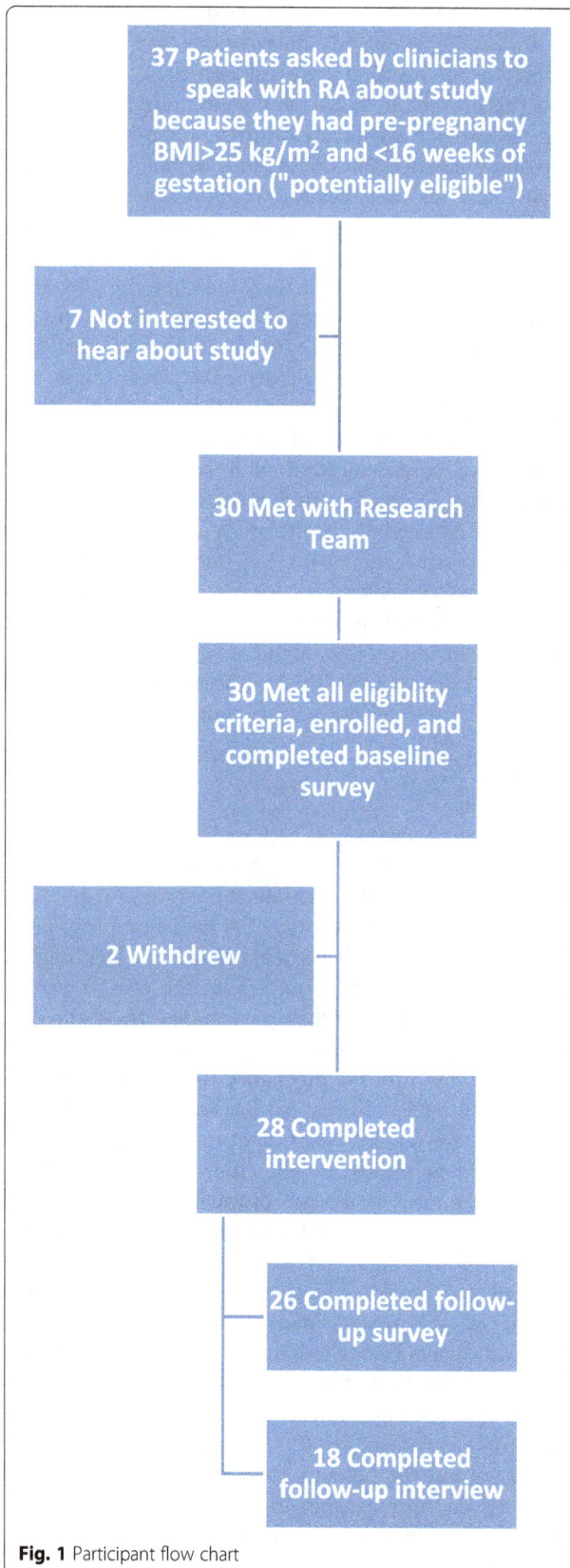

37 Patients asked by clinicians to speak with RA about study because they had pre-pregnancy BMI>25 kg/m² and <16 weeks of gestation ("potentially eligible")

7 Not interested to hear about study

30 Met with Research Team

30 Met all eligiblity criteria, enrolled, and completed baseline survey

2 Withdrew

28 Completed intervention

26 Completed follow-up survey

18 Completed follow-up interview

Fig. 1 Participant flow chart

We gave women a $25 gift card after completing baseline surveys at enrollment, and mailed participants another $25 gift card after completing follow-up phone interviews. This study was approved by the Harvard Pilgrim Health Care Human Studies Committee. All participants provided written informed consent at enrollment.

Study design and sample

Participants completed baseline surveys in person at enrollment, as well as follow-up online surveys and phone interviews at the end of the intervention (36 weeks gestation). Follow-up surveys repeated many of the baseline questions, and additionally asked questions about the intervention. We collected information on demographics, discussions with healthcare providers, attitudes related to weight status and pregnancy, opinions about the intervention, and included general food frequency questions based on surveys used in prior maternal-child health studies conducted at our institution [34]. End of intervention phone interviews followed a guide of open-ended questions to determine insights on what helped achieve goals, motivation, opinions of the health coach intervention, and areas for improvement (Additional file 1: Table S1). A single study staff member (MWS), who had experience with qualitative data collection, conducted all of the individual interviews.

Health coach intervention

We connected participants at enrollment (median gestation of 12.5 weeks, IQR: 11–15) with a trained health coach who called participants every 2–3 weeks until 36 weeks of gestation. During these phone calls, health coaches helped participants adopt and maintain new healthful lifestyle behaviors that were evidence-based, simple, and easy to track (Additional file 1: Table S2). Goals aimed to promote appropriate gestational weight gain by addressing several behavioral domains including diet, physical activity, screen time, and sleep.

During the first call, health coaches invited participants to prioritize these goals according to their level of self-efficacy, readiness to change, preferences, and values. Specifically, participants were asked to evaluate their lifestyle and identify areas they felt they wanted to focus on to improve their health and wellness. Participants were then asked about barriers to meeting these goals, and this allowed health coaches to create conversations about individual participant's readiness to make changes and to discuss other resources that may be available to them to establish a prioritization that would be acceptable for each participant. Throughout the intervention, health coaches used principles of motivational interviewing that relied on a patient-centered approach to enhance readiness to change by exploring ambivalence and resistance to change [35]. At each check in, the health coach would discuss goals established and if goals were being met, per the participant report. If the goals were not being met, the health coach would discuss barriers and modify goals to be more realistic to the participants' individual situation. Health coaches applied several behavioral theories to modify lifestyle including Social Cognitive Theory, Health Belief Model, and Protection Motivation Theory [36–38]. Together, these theoretical bases emphasized the importance of self-regulation, developing specific behavior change plans, monitoring progress towards goals, attaining skills necessary to reach goals, and receiving support through the behavior change process. In addition to setting personal goals adapted to each participant preference and reality, health coaches also presented optimal goals, including targets for ideal cardiovascular health based on the Life's Simple 7 health factors from the American Heart Association (Additional file 1: Table S2) [39].

During follow-up calls, health coaches monitored progress and helped adjust goals when necessary (e.g. too many goals, or the goal was too ambitious). Health coaches also addressed barriers and potential solutions with participants, and helped them target higher goal settings or select new goals when participants attained them. Health coaches sent emails or text messages depending on participant preferences to check-in about progress toward goals or clinical appointments between calls. Research staff (including an MD) met weekly with health coaches to review their conversations with participants, and to address any medical issues to ensure that it would be reported to the primary care provider obstetric team if appropriate. Although this procedure of notifying the medical team was in place throughout the study, no major concerns were raised to health coaches so there was no direct interaction between the health coaches and the medical team.

We accessed electronic medical records (EMR) and calculated GWG based on pre-pregnancy reported weight and the last weight recorded during pregnancy (> 34 weeks). We defined excessive GWG based on IOM definition per categories (> 11.3 kg of GWG in overweight category, > 9.1 kg of GWG in obesity category).

Statistical analyses

We measured feasibility via the ease of recruitment based on the ratio of enrolled women to the number of women approached about the study, and via maintenance of contact with a health coach based on the study participant attrition and follow-up survey completion rates (retention). We measured acceptability via survey items about components of the intervention and through qualitative comments from a semi-structured interview.

Surveys

We performed all analyses using SAS software version 9.4 (SAS Institute Inc., Cary, NC). For most questions, participants chose between four categories: strongly agree, somewhat agree, somewhat disagree, and strongly disagree. For

the group of questions asking about attitudes related to weight status and pregnancy, we pooled answers into "agree" and "disagree" for simplicity (Table 3). We conducted McNemar-Bowker symmetry tests to examine differences between baseline and follow-up survey responses.

Interviews

We transcribed phone interviews verbatim during the calls, and completed content analysis of the transcripts using principles of the immersion-crystallization method [40]. This qualitative technique includes multiple rounds of "immersion" through close readings of transcripts, followed by reflection and the "crystallization" of emerging themes. Three investigators (MWS, DS, and MFH) read the transcripts, and one investigator (MWS) coded the transcripts. The three investigators (MWS, DS, and MFH) had to arrive at a unanimous consensus concerning the emerging themes after reading the verbatim transcripts. We reported the 5 themes that emerged from the analysis with representative quotes.

Results

Participant characteristics

Participants at baseline ($N = 30$) had a median age of 31.5 years (IQR: 28.3–33), a median self-reported pre-pregnancy BMI of 27.3 kg/m^2 (IQR: 25.7–31.1), and 57% (17 of 30) were white, 30% (9 of 30) African-American, and 10% (3 of 30) Asian. Three-quarters (75%, 22 of 29) of participants completed a college degree or higher level of education. Two-thirds (67%, 20 of 30) of participants were married, 23% (7 of 30) were single and living with a partner or a significant other, and 10% (3 of 30) were single. Thirteen percent (4 of 30) reported an annual household income of $40,000 or less, 20% (6 of 30) reported incomes between $40,001 and $100,000, and 60% (18 of 30) reported incomes above $100,000 (Table 1).

Feasibility

Most (81%, 30 of 37) of the women potentially eligible to join the study and 100% (30 out of 30) of women approached by research staff about the study enrolled as participants. Participants completed baseline ($N = 30$) surveys in person at enrollment, as well as follow-up online surveys ($N = 26$) and phone interviews ($N = 18$) at the end of the intervention (36 weeks gestation) (Fig. 1).

Surveys

Trust in information sources about weight-related issues in pregnancy

Large proportions of participants at baseline reported "a lot of trust" in advice related to weight gain during pregnancy given by doctors (93%, 28 of 30), midwives (92%, 24 of 26), and prenatal or childbirth classes (65%, 13 of 20). Fewer participants said they put a lot of trust in husbands

Table 1 Characteristics of participating women at baseline

Characteristics	Median (IQR) or N (%)
	N = 30
Age, years	31.5 (28.3–33.0)
Gestational age at enrollment, weeks	12.5 (11.0–15.0)
Self-reported pre-pregnancy BMI, kg/m^2	27.3 (25.7–31.1)
Primiparous	23 (77)
Race/Ethnicity	
White	17 (57)
Black or African American	9 (30)
Asian	3 (10)
Other	1 (3)
Highest level of education	
High school graduate	2 (7)
Some college	5 (17)
College graduate	12 (41)
Graduate school	10 (34)
Marital Status	
Single	3 (10)
Single & living with partner or significant other	7 (23)
Married	20 (67)
Household Income ($)	
$40,000 or less	4 (13)
$40,001 - $100,000	6 (20)
$100,001 - $150,000	10 (33)
More than $150,000	8 (27)
Don't know	2 (7)

pregnancy books or magazines (26%, 5 of 19), the internet (18%, 3 of 17), husbands or partners (15%, 2 of 13), or friends and family (13%, 2 of 16). No participants reported a lot of trust in advice from the television.

Discussions with healthcare providers about weight and health behaviors during pregnancy

At baseline, half of the participants (50%, 15 of 30) reported that healthcare providers (doctors and/or midwives) had discussed the risks of gaining too much weight during pregnancy, almost all women (97%, 28 of 29) reported healthcare providers had discussed diet, most (80%, 24 of 30) reported healthcare provider discussions concerning physical activity, and half (50%, 15 of 30) concerning sleep. At follow-up, more participants (81%, 21 of 26) reported that their healthcare providers had discussed the risks of gaining too much weight, almost all women (96%, 25 of 26) reported healthcare provider discussions about diet, the vast majority (88%, 23 of 26) about physical activity, and over three-quarters (77%, 20 of 26) about sleep.

Attitudes towards weight-related issues in pregnancy

We found substantial differences between baseline and follow-up surveys for two of the attitudes queried (Table 3). While over three-quarters (77%, 23 of 30) of participants reported in baseline surveys that they worried they may get fat during pregnancy, fewer participants (58%, 15 of 26) reported the same at the end of the intervention ($P = 0.01$). Similarly, although most (83%, 25 of 30) said at baseline that they worried about being able in post-partum to lose the weight that they would gain during pregnancy, under half (46%, 12 of 26) reported the same at follow-up ($P < 0.001$) (Table 3).

Among attitudes that we did not find to have meaningful differences between baseline and follow-up, the vast majority in baseline (83%, 25 of 30) and follow-up (88%, 23 of 26) surveys said they were proud of looking pregnant. All 26 women thought a pregnant woman is beautiful. However, over a third (36%, 9 of 25) said the weight they gained during pregnancy makes them feel

or partners (29%, 6 of 21), friends or family (20%, 4 of 20), and pregnancy books or magazines (8%, 2 of 24). No participants reported a lot of trust in advice from the internet or television (Table 2). We saw similar trends at follow-up: women put a lot of trust in doctors (88%, 21 of 24), midwives (81%, 17 of 21), and prenatal or childbirth classes (73%, 8 of 11). Fewer participants put a lot of trust in

Table 2 Level of trust for various sources of advice related to weight gain during pregnancy reported by participants at baseline

Source	N*	Do not trust at all N (%)	Trust a little N (%)	Trust a lot N (%)
Doctor	30	0 (0)	2 (7)	28 (93)
Midwife	26	0 (0)	2 (8)	24 (92)
Husband/partner	21	2 (10)	13 (62)	6 (29)
Friends and family	20	4 (20)	12 (60)	4 (20)
Pregnancy books or magazines	24	2 (8)	20 (83)	2 (8)
Internet	24	6 (25)	18 (75)	0 (0)
Television	19	11 (58)	8 (42)	0 (0)
Prenatal or childbirth classes	20	1 (5)	6 (30)	13 (65)

*Number of participants who answered each question

Table 3 Attitudes related to weight status and pregnancy reported by participants at baseline (median gestation of 12.5 weeks) and at the end of the intervention (median gestation of 36.0 weeks)

Opinions or Worries	Baseline		End of intervention		P-value**
	N*	Agree, N (%)	N*	Agree, N (%)	
I am proud of looking pregnant	30	25 (83)	26	23 (88)	0.65
I think a pregnant woman is beautiful	30	29 (97)	26	26 (100)	1.00
I like my maternity clothes	29	13 (45)	26	15 (58)	0.48
I worry that I may get fat during this pregnancy	30	23 (77)	26	15 (58)	0.01
The weight that I've gained during this pregnancy makes me feel unattractive	29	10 (34)	25	9 (36)	1.00
I am embarrassed at how big I have gotten during this pregnancy	28	6 (21)	26	3 (12)	0.32
As long as I'm eating a well-balanced diet, I don't care how much I gain	30	9 (30)	26	14 (54)	0.06
If I gain too much weight one month, I try to keep from gaining the next month	30	8 (27)	26	5 (19)	0.53
I tried to keep my weight down so I didn't look pregnant earlier on	30	6 (20)	26	3 (12)	0.18
Just before going to the doctor, I try not to eat	30	2 (7)	26	3 (12)	0.56
I worry that I will have a difficult time losing the weight I've gained during this pregnancy	30	25 (83)	26	12 (46)	0.0009

*Number of participants who answered each question
**P-value calculated from the difference between baseline and end of intervention surveys using the McNemar test

unattractive, and only a few (12%, 3 of 26) said they were embarrassed at how big they got during pregnancy. At the end of pregnancy, over half (54%, 14 of 26) said they did not care how much weight they gain as long as they eat a well-balanced diet (Table 3).

Health coach intervention acceptability and satisfaction

In follow-up surveys, most participants (81%, 21 of 26) reported that the health coach was helpful in selecting and setting goals, and that the health coach was helpful in keeping them motivated. Over three-quarters (77%, 20 of 26) thought the health coach was helpful in measuring and monitoring lifestyle goals. The large majority (85%, 22 of 26) said phone conversations helped them face problems and find solutions, while slightly fewer (70%, 16 of 23) said personalized text messages or emails were helpful reminders (Table 4).

Participants most commonly selected goals to increase vegetable and fruit intake (77%, 20 of 26), increase physical activity (50%, 13 of 26), and increase the number of steps per day (42%, 11 of 26). In self-evaluations of the level of achievement for selected goals, participants did best with dietary goals: the majority fully achieved an increase in vegetables and fruit (60%, 12 of 20), an increase in whole grains (57%, 4 of 7), and a decrease in fast-food (56%, 5 of 9). Participants had the least success with physical activity and sleep goals: about a quarter fully achieved an increase in the number of steps per day (27%, 3 of 11) and more optimal sleep (25%, 2 of 8) (Table 5).

Despite self-reported success achieving dietary goals, we did not find differences between self-reported baseline and follow-up consumption of food, beverages, or fast-food in the overall group (Additional file 1: Table S3-S5). Although we did not measure GWG, we did access EMR weight data and found that 10/28 women who completed the intervention had excessive GWG, as defined by the IOM.

Post-intervention interviews

We conducted 18 individual follow-up phone interviews for a mean of 12 min each (range: 8–20). Several important themes emerged about the quality of the intervention including motivation for personal health and the health of the baby, as well as accountability and support from health coaches. Participants also suggested ways to improve the intervention such as integration with standard clinical care and expressed desire for more visual resources such as mobile apps and tracking tools (Table 6).

Motivation

The majority (11 of 18) cited primarily their own personal health as motivation to achieve lifestyle goals. Most of these women listed "general wellbeing" or "staying healthy and fit" as important drivers. Many participants also mentioned their bodies as motivation: "I want to be able to get my body back once I have the baby," or "I definitely did not want to come out of pregnancy sloppy." One woman said she "didn't want high blood pressure," and another said she is a "happier person when I'm moving and active."

A few (3 of 18) cited principally the health of the baby as motivation: "I just want to have a healthy baby." Another woman stated: "Making sure the baby is healthy to be honest with you. It was my number one motivation. I don't want to deprive him of anything, taking prenatal vitamins every day, and yeah number one was 'what does he need?'" Others (4 of 18) mentioned both personal

Table 4 Opinions about the health coach intervention reported by participants at the end of intervention

	N*	Strongly disagree N (%)	Somewhat disagree N (%)	Somewhat agree N (%)	Strongly agree N (%)
The health coach was helpful in selecting and setting goals for myself.	26	1 (4)	4 (15)	12 (46)	9 (35)
The health coach was helpful to keep me motivated.	26	1 (4)	4 (15)	14 (54)	7 (27)
The health coach was helpful to measure and monitor my lifestyle goals.	26	1 (4)	5 (19)	14 (54)	6 (23)
The phone conversations help me to face problems and find solutions.	26	1 (4)	3 (12)	15 (58)	7 (27)
The personalized text messages or emails were helpful reminders.	23	3 (13)	4 (17)	10 (43)	6 (26)

*Number of participants who answered each question

and maternal sources of motivation: "I wanted to stay healthy for me and the baby."

Accountability
Several women discussed how the health coach intervention made them take responsibility for their lifestyle goals: "It was nice...to have someone that made me accountable...I didn't have to do it on my own." One woman particularly liked how the health coach filled a unique role as an independent source of feedback and described how "it was really good to have a third party outside of family and friends... [The health coach] helped me set goals and helped me keep track of where I stood with those goals." Most women agreed that the health coaches provided helpful check-ins: "It was good having someone there that was sort of checking in on you so that you had that urge to please someone."

Support
Many participants welcomed the help they received from health coaches and thought they were "very supportive." Here is how one woman described her experience with the health coach:

"I liked the fact that I had someone on my team. She never said I was doing something wrong so it was good positive reinforcement. It was great to bounce stuff off...My coach helped me be able to better grasp the need to do these things and I think at this point, the fruit has become a habit that I will keep after the baby. Now I'm loving the fruit. [My husband] comes in with tangerines and now I'm tearing the fruit up!"

One participant described her preference for phone communication over texts or emails from health coaches, she noted that the phone calls allowed the health coach to show "she had a supportive nature and genuinely was concerned." Another woman agreed that this personal touch was important: "I always thought she was like a friend and she would go above and beyond to find answers. We talked about certain goals. I felt like I could go to her even if it wasn't for a call. If had a question I could reach out to her."

Wishes for more integration
When asked about how the intervention could be improved, some women wished the health coach interactions were "more closely tied with the doctor's appointments... It

Table 5 Goals selected during the intervention and self-evaluation on the level of achievement for each selected goal by the participants at the end of intervention

Domain	Goal	Number of participants selecting each goal	Did not achieve N (%)	Somewhat achieved N (%)	Fully achieved N (%)
Diet	Increase vegetables and fruits intake	20	0 (0)	8 (40)	12 (60)
Diet	Increase whole grains intake	7	0 (0)	3 (43)	4 (57)
Diet	Decrease fast-food intake	9	0 (0)	4 (44)	5 (56)
Diet	Decrease sugar-sweetened beverages	6	0 (0)	3 (50)	3 (50)
Diet	Increase low-mercury fish intake	5	0 (0)	3 (60)	2 (40)
Physical Activity	Increase physical activity	13	4 (31)	4 (31)	5 (38)
Screen time	Decrease screen time	6	1 (17)	3 (50)	2 (33)
Physical Activity	Increase number of steps/day	11	2 (18)	6 (55)	3 (27)
Sleep	Optimize sleep duration	8	1 (13)	5 (63)	2 (25)
	Other	3	0 (0)	0 (0)	3 (100)

Table 6 Representative quotes for emerging themes from 18 follow-up phone interviews

Theme	Representative Quote
Motivation	• "I want to be able **to get my body back** once I have the baby." • "I didn't want **high blood pressure**, and thankfully I don't have it anymore." • "Making sure the **baby** is healthy…number one was 'what does he need?'"
Accountability	• "It was nice…to have someone that made me **accountable**…I didn't have to do it on my own." • "It was really good to have a **3rd party** outside of family and friends… [The health coach] helped me set goals and helped me keep track of where I stood with those goals." • "It was good having someone there that was sort of **checking in on you** so that you had that **urge to please someone**"
Support	• "I had **someone on my team**…so it was good positive reinforcement. It was great to bounce stuff off…My coach helped me be able to better grasp the need to do these things and I think at this point, the fruit has become **a habit that I will keep after the baby.** Now I'm loving the fruit. He comes in with tangerines and now I'm tearing the fruit up!" • "She was great and **supportive.**" • "I always thought **she was like a friend and she would go above and beyond to find answers…I felt like I could go to her** even if it wasn't for a call. If had a question I could reach out to her."
Wishes for more Integration	• "…if it was more closely tied with the doctor's appointments…It was **too removed from the medical** side." • "more **integration with the doctors** in general. If you're already going in to see the doc once a month it would be great to see someone [a health coach] there already." • "If the health coach had **access to medical records** she could ask what has happened over the last two weeks if she sees you gained 2 pounds. Sometimes you don't want to admit you gained weight to health coach, so it would be better if she already knew."
Desire for More Resources	• "There's no way to track your goal other than a conversation, so if there was some **study app** that made it a little more automated." • "I want **more resources**, not just a checkin to talk." • "Maybe offering some **guidelines in the beginning**…starting off with 'try these meal planners' or 'try this calorie tracking app.'" • "All the goals are just discussed verbally. Maybe having more concrete goals that are maybe a **worksheet** or something."

Boldface text highlights representative quotes from themes that emerged across all phone interviews

was too removed from the medical side." Another woman agreed that incorporating the intervention into the clinic would be more convenient: "more integration with the doctors in general. If you're already going in to see the doc once a month it would be great to see someone [a health coach] there already." Besides convenience, another

participant explained that more integration would also help keep herself accountable: "If the health coach had access to medical records she could ask what has happened over the last two weeks if she sees you gained 2 pounds. Sometimes you don't want to admit you gained weight to a health coach, so it would be better if she already knew."

Desire for more resources

Although the majority of participants thought the intervention was useful, several women said they "want more resources, not just a check in to talk." Another participant explained that "all the goals are just discussed verbally. Maybe having more concrete goals that are maybe a worksheet or something." One woman suggested "there's no way to track your goal other than a conversation, so if there was some study app that made it a little more automated." Another woman proposed front-loading these additional resources: "Maybe offering some guidelines in the beginning…starting off with 'try these meal planners' or 'try this calorie tracking app.'"

Discussion

In this pilot study, we found that a remote health coach intervention during pregnancy was feasible and that women reported high satisfaction. Surveys showed participants placed a high level of trust in healthcare providers, and 81% (21 of 26) said health coaches motivated them to achieve their goals. Although we did not find differences in food or beverage consumption frequency, fewer participants at follow-up than at baseline worried about being able in post-partum to lose the weight that they gained during pregnancy. In interviews, women primarily cited their own health, sometimes adding the health of the baby, as the main source of motivation to achieve lifestyle goals. Several women liked the supportive approach used by health coaches and most thought health coaches kept them accountable, particularly because coaches served as a third-party resource outside of family/friends and healthcare providers. Participants suggested more integration with clinical care and adding visual materials (e.g. goal worksheets or mobile apps) to improve future remote health coach interventions.

Previous lifestyle interventions have focused on adapting the approach and content (e.g. type of physical activity, diet) of the intervention to the individual [33]. We now see a need to individualize interventions according to participant technology preferences including methods of communication with health coaches, and goal tracking. For example, authors of one RCT designed to reduce behavioral cancer risk factors found that equal proportions of participants chose to receive intervention materials via print and the web [41], and concluded in another study that using just one modality of communication (text messages vs. automated voice responses) with participants may limit efficacy [42]. Although we considered implementing a study mobile app to track goals in this study, we decided against an app based on findings from focus groups prior to our pilot study that such an app would be "not that useful" [43]. However, in the current pilot study, several participants in interviews proposed adding more visual materials and tracking tools (both paper goal worksheets and mobile apps) in future interventions, suggesting that individuals have a wide range of preferences regarding how technology can facilitate behavior change.

In recent large RCTs of lifestyle interventions during pregnancy, just 19% of eligible women in the UPBEAT study and 40% in the LIMIT study decided to enroll. In contrast, while considering this was a pilot study in a selected population, 81% (30 out of 37) of potentially eligible and 100% (30 out of 30) of approached women enrolled in our pilot study. We hypothesize that the flexible modes of remote communication (phone, email, text) with health coaches allowed for a more individualized delivery of the intervention that improved enrollment compared to interventions proposed in UPBEAT and LIMIT trials that requested up to 1.5 h weekly face-to-face sessions [27, 28].

Our surveys support previous qualitative research that pregnant women put a lot of trust in advice about weight-related issues from clinicians [43], yet some (19%, 5 of 26) participants in end of pregnancy surveys reported that none of their healthcare providers (neither doctor nor midwife) discussed GWG with them. Our previous study found that healthcare providers often hesitated to spontaneously offer information about appropriate GWG or about how to make lifestyle changes to achieve appropriate weight gain [43], and other research on clinicians found that many of them are uncomfortable discussing weight with pregnant women [30, 44]. These reports along with our interview findings that the health coach's position as a third-party resource was helpful, suggest that support from a health coach to adopt lifestyles encouraging appropriate GWG could be useful for both pregnant women and clinicians.

Limitations

We conducted this study at one clinic with a high socioeconomic sample of women, so results may vary for other women depending on the clinic and location; however, the ethnicities and ages of study participants were similar to the overall group medical practice. Because this study was a one-arm pilot without a control group, we were unable to determine if differences between baseline and follow-up surveys were responses to the intervention or the results of a progressing pregnancy. A few participants in interviews expressed dissatisfaction with the intervention after some lag time occurred when switching a few participants' health coach due to an unexpected event unrelated to the study.

Future interventions could use multiple health coaches to avoid unanticipated break of continuity in health coach support. Another limitation of the study is that we did not measure GWG. Yet, based on electronic medical record data, we observed that 35.7% (10 of 28) had excessive GWG, which is less than the 62% of overweight women and 56% of women with obesity who had excessive GWG in the national report based on CDC data from 2012 to 2013 [3].

Conclusions

In this remote health coach intervention pilot study, we found that we can recruit very effectively, that the intervention was acceptable, and that participants reported high satisfaction. Although it remains to be tested with a larger study population, the efficient recruitment, remote methods of intervention delivery, and modest research expenses suggest scalability of the intervention. Based on the relatively unsuccessful trials using lifestyle interventions during pregnancy, there is recent interest in targeting at-risk women prior to pregnancy. We feel that some of the lessons learned from this pilot study could be applied to behavioral studies with pregnant women or to pre-pregnancy designs [45, 46]. We propose that future interventions targeting women of reproductive age with excess weight include a supportive, integrated health coach intervention that includes the rest of the health care team to provide one coordinated front to educate and motivate patients. Future interventions should be personalized not only in the approach and content, but also to the women's preferences in mode of communication and technological tools to support goals tracking.

Abbreviation
GWG: Gestational weight gain

Acknowledgements
Thank you to the study participants and to the administrative and clinical staff at the Atrius Copley Obstetric practice for help coordinating the study and recruitment.
The views expressed in this article do not necessarily represent the views of the US Government, the Department of Health and Human Services or the National Institutes of Health.

Funding
This work was supported by an award from the American Heart Association (14CRP20490354). Dr. Oken received additional funding from the National Institutes of Health (P30 DK092924, K24 HD069408). The funding bodies did not participate in the design of the study; collection, analysis, and interpretation of data; or in writing the manuscript.

Authors' contributions
MWS collected data, conducted analyses, and wrote the manuscript. DS contributed to data analyses and revised critically the manuscript for important intellectual content. MFH designed the study, contributed to data interpretation, and revised critically the manuscript for important intellectual content. MR, EO, and MG contributed to data interpretation, and revised critically the manuscript for important intellectual content. All authors read and approved the final manuscript and agreed to be accountable for all aspects of the work related to its accuracy.

Consent for publication

Not applicable.

Competing interests

The authors declare that they have no competing interest.

Author details

[1]Division of Chronic Disease Research Across the Lifecourse, Department of Population Medicine, Harvard Medical School and Harvard Pilgrim Health Care Institute, Boston, MA, USA. [2]Obstetrics & Gynecology, Harvard Vanguard Medical Associates, Boston, MA, USA. [3]Environmental Influences on Child Health Outcomes (ECHO) Program, Office of the Director, National Institutes of Health, Bethesda, MD, USA. [4]Diabetes Unit, Massachusetts General Hospital, Boston, MA, USA.

References

1. Flegal KM, Carroll MD, Kit BK, Ogden CL. Prevalence of obesity and trends in the distribution of body mass index among US adults, 1999-2010. JAMA. 2012;307(5):491–7.
2. Deputy NP, Sharma AJ, Kim SY, Hinkle SN. Prevalence and characteristics associated with gestational weight gain adequacy. Obstet Gynecol. 2015; 125(4):773–81.
3. Deputy NP, Sharma AJ, Kim SY. Gestational weight gain - United States, 2012 and 2013. MMWR Morb Mortal Wkly Rep. 2015;64(43): 1215–20.
4. Nehring I, Schmoll S, Beyerlein A, Hauner H, von Kries R. Gestational weight gain and long-term postpartum weight retention: a meta-analysis. Am J Clin Nutr. 2011;94(5):1225–31.
5. Oken E, Kleinman KP, Belfort MB, Hammitt JK, Gillman MW. Associations of gestational weight gain with short- and longer-term maternal and child health outcomes. Am J Epidemiol. 2009;170(2):173–80.
6. Walter JR, Perng W, Kleinman KP, Rifas-Shiman SL, Rich-Edwards JW, Oken E. Associations of trimester-specific gestational weight gain with maternal adiposity and systolic blood pressure at 3 and 7 years postpartum. Am J Obstet Gynecol. 2015;212(4):499 e491–12.
7. Viswanathan M, Siega-Riz AM, Moos MK, Deierlein A, Mumford S, Knaack J, Thieda P, Lux LJ, Lohr KN. Outcomes of maternal weight gain. Evid Rep Technol Assess (Full Rep). 2008;168:1–223.
8. Fraser A, Tilling K, Macdonald-Wallis C, Sattar N, Brion MJ, Benfield L, Ness A, Deanfield J, Hingorani A, Nelson SM, et al. Association of maternal weight gain in pregnancy with offspring obesity and metabolic and vascular traits in childhood. Circulation. 2010;121(23):2557–64.
9. Hivert MF, Rifas-Shiman SL, Gillman MW, Oken E. Greater early and mid-pregnancy gestational weight gains are associated with excess adiposity in mid-childhood. Obesity (Silver Spring). 2016;24(7):1546–53.
10. Hochner H, Friedlander Y, Calderon-Margalit R, Meiner V, Sagy Y, Avgil-Tsadok M, Burger A, Savitsky B, Siscovick DS, Manor O. Associations of maternal prepregnancy body mass index and gestational weight gain with adult offspring cardiometabolic risk factors: the Jerusalem perinatal family follow-up study. Circulation. 2012;125(11):1381–9.
11. Karachaliou M, Georgiou V, Roumeliotaki T, Chalkiadaki G, Daraki V, Koinaki S, Dermitzaki E, Sarri K, Vassilaki M, Kogevinas M, et al. Association of trimester-specific gestational weight gain with fetal growth, offspring obesity, and cardiometabolic traits in early childhood. Am J Obstet Gynecol. 2015;212(4):502 e501–14.
12. Oken E, Rifas-Shiman SL, Field AE, Frazier AL, Gillman MW. Maternal gestational weight gain and offspring weight in adolescence. Obstet Gynecol. 2008;112(5):999–1006.
13. Oken E, Taveras EM, Kleinman KP, Rich-Edwards JW, Gillman MW. Gestational weight gain and child adiposity at age 3 years. Am J Obstet Gynecol. 2007;196(4):322 e321–8.
14. Parker M, Rifas-Shiman SL, Oken E, Belfort MB, Jaddoe VW, Gillman MW. Second trimester estimated fetal weight and fetal weight gain predict childhood obesity. J Pediatr. 2012;161(5):864–70.
15. Bogaerts AF, Devlieger R, Nuyts E, Witters I, Gyselaers W, Van den Bergh BR. Effects of lifestyle intervention in obese pregnant women on gestational weight gain and mental health: a randomized controlled trial. Int J Obes 2013, 37(6):814–821.

16. Harrison CL, Lombard CB, Strauss BJ, Teede HJ. Optimizing healthy gestational weight gain in women at high risk of gestational diabetes: a randomized controlled trial. Obesity (Silver Spring). 2013; 21(5):904–9.
17. Herring SJ, Cruice JF, Bennett GG, Rose MZ, Davey A, Foster GD. Preventing excessive gestational weight gain among African American women: a randomized clinical trial. Obesity (Silver Spring). 2016;24(1):30–6.
18. Huang TT, Yeh CY, Tsai YC. A diet and physical activity intervention for preventing weight retention among Taiwanese childbearing women: a randomised controlled trial. Midwifery. 2011;27(2):257–64.
19. Renault KM, Norgaard K, Nilas L, Carlsen EM, Cortes D, Pryds O, Secher NJ. The Treatment of Obese Pregnant Women (TOP) study: a randomized controlled trial of the effect of physical activity intervention assessed by pedometer with or without dietary intervention in obese pregnant women. Am J Obstet Gynecol. 2014;210(2):134 e131–9.
20. Vesco KK, Karanja N, King JC, Gillman MW, Leo MC, Perrin N, McEvoy CT, Eckhardt CL, Smith KS, Stevens VJ. Efficacy of a group-based dietary intervention for limiting gestational weight gain among obese women: a randomized trial. Obesity (Silver Spring). 2014;22(9):1989–96.
21. Vesco KK, Karanja N, King JC, Gillman MW, Leo MC, Perrin N, McEvoy CT, Eckhardt CL, Smith KS, Stevens VJ. Efficacy of a group-based dietary intervention for limiting gestational weight gain among obese women: a randomized trial. Obesity. 2014;22(9):1989–96.
22. Guelinckx I, Devlieger R, Mullie P, Vansant G. Effect of lifestyle intervention on dietary habits, physical activity, and gestational weight gain in obese pregnant women: a randomized controlled trial. Am J Clin Nutr. 2010;91(2):373–80.
23. Hawkins M, Hosker M, Marcus BH, Rosal MC, Braun B, Stanek EJ 3rd, Markenson G, Chasan-Taber L. A pregnancy lifestyle intervention to prevent gestational diabetes risk factors in overweight Hispanic women: a feasibility randomized controlled trial. Diabet Med. 2015;32(1):108–15.
24. Hui A, Back L, Ludwig S, Gardiner P, Sevenhuysen G, Dean H, Sellers E, McGavock J, Morris M, Bruce S, et al. Lifestyle intervention on diet and exercise reduced excessive gestational weight gain in pregnant women under a randomised controlled trial. BJOG. 2012;119(1):70–7.
25. Phelan S, Phipps MG, Abrams B, Darroch F, Grantham K, Schaffner A, Wing RR. Does behavioral intervention in pregnancy reduce postpartum weight retention? Twelve-month outcomes of the fit for delivery randomized trial. Am J Clin Nutr. 2014;99(2):302–11.
26. Skouteris H, McPhie S, Hill B, McCabe M, Milgrom J, Kent B, Bruce L, Herring S, Gale J, Mihalopoulos C, et al. Health coaching to prevent excessive gestational weight gain: a randomized-controlled trial. Br J Health Psychol. 2016;21(1):31–51.
27. Dodd JM, Turnbull D, McPhee AJ, Deussen AR, Grivell RM, Yelland LN, Crowther CA, Wittert G, Owens JA, Robinson JS, et al. Antenatal lifestyle advice for women who are overweight or obese: LIMIT randomised trial. BMJ. 2014;348:g1285.
28. Poston L, Bell R, Croker H, Flynn AC, Godfrey KM, Goff L, Hayes L, Khazaezadeh N, Nelson SM, Oteng-Ntim E, et al. Effect of a behavioural intervention in obese pregnant women (the UPBEAT study): a multicentre, randomised controlled trial. Lancet Diabetes Endocrinol. 2015;3(10):767–77.
29. Brown MJ, Sinclair M, Liddle D, Hill AJ, Madden E, Stockdale J. A systematic review investigating healthy lifestyle interventions incorporating goal setting strategies for preventing excess gestational weight gain. PLoS One. 2012;7(7):e39503.
30. Campbell F, Johnson M, Messina J, Guillaume L, Goyder E. Behavioural interventions for weight management in pregnancy: a systematic review of quantitative and qualitative data. BMC Public Health. 2011;11:491.
31. Gardner B, Wardle J, Poston L, Croker H. Changing diet and physical activity to reduce gestational weight gain: a meta-analysis. Obes Rev. 2011;12(7):e602–20.
32. Streuling I, Beyerlein A, von Kries R. Can gestational weight gain be modified by increasing physical activity and diet counseling? A meta-analysis of interventional trials. Am J Clin Nutr 2010, 92(4):678–687.
33. Flynn AC, Dalrymple K, Barr S, Poston L, Goff LM, Rogozinska E, van Poppel MN, Rayanagoudar G, Yeo S, Barakat Carballo R, et al. Dietary interventions in overweight and obese pregnant women: a systematic review of the content, delivery, and outcomes of randomized controlled trials. Nutr Rev. 2016;74(5):312–28.
34. Taveras EM, Gortmaker SL, Hohman KH, Horan CM, Kleinman KP, Mitchell K, Price S, Prosser LA, Rifas-Shiman SL, Gillman MW. Randomized controlled trial to improve primary care to prevent and manage childhood obesity: the high five for kids study. Arch Pediatr Adolesc Med. 2011;165(8):714–22.

35. Hettema J, Steele J, Miller WR. Motivational interviewing. Annu Rev Clin Psychol. 2005;1:91–111.

36. Wurtele SK, Maddux JE. Relative contributions of protection motivation theory components in predicting exercise intentions and behavior. Health Psychol. 1987;6(5):453–66.

37. Janz NK, Becker MH: The health belief model: a decade later. Health Educ Q 1984, 11(1):1–47.

38. Bandura A. Health promotion by social cognitive means. Health Educ Behav. 2004;31(2):143–64.

39. Sacco RL. The new American Heart Association 2020 goal: achieving ideal cardiovascular health. J Cardiovasc Med (Hagerstown). 2011;12(4):255–7.

40. Crabtree BF, Miller WL. Doing qualitative research. 2nd ed. Calif.: Sage Publications: Thousand Oaks; 1999.

41. Greaney ML, Puleo E, Bennett GG, Haines J, Viswanath K, Gillman MW, Sprunck-Harrild K, Coeling M, Rusinak D, Emmons KM. Factors associated with choice of web or print intervention materials in the healthy directions 2 study. Health Educ Behav. 2014;41(1):52–62.

42. Greaney ML, Puleo E, Sprunck-Harrild K, Bennett GG, Cunningham MA, Gillman MW, Coeling M, Emmons KM. Electronic reminders for cancer prevention: factors associated with preference for automated voice reminders or text messages. Prev Med. 2012;55(2):151–4.

43. Criss S, Oken E, Guthrie L, Hivert MF. A qualitative study of gestational weight gain goal setting. BMC Pregnancy Childbirth. 2016;16(1):317.

44. Oken E, Switkowski K, Price S, Guthrie L, Taveras EM, Gillman M, Friedes J, Callaghan W, Dietz P. A qualitative study of gestational weight gain counseling and tracking. Matern Child Health J. 2013;17(8):1508–17.

45. Catalano P, deMouzon SH. Maternal obesity and metabolic risk to the offspring: why lifestyle interventions may have not achieved the desired outcomes. Int J Obes. 2015;39(4):642–9.

46. Rönö K, Stach-Lempinen B, Klemetti MM, Kaaja RJ, Pöyhönen-Alho M, Eriksson JG, Koivusalo SB. Prevention of gestational diabetes through lifestyle intervention: study design and methods of a Finnish randomized controlled multicenter trial (RADIEL). BMC Pregnancy and Childbirth. 2014;14:70.

8

Should prenatal care providers offer pregnancy options counseling?

Nancy F. Berglas[1]* ⓘ, Valerie Williams[2], Katrina Mark[3] and Sarah C. M. Roberts[1]

Abstract

Background: Professional guidelines indicate that pregnancy options counseling should be offered to pregnant women, in particular those experiencing an unintended pregnancy. However, research on whether pregnancy options counseling would benefit women as they enter prenatal care is limited. This study examines which women might benefit from options counseling during early prenatal care and whether women are interested in receiving counseling from their prenatal care provider.

Methods: At four prenatal care facilities in Louisiana and Maryland, women entering prenatal care completed a self-administered survey and brief structured interview ($N = 586$). Data were analyzed through descriptive statistics, bivariate analyses, multivariate multinomial logistic regression, and coding of open-ended responses.

Results: At entry into prenatal care, most women reported that they planned to continue their pregnancy and raise the child. A subset (3%) scored as having low certainty about their decision on the validated Decision Conflict Scale, indicating need for counseling. In addition, 9% of women stated that they would be interested in discussing their pregnancy options with their prenatal care provider. Regression analyses indicated some sociodemographic differences among women who are in need of or interested in options counseling. Notably, women who reported food insecurity in the prior year were found to be significantly more likely to be in need of options counseling ($RRR = 3.20$, $p < 0.001$) and interested in options counseling ($RRR = 5.48$, $p < 0.001$) than those who were food secure. Most women were open to discussing with their provider if their pregnancy was planned (88%) or if they had considered abortion (81%). More than 95% stated they would be honest with their provider if asked about these topics.

Conclusions: Most women are certain of their decision to continue their pregnancy at the initiation of prenatal care. However, there is a subset of women who, despite entering prenatal care, are uncertain of their decision and wish to discuss their options with their health care provider. Screening tools and/or probing questions are needed to support prenatal care providers in identifying these women and ensuring unbiased, non-directive counseling on all pregnancy options.

Keywords: Abortion, Adoption, Pregnancy options counseling, Prenatal care, Screening

Background

Health care providers play an important role in ensuring that women have the information and services they need to make informed decisions about their pregnancies. Pregnancy options counseling is an opportunity for the pregnant woman to consider, in conversation with her provider, whether she wants to continue the pregnancy and parent the child, continue the pregnancy with a plan for adoption, or have an abortion. Nearly half of pregnancies in the U.S. are unintended, [1] indicating there may be a substantial number of women who might benefit from options counseling in early pregnancy.

A number of leading professional societies have produced guidelines on offering information and referrals for prenatal care, adoption services, and abortion services to pregnant patients [2–5]. These guidelines describe a provider's professional and ethical obligation to provide unbiased, non-directive counseling on all

* Correspondence: nancy.berglas@ucsf.edu
[1]Advancing New Standards in Reproductive Health, Department of Obstetrics, Gynecology and Reproductive Sciences, University of California, San Francisco, 1330 Broadway, Suite 1100, Oakland, CA 94612, USA
Full list of author information is available at the end of the article

available pregnancy options or, if he or she cannot due to personal beliefs, make a timely referral to another provider. This obligation is framed as fundamental to respecting patients' autonomy.

Patient-centered care—respectful and responsive to individual patient preferences, needs and values [6]—requires understanding of patient experiences, and yet there is little research that elicits women's own views on pregnancy options counseling. In one qualitative study with 28 women at prenatal and abortion clinics in Nebraska, most women voiced support for offering options counseling to all pregnant women. [7] They expressed the need for comprehensive, unbiased information given with respect for their autonomy, free from assumptions about their preferred outcome for the pregnancy, and tailored to their medical and social circumstances.

Assessing women's certainty about her decision to have an abortion has become a regular component of abortion care [8]. However, the availability and timing of pregnancy options counseling beyond the context of abortion is not routine and has not been widely explored. It is not clear whether counseling should be provided to all women, directed at some women, or given only if requested. It is also unclear at what point in care that options counseling should be provided. The pregnancy test visit may be an opportune time to open this discussion, [9] but many women determine that they are pregnant outside of the health care system using home pregnancy tests. Many choose not to address an unintended pregnancy with their regular gynecologist before seeking abortion [10]. Furthermore, the availability of counseling varies by provider and setting. Many primary care providers do not address all pregnancy options as part of routine care, even when they support the availability of counseling in concept [11]. For women who receive pregnancy tests at publicly-funded family planning clinics, the availability of options counseling varies by type of facility [12].

For all these reasons, the initial visit to a prenatal care provider may be a woman's first opportunity to speak with a provider about her pregnancy options. The first prenatal visit tends to be longer than subsequent visits, offering time for in-depth conversation that allows the provider to understand a woman's individual circumstances, the context of her pregnancy, and her need for additional support and resources [13]. However, through training and at the guidance of their professional societies, providers are tasked with completing many required practices as part of prenatal care, including medical screening and treatment, promotion of positive health behaviors, and psychosocial support [14]. Time is limited, and it is important for providers to be able to prioritize care based on scientific evidence in concert with individual patient needs. To that end, it needs to be determined whether universal

pregnancy options counseling is a necessary and beneficial part of early prenatal care.

In this exploratory study, we aim to understand which pregnant women, if any, might benefit from pregnancy options counseling upon entry into prenatal care. We base our determination on a validated measure of decision certainty about the pregnancy (as an objective indication of clinical need), as well as a direct question of interest in receiving counseling from their provider (as an indication of patient preference). We also seek to understand women's level of comfort discussing their pregnancy intentions and options with their provider, as an indication of potential harm should providers raise the topic of pregnancy options during a visit.

Methods

Study design and setting

The current analysis is part of a large cross-sectional study, the Multistate Abortion Prenatal Study (Roberts SCM, Kimport K, Kriz R, Holl J, Mark K, Williams V: Consideration of and reasons for not obtaining abortion among women entering prenatal care in Southern Louisiana and Baltimore, Maryland, forthcoming). We recruited English- and Spanish-speaking women ages 18 and older who presented for their first prenatal visit at four prenatal care facilities in Southern Louisiana and Baltimore, Maryland between June 2015 and July 2017. These locations were selected for their similar demographic profiles in terms of race/ethnicity, poverty and birth rate, but different reproductive health policy environments. The prenatal care facilities were affiliated with local universities and served primarily low-income pregnant women, many of whom were eligible for Medicaid for their prenatal care. The institutional review boards of the University of California, San Francisco (UCSF) and Louisiana State University approved the study protocol. The University of Maryland's institutional review board relied on the approval of the UCSF institutional review board.

Participants

At each facility, an onsite research coordinator approached eligible women and invited them to participate in the study. Women were eligible if they were at least 18 years old, were pregnant, were presenting for their first prenatal care visit, and spoke and read English or Spanish. Women who were younger than 18, were not pregnant, were there for a subsequent prenatal care visit, did not speak and read English or Spanish, or were incarcerated were ineligible. After participants provided written consent, the research coordinator demonstrated how to complete a self-administered iPad survey and left them to complete it independently. The research coordinator then conducted a brief (5 to 15 min) structured interview in a private space. Women received a $30 gift card for their participation.

Measures

On the self-administered survey, participants were asked their current preferred outcome for this pregnancy: having the baby and raising it, adoption or having someone else raise it, or abortion. Participants were also asked on both the self-administered survey and during the in-clinic interview if they had considered abortion at any point ("for just one second") during their pregnancy. We considered a participant as having considered abortion if they responded affirmatively either on the survey or during the interview.

Participants completed the Decisional Conflict Scale (DCS) based on their preferred pregnancy outcome. The DCS is a validated scale used to assess individuals' perceptions of certainty in the context of health care decisions [15]. The DCS includes 16 items, answered on a 5-point Likert scale to indicate level of agreement (strongly disagree to strongly agree). Scores are transformed to range from 0 to 100, with lower scores reflecting lower levels of conflict and greater certainty about a decision. Scores greater than 37.5 have been found to be associated with delay and difficulty implementing a decision, and are considered to be of clinical concern [16]. These were categorized dichotomously as "low decision certainty." We considered these women as being *in need of pregnancy options counseling*.

During the interview, participants were asked whether they would like to discuss their pregnancy options with a doctor or nurse. Participants could indicate if they wanted counseling, did not want counseling, and/or had already received counseling during this pregnancy. Although participants could provide more than one response, the categories were mutually exclusive in this sample, resulting in a categorical variable. We considered women who responded that they "wanted counseling" as *interested in pregnancy options counseling*.

Participants were asked whether their provider could ask them about sensitive health topics, including whether this pregnancy was planned and if they had considered abortion. Participants were also asked how honest they would be if their provider asked whether their pregnancy was planned and if they had considered abortion. Participants answered each item on a 5-point Likert scale. Women who disagreed or strongly disagreed were asked open-ended questions about the reasons they might not want to talk to their provider about these topics.

Other variables on the self-administered survey included age, race/ethnicity, highest level of education, employment status, use of public assistance in the last 12 months, food insecurity in the last 12 months, gestational age of the pregnancy, trimester entering prenatal care, pregnancy intentions (measured using the London Measure of Unplanned Pregnancy (LMUP) [17]), and pregnancy history.

Analysis

Data were analyzed through descriptive statistics, χ^2 and t-tests, multivariate logistic regression, and coding of open-ended responses using Stata version 15 software (College Station, TX). To examine predictors of need for or interest in options counseling, we first assessed bivariate relationships with patient characteristics using χ^2 tests for categorical variables and t-tests for continuous variables. We used multivariate multinomial logistic regression with a three-category outcome variable (needing options counseling, interested in options counseling, or not needing or interested in options counseling) to understand whether the predictors differed for each group. Four women were both in need of and interested in options counseling; they were categorized as interested in counseling in the model. A sensitivity analysis, categorizing these four women as in need of counseling, yielded similar patterns of results and are not reported. We adjusted for participant characteristics that were significant in bivariate analyses and used clustered standard errors (using Stata's vce cluster command) to account for non-independent observations within recruitment facility. We calculated predictive probabilities based on the regression model (using Stata's margins command).

Results

Sample description

Onsite research coordinators approached 753 women at the four prenatal care facilities; 91% ($n = 685$) were found to be eligible for the study. Of those eligible, 86% ($n = 589$) consented to participate. The final sample included 586 women who initiated the self-administered survey and in-clinic interview.

The mean age of participants was 27 years, ranging from 18 to 44 (Table 1). Most participants were African American (79%), had completed high school (80%), and had received public assistance in the past year (75%). About half reported being unemployed (49%) and having food insecurity in the past year (47%). Most had been pregnant before (80%), and about one-quarter had previously had an abortion (28%). Most (72%) were in the first trimester of pregnancy upon entry into prenatal care.

Preferred pregnancy outcome

Nearly all women (97%, $n = 564$) reported their preferred pregnancy outcome as having and raising the child. Two percent of women ($n = 10$) reported preferring for the child to be adopted, and 1% ($n = 8$) reported preferring to have an abortion. Among the eight women who currently preferred abortion, all were in their first trimester of pregnancy, within the gestational limit for abortion in their state. Among all women in the sample, nearly one-third (31%, $n = 182$) reported considering abortion at some time during this pregnancy.

Table 1 Description of sample of pregnant women at first prenatal visit ($N = 586$)

Variable	n (%) or mean ± SD
Age, in years (M, SD)	27.0 ± 5.6
Race/ethnicity	
White	45 (7.7)
Black or African American	461 (78.8)
Hispanic/Latina	55 (9.4)
Other/Multiple	24 (4.1)
Highest level of education	
Less than high school	120 (20.5)
Completed high school or GED	286 (48.9)
Some or completed college	179 (30.6)
Employment	
Employed full time	176 (30.2)
Employed part time	122 (20.9)
Unemployed	285 (48.9)
Public assistance in last 12 months	431 (75.5)
Food insecurity in last 12 months	271 (46.9)
Prior pregnancy	467 (80.1)
Prior birth	401 (68.6)
Prior abortion	165 (28.3)
Trimester entered prenatal care	
1st trimester	417 (72.2)
2nd trimester	130 (22.5)
3rd trimester	31 (5.4)
Gestational age of pregnancy, in weeks (M, SD)	11.3 ± 8.1
London Measure of Unplanned Pregnancy score (M, SD)	7.0 ± 2.9

Decision certainty (needing options counseling)

Overall, DCS scores were low (mean 10.3, median 3.1), indicating high decision certainty among women at the first prenatal care visit. Mean DCS scores were significantly higher (indicating lower certainty) for women currently preferring adoption or abortion, compared to woman preferring to raise the child (27.2 adoption, 23.9 abortion, 9.9 raise child, $p < 0.001$). Twenty women (3%) were categorized as having low decision certainty (DCS > 37.5), indicating need for pregnancy options counseling.

In bivariate analyses, low decision certainty was significantly associated with participants' state of residence, race/ethnicity, education, food insecurity, and LMUP score.

Interest in options counseling

Most women (88%, $n = 499$) reported that they were not interested in discussing their pregnancy options with their provider at their prenatal care visit. Nine percent

($n = 49$) stated that they would like to discuss their pregnancy options, and 3% ($n = 20$) reported that they had already discussed their options with a provider. Women who currently preferred adoption or abortion were significantly more likely to be interested in discussing their pregnancy options with their provider, compared to women preferring to raise the child (30% adoption, 38% abortion, 8% raise child, $p < 0.001$).

In bivariate analyses, interest in pregnancy options counseling was significantly associated with participants' state of residence, age, race/ethnicity, food insecurity, and pregnancy history.

Need for vs. interest in pregnancy options counseling

There was little overlap between the 20 women who reported low decision certainty and 49 women who expressed interest in options counseling. Only four women were categorized as both in need of and interested in options counseling.

Predictors of needing or being interested in pregnancy options counseling

The results of the multivariate regression model are presented in Table 2; the base outcome for the model is women who reported neither needing nor being interested in counseling. Compared to these women, women interested in options counseling were more likely to be living in Louisiana (RRR = 4.95, $p < 0.001$) and Hispanic/Latina (RRR = 3.00, $p < 0.05$). As might be predicted, higher LMUP scores – indicating more planned pregnancies – were associated with less need for (RRR = 0.77, $p < 0.01$) or interest in (RRR = 0.90, $p < 0.001$) options counseling.

Notably, the model indicates significant differences by food insecurity. Women who reported food insecurity in the prior year were three times more likely to be in need of options counseling (RRR = 3.20, $p < 0.001$) and five times more likely to be interested in options counseling (RRR = 5.48, $p < 0.001$) than those who had not experienced food insecurity. The predicted probabilities of needing or being interested in pregnancy options counseling by food insecurity status are presented in Fig. 1.

Provider questions about pregnancy intentions and abortion

Most women agreed that their providers can ask if their pregnancy was planned (88% agree/strongly agree, $n = 498$) and whether they had considered having an abortion during their pregnancy (81% agree/strongly agree, $n = 462$).

Among women who stated that providers should not ask if their pregnancy was planned (5% disagree/strongly disagree, $n = 31$), all planned to raise the child. Among women who stated that providers should not ask

Table 2 Multivariate multinomial logistic regression model predicting in need of or wanting pregnancy options counseling among pregnant women at their first prenatal visit (n = 570)

	Relative Risk Ratio	p-value	95% Confidence Interval	
In need of options counseling				
State				
Maryland	Reference			
Louisiana	1.29	n.s.	0.97	1.72
Age (cont.)	0.98	n.s.	0.94	1.02
Race/Ethnicity				
Black or African American	Reference			
White	1.02	n.s.	0.10	10.14
Hispanic/Latina	3.41	n.s.	0.32	36.30
Other/Multiple	2.01	n.s.	0.15	26.14
Education				
Did not complete high school	Reference			
High school or GED	0.38	*	0.18	0.82
Some or completed college	0.17	n.s.	0.01	2.11
Food insecurity in past 12 months	3.20	***	2.50	4.08
Previous abortion	0.83	n.s.	0.38	1.83
Previous pregnancy	0.41	n.s.	0.09	1.87
Gestational age (cont.)	1.01	n.s.	0.97	1.05
LMUP score (cont.)	0.77	**	0.64	0.91
Wanting options counseling				
State				
Maryland	Reference			
Louisiana	4.95	***	3.50	7.00
Age (cont.)	0.94	*	0.88	0.99
Race/Ethnicity				
Black or African American	Reference			
White	1.05	n.s.	0.43	2.57
Hispanic/Latina	3.00	*	1.10	8.22
Other/Multiple	0.75	n.s.	0.13	4.36
Education				
Did not complete high school	Reference			
High school or GED	1.45	n.s.	0.93	2.28
Some or completed college	1.22	n.s.	0.45	3.30
Food insecurity in past 12 months	5.48	***	2.49	12.03
Previous abortion	0.37	*	0.16	0.88
Previous pregnancy	0.76	n.s.	0.24	2.40
Gestational age (cont.)	1.00	n.s.	0.97	1.03
LMUP score (cont.)	0.90	***	0.86	0.95

*p < 0.05, **p < 0.01, ***p < 0.001, n.s. = not significant
Base outcome: Women not in need of or wanting pregnancy options counseling. Four women reporting both in need of and wanting counseling were categorized in model as wanting pregnancy options counseling. LMUP = London Measure of Unplanned Pregnancy

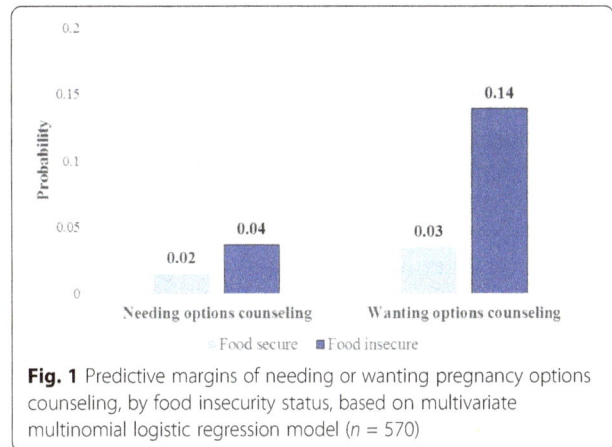

Fig. 1 Predictive margins of needing or wanting pregnancy options counseling, by food insecurity status, based on multivariate multinomial logistic regression model (n = 570)

whether they had considered abortion (9% disagree/strongly disagree, n = 66), 95% planned to raise the child. Among the 20 women with low decision certainty, most were comfortable with their provider asking if their pregnancy was planned (n = 19) or if they had considered abortion (n = 17).

Nearly all women reported that they would answer honestly if their providers asked if their pregnancy was planned (97% agree/strongly agree, n = 552) and whether they had considered having an abortion (95% agree/strongly agree, n = 539).

Discussion

Upon entry into prenatal care, most women felt certain about their decision to continue their pregnancy and raise the child, and most indicated that they were not interested in discussing their pregnancy options at this time. However, a not-insignificant minority of women felt less sure about their pregnancy. Women who preferred adoption had particularly high rates of low decision certainty. A few women preferred to terminate their pregnancy but presented for prenatal care despite being within the gestational limit for abortion in their state of residence. This indicates that the mere act of presenting to a prenatal care visit does not necessarily imply that the woman is certain of her plan to continue the pregnancy. Moreover, 9% of women expressed interest in options counseling at their first prenatal visit, even if they were not considered clinically "in need."

Our analyses indicate that women in need of and/or interested in pregnancy options counseling differ from other pregnant women entering prenatal care. Not surprisingly, their pregnancies were less likely to be intended. Those who requested options counseling were more likely to be younger, Latina, and living in Louisiana – where women may face more policy barriers to accessing abortion. Most notably, food insecurity with the past year was highlighted as a significant predictor of both need for and interest in options counseling. Even within a relatively low-income population of women, those experiencing immediate economic insecurities were in greater need of support from their provider. Their needs are clearly material, but their interest in discussing their pregnancy options indicates that they are looking to providers for less tangible support as well.

It is worth noting that these interviews were conducted at women's first prenatal care visits and not at the time that they obtained a positive pregnancy test. As many women take home pregnancy tests, it is possible that presenting to a prenatal care provider is the only way that they are familiar with to engage in the health care system and/or discuss options for their pregnancy. It stands to reason that women would be most comfortable speaking to their provider about their pregnancy options, just as is expected with other medical decision-making. If their provider assumes that their engagement in prenatal care implies their intent to continue the pregnancy, an opportunity may be missed to provide women with the counseling and autonomy that they need to fully understand and consider all of their options.

This study's findings about food insecurity make clear how much these broader circumstances play a role in pregnancy decision-making and outcomes. Women who were food insecure were much more likely to be uncertain of their decision to continue pregnancy and be interested in pregnancy options counseling. This elucidates the fact that pregnancy options counseling does not consist solely of explaining the three seemingly obvious options (raising a child, adoption, or abortion), but that it should also include a more comprehensive discussion of how to best provide the support a woman needs to attain her desired pregnancy outcome. The question remains how to identify those women who are most in need of support, and then how to ensure that they are connected with necessary services. Screening tools and/or probing questions are needed to support prenatal care providers in identifying these women and ensuring unbiased, non-directive counseling on all pregnancy options.

This study has limitations. First, women's reports about their preferences for abortion or adoption may be underreported due to stigma [18, 19]. We note, however, that more than 30% of women disclosed they had considered abortion during this pregnancy, indicating that our study procedures did encourage women to disclose. Nonetheless, to the extent that women may be unwilling to disclose their preference for their pregnancy, we may not fully understand which women might benefit from options counseling at the first prenatal visit. Second, we did not recruit participants younger than age 18; thus, the results may not represent the need for options counseling among pregnant minors. The American Academy

of Pediatrics' guidelines on options counseling may prove useful to providers working with younger patients [5]. Third, the women in this sample are primarily African American, low-income, and living in more urban settings, and all were recruited at large prenatal clinics. Although women were recruited from all levels of prenatal care, including midwifery, low-risk obstetrics and high-risk obstetrics, their experiences and needs may not be representative of all women entering prenatal care. The current body of research on the value of including pregnancy options counseling in early prenatal care is limited to this study and one other [7]. Both quantitative and qualitative research are needed to understand the value and potential impact of options counseling for different populations of women living in varied contexts.

Conclusions

Our study finds that most women are certain of their decision to continue their pregnancy at the initiation of prenatal care. These results mirror research indicating that most women are certain of their decision when they present for an abortion [20–22]. In both settings, the options for the pregnancy are generally well known and women's decisions about whether to proceed with an unintended pregnancy are typically made prior to reaching the health care system. However, there is a subset of women who, despite entering prenatal care, are uncertain of their decision and wish to discuss their options with their provider.

Acknowledgements
The authors thank Finley Baba, Elise Belusa, Anna Bernstein, Mattie Boehler-Tatman, Ivette Gomez, Heather Gould, Heather Lipkovich, Nicole Nguyen, Brenly Rowland, Alison Swiatlo, Ushma Upadhyay, and Erin Wingo for research and project assistance and the facilities in Louisiana and Maryland for their collaboration.

Funding
This study was funded by the David and Lucile Packard Foundation and an anonymous foundation. The sponsors had no involvement in study design; in the collection, analysis and interpretation of data; in the writing of the report; or in the decision to submit the article for publication.

Authors' contributions
SCMR conceptualized the study design. VW and KM provided clinical research expertise and oversight of study implementation at local recruitment sites. NFB analyzed and interpreted the data. NFB drafted the manuscript. All authors read and approved the final manuscript.

Competing interests
The authors declare that they have no competing interests.

Author details
[1]Advancing New Standards in Reproductive Health, Department of Obstetrics, Gynecology and Reproductive Sciences, University of California,

San Francisco, 1330 Broadway, Suite 1100, Oakland, CA 94612, USA.
[2]Department of Obstetrics and Gynecology, Louisiana State University Health Sciences Center New Orleans, 1542 Tulane Avenue, Box T5-2, New Orleans, LA 70112, USA. [3]Department of Obstetrics, Gynecology and Reproductive Sciences, University of Maryland School of Medicine, 655 W. Baltimore Street, Baltimore, MD 21201, USA.

References

1. Finer LB, Zolna MR. Declines in unintended pregnancy in the United States, 2008-2011. N Engl J Med. 2016;374(9):843–52.
2. American Academy of Family Physicians: Reproductive Decisions. In.; 2017.
3. American College of Nurse-Midwives: Access to Comprehensive Sexual and Reproductive Health Care Services In.; 2016.
4. American College of Obstetricians and Gynecologists. The American College of Obstetricians and Gynecologists. In: Guidelines for women's health care : a resource manual, Fourth edition. Washington, DC: Women's Health Care Physicians; 2014.
5. Hornberger LL, AAP Committee on Adolescence. Options counseling for the pregnant adolescent patient. Pediatrics. 2017;140(3):e2017224.
6. Institute of Medicine. Crossing the quality chasm: a new health system for the 21st century. Washington, DC: National Academy Press; 2001.
7. French VA, Steinauer JE, Kimport K. What women want from their health care providers about pregnancy options counseling: a qualitative study. Womens Health Issues. 2017;27(6):715–20.
8. Gould H, Perrucci A, Barar R, Sinkford D, Foster DG. Patient education and emotional support practices in abortion care facilities in the United States. Womens Health Issues. 2012;22(4):e359–64.
9. Gavin L, Moskosky S, Carter M, Curtis K, Glass E, Godfrey E, Marcell A, Mautone-Smith N, Pazol K, Tepper N, et al. Providing quality family planning services: recommendations of CDC and the U.S. Office of Population Affairs. MMWR Recomm Rep. 2014;63(RR-04):1–54.
10. Chor J, Tusken M, Lyman P, Gilliam M. Factors shaping Women's pre-abortion communication with their regular gynecologic care providers. Womens Health Issues. 2016;26(4):437–41.
11. Holt K, Janiak E, McCormick MC, Lieberman E, Dehlendorf C, Kajeepeta S, Caglia JM, Langer A. Pregnancy options counseling and abortion referrals among US primary care physicians: results from a National Survey. Fam Med. 2017;49(7):527–36.
12. Hebert LE, Fabiyi C, Hasselbacher LA, Starr K, Gilliam ML. Variation in pregnancy options counseling and referrals, and reported proximity to abortion services, among publicly funded family planning facilities. Perspect Sex Reprod Health. 2016;48(2):65–71.
13. Meiksin R, Chang JC, Bhargava T, Arnold R, Dado D, Frankel R, Rodriguez KL, Ling B, Zickmund S. Now is the chance: patient-provider communication about unplanned pregnancy during the first prenatal visit. Patient Educ Couns. 2010;81(3):462–7.
14. American Academy of Pediatrics, American College of Obstetricians and Gynecologists: Guidelines for perinatal care, Eighth edition. edn. Elk Grove Village, IL and Washington, DC: AAP and ACOG; 2017.
15. O'Connor AM. Validation of a decisional conflict scale. Med Decis Mak. 1995; 15(1):25–30.
16. O'Connor AM. User manual - decisional conflict scale. In. Ottawa: Ottawa Hospital Research Institute; 2010.
17. Barrett G, Smith SC, Wellings K. Conceptualisation, development, and evaluation of a measure of unplanned pregnancy. J Epidemiol Community Health. 2004;58(5):426–33.
18. Jagannathan R. Relying on surveys to understand abortion behavior: some cautionary evidence. Am J Public Health. 2001;91(11):1825–31.
19. Rice WS, Turan B, Stringer KL, Helova A, White K, Cockrill K, Turan JM. Norms and stigma regarding pregnancy decisions during an unintended pregnancy: development and predictors of scales among young women in the U.S. south. PLoS One. 2017;12(3):e0174210.
20. Cameron ST, Glasier A. Identifying women in need of further discussion about the decision to have an abortion and eventual outcome. Contraception. 2013;88(1):128–32.
21. Goenee MS, Donker GA, Picavet C, Wijsen C. Decision-making concerning unwanted pregnancy in general practice. Fam Pract. 2014;31(5):564–70.
22. Ralph LJ, Foster DG, Kimport K, Turok D, Roberts SCM. Measuring decisional certainty among women seeking abortion. Contraception. 2017;95(3):269–78.

9

Missed opportunities in antenatal care for improving the health of pregnant women and newborns in Geita district, Northwest Tanzania

Eveline Thobias Konje[1,2*] (iD), Moke Tito Nyambita Magoma[3], Jennifer Hatfield[2], Susan Kuhn[4], Reginald S. Sauve[2] and Deborah Margret Dewey[2,4,5]

Abstract

Background: Despite the significant benefits of early detection and management of pregnancy related complications during antenatal care (ANC) visits, not all pregnant women in Tanzania initiate ANC in a timely manner. The primary objectives of this research study in rural communities of Geita district, Northwest Tanzania were: 1) to conduct a population-based study that examined the utilization and availability of ANC services; and 2) to explore the challenges faced by women who visited ANC clinics and barriers to utilization of ANC among pregnant women.

Methods: A sequential explanatory mixed method design was utilized. Household surveys that examined antenatal service utilization and availability were conducted in 11 randomly selected wards in Geita district. One thousand, seven hundred and nineteen pregnant women in their 3rd trimester participated in household surveys. It was followed by focus group discussions with community health workers and pregnant women that examined challenges and barriers to ANC.

Results: Of the pregnant women who participated, 86.74% attended an ANC clinic at least once; 3.62% initiated ANC in the first trimester; 13.26% had not initiated ANC when they were interviewed in their 3rd trimester. Of the women who had attended ANC at least once, the majority (82.96%) had been checked for HIV status, less than a half (48.36%) were checked for hemoglobin level, and only a minority had been screened for syphilis (6.51%). Among women offered laboratory testing, the prevalence of HIV was 3.88%, syphilis, 18.57%, and anemia, 54.09%. In terms of other preventive measures, 91.01% received a tetanus toxoid vaccination, 76.32%, antimalarial drugs, 65. 13%, antihelminthic drugs, and 76.12%, iron supplements at least once. Significant challenges identified by women who visited ANC clinics included lack of male partner involvement, informal regulations imposed by health care providers, perceived poor quality of care, and health care system related factors. Socio-cultural beliefs, fear of HIV testing, poverty and distance from health clinics were reported as barriers to early ANC utilization.

Conclusion: Access to effective ANC remains a challenge among women in Geita district. Notably, most women initiated ANC late and early initiation did not guarantee care that could contribute to better pregnancy outcomes.

Keywords: Antenatal care, Missed opportunity, Tanzania, Sequential explanatory mixed method

* Correspondence: etkonje@ucalgary.ca
[1]Department of Biostatistics & Epidemiology, School of Public Health, Catholic University of Health and Allied Sciences, P.O. box 1464 Bugando Area, Mwanza, Tanzania
[2]Department of Community Health Sciences, Cumming School of Medicine, University of Calgary, 3280 Hospital Drive, NW, Calgary, AB, Canada
Full list of author information is available at the end of the article

Background

To reduce preventable maternal and newborn mortality and morbidity, the provision of quality antenatal care (ANC), accessible obstetrics care, and life-saving interventions are essential services [1–5]. In 2015, approximately 303,000 maternal deaths occurred worldwide with sub-Saharan Africa accounting for 66% of all maternal deaths [6]. Although some developing countries have achieved up to a 75% reduction in the maternal mortality ratio (MMR) since 1990, Tanzania has made little progress over the past 25 years [2, 6]. In 1990, the MMR was 529 maternal deaths per 100,000 live births and in 2015/16 it was 545 maternal deaths per 100,000 live births [7]. Most developing countries have achieved a reduction in mortality among under five children; however, the proportion of neonatal deaths and stillborn babies remains unacceptably high [2, 8]. Globally, it was estimated in 2015 that there were 18.4 stillbirths per 1000 births with rural populations accounting for 60% of all stillborn babies [8]. Tanzania ranked ninth in the world among the ten countries with the highest number of stillbirths in 2015 with an estimated 47,000 stillbirths [8]. Most of these stillbirths occurred during labor and delivery and were considered to be due to preventable or manageable health conditions [8, 9].

The sustainable development goal 3.1, emphasizes reducing the MMR to less than 220 per 100, 000 live births for countries with an MMR above the average global level [10]. To end preventable causes of maternal deaths due to pregnancy related complications, scaling up of existing interventions during pregnancy and delivery is crucial [5]. The main causes of maternal deaths are hemorrhage, hypertensive disorder, and infection [11]. Newborn deaths and stillbirths are mainly due to asphyxia, prematurity, and infections [8, 9] and most are preventable with existing evidence-based interventions either directly or indirectly during pregnancy, labor, delivery, and post delivery [1, 3, 5].

Safe motherhood initiative programs recognize the significance of the provision of quality care from preconception to the postnatal period for women and newborn babies. They consist of four pillars, namely, family planning, ANC, clean and safe delivery, and essential obstetric care services [3]. ANC is recognized and emphasized due to its influence on the wellbeing of pregnant women and their unborn babies [1, 3, 5]. In 2002, Tanzania adopted the Focused ANC (FANC) model recommended by the World Health Organisation (WHO). It is still utilized although the WHO introduced a new ANC model in 2016 [1, 12]. The FANC model emphasizes individualized care for all pregnant women as any pregnancy could face complications. It suggests a minimum of 4 visits for uncomplicated pregnancies with the initial visit occurring before 16 weeks gestation, the second visit between 20 and 24 weeks, a third visit between 28 and 32 weeks, and a fourth visit at 36 weeks [13].

Although universal coverage of ANC services is reported globally and at the country level [2, 7, 10, 14], in developing countries, many pregnant women fail to benefit from comprehensive ANC due to factors such as late initiation and the poor quality of ANC services [2, 14–17]. Early initiation during the first trimester and quality ANC over the pregnancy period has been recognized as improving pregnancy outcomes and increasing newborn survival [18, 19]. However, in developing countries, only 25% of pregnant women initiated ANC before 14 weeks gestation and 48% of pregnant women did not complete 4 ANC visits [2, 15]. Several factors have been associated with late initiation including: older age, higher parity/multiparity, lower education level, hidden costs, lack of male support, pregnancy-related cultural beliefs, unplanned pregnancy, and health system related issues such as shortages of supplies and drugs [14, 20–24]. However, most of the studies that have reported on the timing and frequency of ANC utilization were retrospective in nature and included women who had a live birth in the 2–5 years prior to the conduct of the study. The results of these studies could be influenced by survival and recall bias, as the information obtained was from women who survived their pregnancy and were able to provide a self report [14, 20–22, 25, 26]. In addition, these studies were health facility-based, and as a result may suffer from selection bias as attendees were likely to be women with better health care seeking behavior than non-attendees, particularly in rural low income settings, leading to an over estimation of early initiation and utilization of ANC during pregnancy [20, 21, 25].

In Tanzania, early initiation of ANC (i.e., attending antenatal care in the first trimester) is reported to be 24%, and only 51% of women had more than 4 antenatal care visits in 2015/16 [7]. Northwest Tanzania is a region with a low rate of utilization of ANC services despite the existing high fertility rate in this region [7]. The primary objectives of this research study in rural communities of Geita district, Northwest Tanzania were: 1) to conduct a population-based study that examined the utilization and availability of ANC services, and 2) to explore the challenges faced by women who visited ANC clinics and barriers to utilization of ANC among pregnant women.

Methods

Study setting

The study was conducted at Geita district, one of the six districts in Geita region Northwest Tanzania. The district has 35 wards with a district hospital, 5 health centers, and 38 dispensaries. Eleven wards (31%) were randomly selected for inclusion in the study, namely: Lwamgasa, Nyaruyeye, Bukoli, Nyarugusu, Nyakamwaga, Butundwe, Chigunga, Nyamiluluma, Bukondo, Nzera, and Lwenzera. Random selection was accomplished by first alphabetically ordering the wards and numbering them from 1 to 35. Then a random numbers table was used to select eleven wards. Based on the Tanzania Demographic and Health Survey (TDHS) 2015/16, Geita performed poorly on components of ANC and more than a half (52.3%) of pregnant women delivered at home [7].

Study design

This study is part of a large cohort study that is investigating utilization of maternal and child health services, pregnancy outcomes, birth-related complications, and maternal and child mortality and morbidity up to 4 months postpartum. The study utilized a sequential explanatory mixed method approach. This method has two phases. The first phase is characterized by the collection and analysis of quantitative data. The second phase involves the collection and analysis of qualitative data. This method uses the qualitative findings to further explain and interpret the findings of the quantitative data and was selected as it allowed exploring in detail the challenges pregnant women faced when accessing ANC services and the barriers to utilization of ANC services.

Quantitative data collection process

A household survey using a cross sectional design involving pregnant women in the third trimester was conducted between September 2016 and August 2017. Based on 2015 total deliveries for the entire district (36,101), we assumed that approximately 10,000 (28%) pregnant women would be residing in the study area with at least 20% (2000) of them being in their third trimester of pregnancy. The study reached 1805 (90%) of the expected pregnant women in the selected wards, of whom 1719 participated in the survey. Of those who were contacted but not included in our final sample, 81 were not residents of a study area, two had had miscarriages, one woman was in the second trimester of her pregnancy based on her last menstruation period, and two women refused to participate because they were not feeling well.

The household survey consisted of a face-to-face interview. During the conduct of the household survey interview, only pregnant women in their 3rd trimester who voluntarily consented were invited to participate in the study. In the situation that a pregnant woman was not at home during the time the household survey was conducted, that household was re-visited up to three times to see if the woman was interested in participating.

Village leaders, community health workers, and traditional birth attendants assisted in the identification of households with pregnant women. Trained research assistants who were registered nurses, and intern medical doctors conducted the household survey. The research assistants were not health care providers at health facilities in the study areas (they were from college/university and were not employed as health care providers); hence, interview bias was expected to be minimal. The principal investigator (EK) supervised the conduct of the survey.

For the household survey, a structured pretested questionnaire was utilized to capture baseline information including socio-demographic characteristics, gestational age, parity, gravidity, obstetric history, immunization status, intermittent preventive treatement status, deworming status, and the use of iron and folate supplements. The questionnaire also captured information on birth preparedness, an anticipated place for delivery, social support after delivery, money saving for any emergency during pregnancy, and the purchase baby's items, which are included as part of the health education provided through ANC services (seeAdditional file 1). For women who had attended ANC clinics, responses to the household survey questions were crosschecked with their antenatal cards, which are provided to pregnant women who attend ANC clinics. During the household survey, the pregnant women's blood pressure was checked, weight and height were measured, an identification card for follow-up purposes was provided, and counselling regarding the utilization of ANC services was provided. The household surveys were conducted in the homes of the pregnant women unless otherwise specified by the participant. In those rare cases (only four women), the interview was scheduled at a convenient location identified by the participant, usually at their farm or at a friend's house.

Qualitative data collection process

A case study was conducted to explore in depth barriers to utilization of antenatal care services among women in the study area. Women and community health workers from six wards namely Lwenzera, Nzera, Nyarugusu, Bukoli, Lwamgasa, and Bukondo were invited to participate in focus group discussions. Using the results from the analyses of the household survey data, study wards were selected based on the criterion of having a significant number of women who initiated ANC late or who never attended ANC. Community health workers (CHWs) were also invited to participate because of the nature of their work in bridging the community with the health care system. Hence, participants were purposively selected for the focus group discussions (FGDs). FDGs provided the women with a safe environment in which they could present their views and opinions and provided the participants with the opportunity to see that the challenges and barriers that they experienced were similar those of other women. The FGDs also promoted open discussion and sometimes disagreement, and allowed us to observe the group dynamics. Finally, FGDs allowed us to observe whether there was consensus of group members on the challenges faced by women who visited ANC clinics and the barriers to utilization of ANC among pregnant women.

We conducted six FGDs with women who had recently delivered babies, many of whom had not utilized ANC and delivery services. Thirty-five women from the selected wards participated in the FGDs with an average of five to six women in each group. Six focus groups were also conducted with CHWs, one in each of the six wards. On average, five to six CHWs, both male and female participated from each ward making 32 CHWs. A semi-structured interview guide was used to facilitate discussion among participants. The key issues explored were: 1) What do you know about maternal and child health services available to you during pregnancy or to pregnant women? 2) What has been your experience with ANC services in your community? and 3) Why do some pregnant women not utilize the ANC services available in their communities or are late in utilizing these services?

The research team conducted the FDGs in the Swahili language and where necessary in the local language (Sukuma). Members of the research team who were fluent in Sukuma assisted with translation during discussions. None of the research team members involved in conducting the FGDs provided directed medical care to the participants through the local community health centers. Voice recordings were transcribed, translated into English, and back translated into Swahili to ensure content consistency. Field notes were taken by EK and some of the FGDs were supervised by DD. For the purposes of confidentiality, privacy, and friendly environment, FGDs typically occurred at the village leaders' offices or at primary schools. However, in some cases, (two focus groups), they took place at the local health clinic. Each FGD took approximately one hour and thirty minutes.

Data management and analysis

ANC service utilization was the outcome of interest. Three levels were examined, namely no attendance at ANC services, attendance within the first trimester, and attendance in the second or third trimester. Epi-Data version 3.1 software was used for data entry with the double entry system feature to reduce data entry errors. This feature allows double entry of the same questionnaire data by two different clerks. During dataset validation, inconsistencies were resolved by reviewing the original questionnaires and editing accordingly. Cleaned

data were exported and analyzed using STATA version 13 [27]. The 95% confidence intervals and p values reported were based on a 5% level of statistical significance. Chi-squared tests were used to examine associations between categorical variables.

Qualitative data were transcribed and translated into English by two RAs fluent in Swahili and English and cross-checked by EK for discrepancies. Thematic analysis was conducted by EK and reviewed by DD. It involved familiarization with data, identification of the main themes, indexing, charting, mapping, and interpretation. Line by line coding was done manually and identified themes were compared with written field notes for convergence or divergence of ideas. The identified themes were used to gain a deeper understanding of the quantitative results. The data source triangulation was done by having group discussions with community health workers and women in order to confirm the perceived challenges and barriers. The contiguous approach was adapted for data integration at the interpretation and reporting level.

Results
Household survey participant characteristics

Of the 1805 pregnant women visited at their homes, 1719 were eligible for this study. The average age of the participants was 25.7 years (see Table 1). Almost all of the participants (94.71%) were married and the majority of the women reported having a primary school education (68.59%); however, a considerable proportion (23.61%) reported no formal schooling.

Household survey
Antenatal services utilization and availability

Overall, antenatal attendance with at least one visit was 86.74% (1491/1719); however, a considerable proportion of participants 13.26% (228/1719) had not initiated ANC at the time of the household survey. Of the 1491 pregnant women who visited an antenatal clinic at least once, only 3.62% (54/1491; 95% CI 2.67–4.57) initiated ANC at the first trimester while the rest of the participants initiated ANC either in the 2nd or 3rd trimester. Further, although more than three quarters of participants attended antenatal clinics, provision of laboratory and preventive services were not common to all pregnant women. As per the FANC model, pregnant women should receive services related to disease prevention, health promotion, detection and treatment of existing disease, and information on developing a birth preparedness plan. Laboratory testing was limited to 82.96% women for HIV, 48.36% women for hemoglobin level (Hb in g/dL), and 6.51% for syphilis (see Table 2). The prevalence of existing conditions based on the records from antenatal cards was 3.88% for HIV infection,

Table 1 Socio-demographic characteristics of 1719 pregnant women in rural Geita by ANC attendance

Characteristic	Overall		Women attended ANC at least once (N = 1491)		Women not attended ANC (N = 228)	
	Mean(SD)	n (%)	n (%)	Mean (SD)	n (%)	Mean (SD)
Maternal age (in years)	25.73 (6.60)			25.51 (6.52)		27.28 (6.96)
Maternal height (in cm)	155.66 (6.90)			155.77 (6.73)		154.89 (7.92)
Maternal weight (in Kg)	59.49 (8.39)			59.71 (8.38)		57.97 (8.31)
Marital status						
Currently single		91 (5.29)	83 (5.57)		8 (3.51)	
Currently married		1628 (94.71)	1408 (96.43)		220 (96.49)	
Education level						
No formal education		406 (23.61)	347 (23.27)		59 (25.88)	
Primary		1179 (68.59)	1024 (68.68)		155 (67.98)	
Secondary & above		134 (7.80)	120 (8.05)		14 (6.14)	

Table 2 Antenatal care services received and prevalence of screened conditions among 1491 women

Characteristic	Services received at clinics n (%)	Prevalence n (%)	95% CI
HIV Status			
-Total Screened	1237 (82.96)		
-Tested Positive		48 (3.88)	2.80–4.95
-Tested Negative		1189 (96.12)	
Hemoglobin level			
-Total screened	721 (48.36)		
-Hb level < 10.9 g/dL		390 (54.09)	50.45–57.74
-Hb level > =10.9 g/dL		331 (45.91)	
Syphilis status			
-Total Screened	97 (6.51)		
- Tested Positive		18 (18.57)	10.68–26.43
- Tested Negative		79 (81.43)	
Iron supplements	1135 (76.12)		
Antihelminthic drugs			
- None	520 (34.87)		
- One Dose	475 (31.86)		
- Two Doses	496 (33.27)		
Intermittent preventive treatment			
- None	353 (23.68)		
- One Dose	518 (34.74)		
-Two Doses	620 (41.58)		
Tetanus toxoid vaccine			
- None	134 (8.99)		
- One Dose	229 (15.36)		
-Two or more doses	1128 (75.65)		

54.09% for anemia, and 18.57% for syphilis infection. Regarding preventive measures, 91.01% of participants received a tetanus toxoid vaccination, 76.32%, antimalarial drugs, 65.13%, antihelminthic drugs, and 76.12%, iron supplements at least once.

During the household survey the women were asked about their intentions to deliver at the health facility; plans for transport to the health facility, and saving money for possible emergencies during pregnancy or delivery. They were also asked if they had bought any items for their baby (i.e., basin, clothes, soap), and any social support after the delivery of the baby (i.e., their birth preparedness plan). More than half (54.33%) of the participants indicated that they did not intend to deliver at a health facility. The majority (71.5%) had no plan for transport during labour and 64.39% had not purchased baby items. However, half of the participants had saved money (49.74%) for an emergency during pregnancy or delivery. Significant differences (p value < 0.05) were observed between women who attended ANC clinics at least once and those who did not attend ANC on all components of birth preparedness except social support. ANC clinic attendees were more likely to plan for transport, save money, buy items for their baby, and indicate that they intended to deliver at a health facility compared to those who had not attended an ANC clinic (Table 3).

General characteristics of participants in FGDs

The women who participated in six FGDs (n = 35) were multiparous and had attended ANC clinics at least once in previous pregnancies or the current pregnancy. Of the 32 CHWs who participated in the FGDs, all had at least a year of experience working as a CHW and over half (53%) were male. In terms of the dynamics of the FGDs, the women and the CHWs were very open and forthcoming in their responses to the questions asked by research team members, most women and CHWs contributed to the discussion and participation by all participants was encouraged by the researchers.

Perceived barriers for antenatal care services

This section discusses the perceived barriers that women identified as hindering their utilization of ANC services. It focuses on the issues that women perceived to hinder their utilization of available ANC services. Focus group discussions with women and CHWs were used to identify themes related to perceived barriers to utilization of ANC services in rural Geita district. Women indicated that they do not initiate ANC at all due to the following reasons: poverty, fear of HIV testing, and socio-cultural beliefs (Table 4).

Poverty may influence the health care seeking behavior of pregnant women negatively. Many women have no source of income in the family; therefore, any cost related to health care is a financial burden for the entire family. Fares for transport to ANC clinics, a maternity dress, or other hidden costs can act as a barrier for some women in the rural communities.

Having no income in the family, and [the] health facility being far may lead to women not attending ANC services at all considering the family does not have even a bicycle. Female participant 1

It could be poverty, since nurses here emphasize clean clothes and proper dress such as a maternity dress when a woman wants to attend clinic. If you don't have a maternity dress you may not go. Female participant 5

Participants also identified men's lack of interest and their unwillingness to participate during pregnancy, which resulted in some women not attending ANC clinics. For HIV prevention of mother-to-child transmission, couples are required to go together to the first antenatal visit. This practice aims at providing counselling and HIV testing to both partners. However, some health providers deny ANC services to pregnant women who attended without their male partners. Fear of HIV testing by both female and male partners was also perceived to be a barrier to ANC for couples that were unwilling to participate in HIV testing together.

Table 3 Birth preparedness planning among 1719 pregnant women in rural Geita district

Characteristic		Overall	Women who attended ANC at least once N = 1491	Women who had not attended ANC N = 228	Difference in proportions P value (chi^2 test)
		n (%)	n (%)	n (%)	
Health facility delivery	Yes	785 (45.67)	730 (48.96)	52 (24.12)	< 0.05
Transport preparation	Yes	490 (28.50)	448 (30.05)	42 (18.42)	< 0.05
Saving money	Yes	855 (49.74)	783 (52.52)	72 (31.58)	< 0.05
Purchase baby items	Yes	574 (33.39)	531 (35.61)	43 (18.86)	< 0.05
Social support	Yes	1438 (83.65)	1254 (84.10)	184 (80.70)	0.20

Some women stay at home throughout their pregnancy period because men are not ready to accompany them to the clinic. It is a "must to go" with your husband on the first visit. Female participant 1

Yes, men not escorting their women is a main problem I can say. When a pregnant woman attends clinic for the first time, the health provider must asks where is your husband, and if you don't have your male partner the possibility of being seen in the clinic is very small and you may end up being scolded. To avoid being harassed, pregnant women may not attend the ANC clinic. Male CHW 1

In the rural settings, parents or in-laws make decisions for couples who live with them. Decisions related to health care seeking may depend upon the attitudes of parents/in-laws towards ANC services and their experiences with the health care system. Men who escort their wives are considered weak in this male dominant society. Participants indicated that parents/in-laws might hinder pregnant women from attending ANC clinics and it becomes a barrier when the couple depends on their parents/in-laws financially.

It is a habit based on parents' experiences. Men do think if my mother did not attend clinic at all or attended only once and gave birth without any problem why bother now. It is common with couples that stay with their parents. If your wife mentions about escorting her to the clinic, your father may say in our times, we did not go with women to their services, why do you want to do it now. This is being weak, your mother did not go and all went well. Then you think no need for my wife to attend clinic. Male CHW 5

Sometimes, a few men may prevent women from attending ANC arguing, do women who miss out ANC face any problems during delivery? But there are those who attended and still experienced complications. So you will stay at home, all will be well. With this response, some women decide not to attend at all. Female participant 6

For those families that stay with their in-laws, since the mother-in-law did not attend clinic, a pregnant woman will find it difficult to attend ANC clinic. Since her mother-in-law will discourage her saying, "We did not go to ANC clinic in those years why do you want to go there?" It becomes more difficult if a man depends on his parent financially. Female CHW 6

Challenges faced by women in visiting ANC clinics
This section highlights the challenges faced by pregnant women who attended an ANC clinic at least once. These challenges included poverty, perceived poor quality of ANC services, and lack of male involvement that hindered pregnant women's timely utilization of ANC services (Table 4).

Participants stated clearly that poverty delayed pregnant women from accessing ANC services in a timely manner. Due to the distance to health facilities and lack of transportation, many pregnant women decided to wait until their third trimester to initiate visits to an ANC clinic. Early ANC initiation meant spending a lot of money on transport, and many women had no source of ongoing income and lacked a bicycle or motorcycle for transport. Factor such as distance may act as both a barrier as well as a challenge to the utilization of ANC services. For some women distance to the ANC clinic could delay their attendance until the third trimester. As a result, they would only make a single visit during their pregnancy for a general check-up.

Due to distance and other issues, instead of visiting to the clinic every month a woman opts to attend only once to avoid the frequency of going to the clinic every month by attending in the last months of the pregnancy from seventh month. Female CHW 1

Sometimes you may feel weak and lazy to walk every month, remember we cannot afford paying for boda boda because we don't have money. Then you decide to wait till you approach the 8th or 9th month so that you have one visit to get an ANC card. Female participant 3

Long distance for some of the villages discourages most of the pregnant women to attend ANC clinics early. Some villages are far away from dispensaries, approximately more than 7 kilometers, making it difficult for pregnant women to walk that long distance. This is worse when the household does not have a bicycle or a motorcycle or money for fare. Even if they know the importance of ANC services, still they may not attend early. Male CHW 1

Women appeared to have some knowledge of the benefits of initiating early ANC services; however, perceived poor quality of ANC services in this community discouraged timely initiation of care. Pregnant women are supposed to receive comprehensive ANC when attending clinics, but in these communities, the absence of health care providers and shortages of supplies and drugs were identified as common challenges.

Most of the services such as antimalarial drugs, iron tablets, mosquito nets are not always available, and laboratory supplies are on and off because our clinics serve a large population, which is not proportional to the available supplies and drugs. Female CHW 1

When you go for ANC they send you back several times because health providers are not there or have gone for seminars. You may go to clinic several times with no luck of receiving any ANC services till you get tired and give up. You may miss the services for several visits because the health providers have gone for seminars or training. Female participant 5

This practice of sending back pregnant women without services has been common in our dispensary and it discourages pregnant women. For example, recently there were no ANC services for the entire week because of the shortage of health providers. There was only one health provider attending only out patients and other emergency care services. Male CHW 6

Lack of male involvement and participation during pregnancy was also a challenge for women who attended ANC clinics in the rural communities. Participants noted that the lack of men's involvement or interest was associated with cultural beliefs, the influence of in-laws, and the environment at the health facilities, which was not male friendly. HIV testing is crucial for both partners; however, and both partners need to agree to HIV testing after proper counselling and health education. In this community, HIV testing was associated with fear by the women as the laboratory test was done in the presence of the male partner. Furthermore, the existing health facilities provided no privacy for the couple during the counselling or the conduct of HIV testing.

Actually, most women in this community go late for antenatal services because of the fear of HIV testing while some men refuse to escort their women for fear of HIV testing. Female participant 4

It is really challenging in this community because of the high rates of HIV infection. The habit of HIV testing among men is not there. Escorting women to the clinic requires men to be ready for HIV testing and results. They think how I can go there when I am not ready to take an HIV test. It is better I just send my wife and I will know if I am safe or not through my wife's HIV result. They believe if a woman is HIV negative they are also negative so there is no need of going there. Male CHW 4

We do not have a friendly environment. For example, with our health facility there is no infrastructure for a reproductive and child health unit. Currently, all patients who come for TB and HIV drugs, out

patients, and pregnant women and under-five children are gathered in one place. There is no privacy and friendly environment for the couple. Male CHW 3

Some cultural beliefs in relation to pregnancy were perceived as causing delays in visiting ANC clinics. For example, in the first trimester, women do not disclose their "invisible" pregnancy to people including health providers for the fear of being witched. In addition, there were misconceptions about use of hematinics as many women thought that iron supplements prolonged the period of pregnancy, tended to exaggerate morning sickness symptoms, and sometimes even cause adverse outcomes. To avoid prolonged use of hematinics, they delay the initiation of ANC care.

We wait for a visible pregnancy for us to start clinic. You cannot start attending clinic with an invisible pregnancy; our fellow women may scold you when we go to fetch water. We do not mention to everyone that you are pregnant. We do this because we fear being witched since you cannot know who your enemy is. Female participant 6

You may visit the household with the aim of identifying a pregnant woman. Nobody in the family would dare to disclose that. To your surprise a few months late, you may meet the same woman with a newborn baby. Misconceptions on haematinics are also a challenge because pregnant women think when you use iron or folate you may experience abortion, fetus progress delay, and annoying side effects. Male CHW 5

Misconception regarding use of iron tablet/syrup exists among women thinking that when you use these drugs you delay the growth of the pregnancy while others complain about the side effects of the drugs such as nausea. So they prefer to visit clinic late to avoid continued use of these drugs. Female CHW 4

How women cope with existing ANC requirements

In these communities, some women circumvent ANC requirements during the first antenatal visit. Since attendance of male partners and HIV testing are mandatory during the first visit, participants reported visiting a clinic away from their ward, and carrying a letter from village leaders confirming that their husband was not present. In addition, some pregnant women paid for men who were willing to escort them and take the HIV test with them, a so-called "husband for hire" Table 4.

Husband for hire do exist in our villages. These are boda boda men. When a woman gets a boda boda to

Table 4 Identified themes and subthemes from FGDs

Key issues	Themes	Sub themes
Perceived barriers to utilization of ANC services	Poverty	• Health facility was far from home and pregnant women feeling tied to walking long distances
		• Women or family not having income to afford transport
		• Having no fare for hiring a bicycle or paying for a boda boda
		• Not having a maternity dress
	Fear of HIV testing	• Pregnant women's fear of HIV testing
		• Male partner fear of HIV testing results
		• Misconception regarding HIV testing
		• Self stigmization arising from HIV results
		• Infidelity among men/risk behaviors in fishing community and mining community
	Socio-cultural beliefs	• Men's refusal to escort women/men feel no need to be involved
		• Normal practices or habits because no history of pregnancy related complications
		• Parental influence especially among those couples who live with their parents
Challenges faced by women when utilizing the ANC services	Lack of male involvement	• Unfriendly male environment
		• Men not willing to escort women
		• Attended ANC clinic but not provided services as male partner did not attend
	Perceived poor quality of care	• Services not available because supplies and/or drugs are out of stock
		• No services available most of the times
		• Long waiting times for services
		• Frequent shortages of health providers
	Informal regulation	• HIV testing is no longer voluntarily
		• Male partner must be there during the first ANC visit
		• Not receiving HIV testing since a man is not with you
Coping strategies for existing ANC requirements	Men for hire	• Husband for hire do exist in our villages
		• Men will not accept escorting their wives
		• Boda boda men are willing to accompany women if they are provided with a little money for escorting you
	Letter from village leaders	• To avoid being scolded and to obtain services you get a letter from village leader to present to the CHWs
		• If your partner refuses to escort you state that he is away
	Health facility	• Attend a health facility that is far away from your home
		• Where health providers do not know you or your husband

take her to the health facility, she also requests if the man is willing to escort her for HIV testing just to pretend being a husband. *Female CHW 6*

Since men will not accept escorting their wives to the antenatal clinic for fear of HIV testing, women decide to go to the village leaders for the letter explaining that the husband for this woman is not present in the village and may be working outside the district. They get a letter because health

providers insist if you come without your husband you will not get any service. *Female CHW 5*

Your husband must be there when you go to the clinic for the first visit. This is a big challenge for women. Therefore, for those who cannot get their husband to escort them [they] may go to a clinic far from this ward because nobody knows their husband there. The boda boda driver usually can pretend to be your husband and you pay him something small. *Female participant 1*

Discussion

Antenatal care is one of the pillars in the Safe Motherhood Initiative for promoting and improving maternal and child health through interventions such as health promotion, treatment of existing diseases, early detection and management of pregnancy-related complications, and disease prevention [3]. Initiating ANC in the first trimester provides opportunities for timely optimal care and treatment of existing conditions [3, 5, 13]. Our findings revealed that the timely attendance at the ANC clinic in the first trimester of pregnancy was low with more than three quarters of participants first attending either in the second or third trimester. This is a significant missed opportunity for improving maternal and child health in Geita district, Northwest Tanzania. The extremely low attendance (3.62%) of women in Geita district, Northwest Tanzania in the first trimester is not consistent with the levels of attendance in Tanzania (24%) and globally (58.6%) [7, 15]. It is important to note that in contrast to previous retrospective studies, this household survey involved pregnant women in their third trimester. Hence, social desirability and recall biases that could have influenced the estimates reported in earlier studies [7, 15] were less likely to bias our results.

We also observed that a considerable proportion of women failed to utilize ANC services fully during their pregnancy due to several reasons including lack of male involvement or lack of men's interest in ANC, perceived poor quality of care, poverty and socio-cultural beliefs. Other studies have documented similar issues that may hinder utilization of ANC [22, 25, 26, 28]. For example, to achieve reduction and elimination of HIV infection through mother to child transmission, male involvement has been observed to increase women's adherence to interventions [29]. In low incomes countries, especially in the rural settings, a shortage of skilled health personnel, lack of drugs and supplies, and long waiting times are common challenges encountered in the health facilities [16, 30–33]. Women in the study area reported similar concerns. Further, ANC requirements such as the male partner being present during the first visit for HIV testing, which is emphasized as one strategy for the prevention of maternal to child transmission (PMTCT) of HIV infection, may lead to unintended consequences as documented in this paper. Although the strategy is intended to promote male involvement for positive pregnancy outcomes, it was reported to impede women from initiating ANC in a timely manner or in some cases women may not initiate ANC. Thus, there is a need to revisit such ANC requirements as they may result in unintended harms to maternal and child health.

While ANC improves and promotes maternal and child health, its effectiveness depends in part on the availability and quality of services provided regardless of the antenatal model implemented in the country [3–5, 19, 34, 35]. However, women in the study setting did not receive all the components of ANC services as per national guidelines. Notably, HIV screening was almost universal but far fewer women were screened for syphilis and anaemia, despite evidence for high rates of syphilis sero-prevalence and anaemia. Low coverage for laboratory services has been mentioned in other studies as a public health challenge in most developing countries [16, 30, 31, 36]. In rural settings, laboratory services for measuring Hb level, syphilis, and HIV infections may not be available in public health facilities due to lack of supplies and limited expertise among health care workers to conduct the tests. Further, in private health facilities, these tests may not be free of charge and many women, particularly in rural districts, may not have the funds to pay for these tests. Strengthening laboratory services in primary care facilities is paramount for quality ANC services and prevention of adverse outcomes such as congenital syphilis, stillbirths, prematurity, low birth weight, and perinatal deaths. Concurrently, early initiation of ANC should be emphasized so that women and their unborn babies will reap the full benefits of ANC.

Normative behaviour and traditional beliefs surrounding pregnancy, labour and delivery must also be addressed, as they appear to shape health-seeking behavior and could negatively affect the well-being of pregnant women and their unborn babies. Importantly, the beliefs that the experience of the mother-in-law applies to her son's wife and that the risk of adverse pregnancy outcomes may not be mitigated by ANC need to be addressed urgently through appropriate channels. In addition, health system factors such as shortages in service providers and important components of ANC (i.e., laboratory tests, vaccines, drugs, supplements), and the demands attached to the prevention of mother to child transmission services such as mandatory partner attendance at ANC initiation, need to be revisited and addressed. ANC clinics are considered "women spaces", and the existing infrastructure does not provide any privacy for couples. Women also live in a cultural atmosphere with norms and gender roles that shape and influence their health care decision-making. In the African context, women and young married couples may lack autonomy on health-related issues. The male dominant social structure gives men autonomy over their female partners on different aspects of life including health care issues. Thus, parents, in-laws, or men in the community influencing or making decisions for young couples or women is common in developing countries like Tanzania. Previous research has documented the existence of male dominated social structures and male partners playing significant decision making roles in developing countries [37, 38].

The integration of the quantitative and qualitative data assisted us in understanding the challenges and barriers that these women experience in attaining timely ANC by shedding light on community and health system related factors that need to be addressed. There is a need to understand how social structures, culture and beliefs could enhance or hinder utilization of health services. The imposed informal regulation on male partner involvement in the initial ANC visit that has been implemented to reduce the prevention of maternal to child transmission (PMTCT) of HIV needs to be re-examined using a participatory approach that emphasizes community involvement and engagement. As observed in this study, "husband for hire" and village leaders' written memos used to navigate the ANC requirements imposed on pregnant women, may fail to achieve their intended purpose. If women are checked for HIV infection with their fake male partners, the goal of promoting safer sex, adherence to PMTCT interventions, and HIV status disclosure between partners will not be realized. Hence, this study highlights the *missed opportunities* associated with early initiation of ANC for promoting health seeking behavior and preventing health conditions that directly or indirectly affect maternal and child health in rural settings in Tanzania.

Study strengths and limitations

The study design accounted for possible biases inherent in previous retrospective studies. In addition, the study was strengthened by triangulation in data collection and the fact that almost all FGD interviews were conducted outside the health facility environment. Finally, a significant strength of this study is that it explored the perspectives of *women who used* ANC services, *women who did not use ANC* services and *health care providers* regarding the challenges and barriers to ANC services in this area of Tanzania. A potential limitation of this study was the use of information/data from the antenatal cards. This could have led to biased estimates of the prevalence of existing conditions such as anemia, syphilis, and HIV. These parameters depend on the quality and completeness of the records of the pregnant women who attended ANC clinics at least once.

Conclusion and recommendations

The study highlights the low attendance of pregnant women at ANC clinics in the first trimester in Geita district, Northwest Tanzania and the limited antenatal services provided to women who utilized ANC services at least once. The goal of improving and promoting maternal and child health through ANC remains elusive in this rural setting. Importantly, not all components of ANC are available to pregnant women even when they initiate ANC early. The critical shortage of human

resources, particularly when an ANC provider is invited to attend training away from the health facility further limits women's access to timely ANC services. Based on the findings, in-job training of health providers should be well planned to avoid inconvenience and delays in the provision of care. Improving human resources and timely availability of all essential components of ANC, and a friendly environment for male partners will ensure acceptability and quality services in this and similar rural settings. Further, supportive supervision to health workers during the provision of ANC services and training that specifically focuses on providing services to pregnant women and their partners in an open and sensitive manner needs to be implemented to improve the uptake of ANC services in rural communities. HIV screening for prevention of PMTCT should be conducted voluntarily after provision of health education and counselling and health workers need to ensure that they observe all ethics around ANC services. Finally, community male champions need to be identified. These individuals would take a leading role in exploring and promoting male involvement in maternal and child health services in local communities through family visits, community meetings, and cultural and religious gatherings. Such initiatives are essential for improving the health and outcomes of mothers and newborns.

Abbreviations
ANC: Antenatal care; CHW: Community health worker; FANC: Focused antenatal care; FGD: Focused group discussion; HIV: Human immunodeficiency virus; MMR: Maternal Mortality Ratio; PMTCT: Prevention of mother to child transmission; RCH: Reproductive and Child Health; TDHS: Tanzania Demographic and Health Survey; WHO: World Health Organisation

Acknowledgements
We would like to extend our warm gratitude to the District Medical Officer (DMO-Geita district), the District Reproductive and Child Health coordinator (DRCHco-Geita district), ward leaders, village leaders, community health workers, health providers, and traditional birth attendants who assisted us with this study. Furthermore, we would like to thank all of the women who generously donated their time to participate in this research study. Lastly, thanks to the University of Calgary and the Catholic University of Health and Allied Sciences for their financial support.

Funding
This study received some funding through a grant provided to DD by the Department of Paediatrics, University of Calgary, and a grant provided to EK from the Catholic University of Health and Allied Sciences – CUHAS Bugando, Mwanza, Tanzania (Ph.D. Research Funds). Funding institutions played no role in the study design, data collection, analysis, interpretation of the results, and in writing of the manuscript.

Authors' contributions
ETK conceptualized the idea and MTNM, JH, SK, RS, DMD participated in the design of the study. EK supervised the household survey, DMD supervised focused group discussions, ETK carried out data analysis, wrote the

manuscript, and MTNM, JH, SK, RS, and DMD reviewed the manuscript. All authors read and approved the final manuscript.

Competing interests
MM declares that he is an associate editor of the BMC Pregnancy and Childbirth in Low and Middle-Income Countries' series. All other co-authors declare that they have no competing interests.

Author details
[1]Department of Biostatistics & Epidemiology, School of Public Health, Catholic University of Health and Allied Sciences, P.O. box 1464 Bugando Area, Mwanza, Tanzania. [2]Department of Community Health Sciences, Cumming School of Medicine, University of Calgary, 3280 Hospital Drive, NW, Calgary, AB, Canada. [3]Options Tanzania Ltd 76 Ali Hassan, Mwinyi Road, P.O. Box 65350, Dar es Salaam, Tanzania. [4]Department of Paediatrics, University of Calgary, 2888 Shaganappi Tr. NW, Calgary, AB, Canada. [5]Owerko Centre at the Alberta Children's Hospital Research Institute, Cumming School of Medicine, University of Calgary, 2500 University Dr. NW, Calgary, AB, Canada.

References
1. Tunçalp Ö, Pena-Rosas JP, Lawrie T, Bucagu M, Oladapo OT, Portela A, Gülmezoglu AM. WHO recommendations on antenatal care for a positive pregnancy experience - going beyond survival. BJOG. 2017;124:860–2. https://doi.org/10.1111/1471-0528.14599.

2. United Nations Economic Commission for Africa, African Union, African Development Bank, United Nations Development Programme: MDG Report 2015: Assessing progress in Africa toward the millennium development goals. Addis Ababa: The ECA Printing and Publishing Unit; 2015.

3. WHO, editor. Mother baby package: implementing safe motherhood in countries (practical guide), vol. 360. Geneva: WHO. p. 1994.

4. Tunçalp Ö, Were W, MacLennan C, Oladapo OT, Gülmezoglu AM, Bahl R, Daelmans B, Mathai M, Say L, Temmerman M, et al. Quality of care for pregnant women and newborns - the WHO vision. BJOG. 2015;122:1045–9. https://doi.org/10.1111/1471-0528.13451.

5. Bhutta Z, Das J, Bahl R, Lawn J, Salam R, Paul V, Sankar M, Blencowe H, Rizvi A, Chou V, et al. Can available interventions end preventable deaths in mothers, newborn babies, and stillbirths, and at what cost? Lancet. 2014; 384(9940):347–70. https://doi.org/10.1016/S0140-6736(1014)60792–60793.

6. WHO, UNICEF, UNFPA, World Bank Group, The United Nations Population Division. Trends in Maternal Mortality: 1990 to 2015. Geneva: World Health Organization; 2015.

7. Ministry of Health, Community Development, Gender, Elderly and Children (MoHCDGEC) [Tanzania Mainland], Ministry of Health (MoH) [Zanzibar], National Bureau of Statistics (NBS): Tanzania Demographic and Health Survey and Malaria Indicator Survey 2015–16. In. Edited by OCGS, ICF. Dar es Salaam, Tanzania and Rockville, Maryland, USA; 2016.

8. Blencowe H, Cousens S, Jassir F, Say L, Chou D, Mathers C, Hogan D, Shiekh S, Qureshi Z, You D, et al. National, regional, and worldwide estimates of stillbirth rates in 2015, with trends from 2000: a systematic analysis. Lancet Glob Health. 2016;4:e98–108. https://doi.org/10.1016/s2214-1109x(1015)00275–00272.

9. McClure EM, Goldenberg RL. Stillbirth in Developing Countries: A review of causes, risk factors and prevention strategies. J Matern Fetal Neonatal Med. 2009;22(3):183–90. https://doi.org/10.1080/14767050802559129.

10. WHO: Health in 2015: From MDGs, Millennium Development Goals to SDGs, Sustainable Development Goals. 2015. http://www.who.int/iris/handle/10665/200009. (Accessed 9 May 2017).

11. Say L, Chou D, Gemmill A, Tunçalp Ö, Moller A, Daniels J, Gülmezoglu AM, Temmerman M, Alkema L. Global causes of maternal death: a WHO systematic analysis. Lancet Glob Health. 2014;2:e323–33. https://doi.org/10.1016/s2214-1109x(1014)70227-x.

12. WHO. Antenatal Care Randomized Trial. Manual for the implementation of the new model. Geneva: Department of Reproductive Health and Research, Family and Community Medicine, World Health Organization; 2002.

13. Maternal Health Task Force. Focuses antenatal Care in Tanzania: delivering individualized, targeted, high-quality care. Harvard: HARVARD, School of Public Health, Department of Global Health and Population; 2002.

14. Yaya S, Bishwajit G, Ekholuenetale M, Shah V, Kadio B, Udenigwe O. Timing and adequate attendance of antenatal care visits among women in Ethiopia. PLoS One. 2017;12(9):e0184934.

15. Ann-Beth M, Petzold M, Chou D, Say L. Early antenatal care visit: a systematic analysis of regional and global levels and trends of coverage from 1990 t0 2013. Lancet Glob Health. 2017;5:e977–83.

16. Kanyangarara M, Munoa M, Walker N. Quality of antenatal care services provision in health facilities across sub-Saharan Africa: Evidence from nationally representative health facility assessments. J Glob Health. 2017;7(2). https://doi.org/10.7189/jogh.7107.021101.

17. Conrad P, Schmid G, Tientrebeogo J, Moses A, Kirenga S, Neuhann F, Muller O, Sarker M. Compliance with focused antenatal care services: Do health workers in rural Burkina Faso, Uganda and Tanzania perform all ANC procedures? Trop Med Int Health. 2012;17(3):300–7. https://doi.org/10.1111/j.1365.3156.2011.02923.x.

18. Hawkes SJ, Gomez GB, Broutet N. Early antenatal care: does it make a difference to outcomes of pregnancy associated with syphilis? A systematic review and meta-analysis. PLoS One. 2013;8(2). https://doi.org/10.1371/journal.pone.0056713.

19. Arunda M, Emmelin A, Asamoah BO. Effectiveness of antenatal care services in reducing neonatal mortality in Kenya: Analysis of national survey data. Glob Health Action. 2017;10. https://doi.org/10.1080/16549716.16542017.11328796.

20. Gross K, Alba S, Glass TR, Schellenberg JA, Obrist B. Timing of antenatal care for adolescent and adult pregnant women in South-Eastern Tanzania. BMC Pregnancy Childbirth. 2012;12(16). https://doi.org/10.1186/1471-2393-1112-1116.

21. Exavery A, Kant'e AM, Hingora A, Mabaruku G, Pemba S, Phillips JF. How mistimed and unwanted pregnancies affect timing of antenatal care initiation in three districts in Tanzania. BMC Pregnancy Childbirth. 2013; 13(35). https://doi.org/10.1186/1471-2393-13-35 .

22. Gupta S, Yamada G, Mpembeni R, Frumence G, Callaghan-Koru JA, Stevenson R, Brandes N, Baqui AH. Factors associated with four and more antenatal care visits and its decline among pregnant women in Tanzania between 1999 and 2010. PLoS One. 2014;9(7):e101893. https://doi.org/10.1371/journal.pone.0101893.

23. Magadi MA, Madise NJ, Rodrigues RN. Frequency and timing of antenatal care in Kenya: explaining the variations between women of different communities. Soc Sci Med. 2000;51:551–61.

24. Ndidi EP, Oseremen IG. Reasons given by pregnant women for late initiation of antenatal care in the Niger Delta, Nigeria. Ghana Med J. 2010;44(2).

25. Simkhada B, van Teijlingen ER, Porter M, Simkhada P. Factors affecting the utilization of antenatal care in developing countries: systematic review of the literature. J Adv Nurs. 2008;61(3):244–60. https://doi.org/10.1111/j.1365-2648.2007.04532.x.

26. Finlayson K, Downe S. Why do women not use antenatal services in low and middle income countries? A meta-synthesis of qualitative studies. PLoS Med. 2013;10(1):e1001373p.

27. StataCorp. Stata Statistical Software: Release 13. College Station: StataCorp LP; 2013.

28. Hagen JP, Rulisa S, Pe'rez-Escamilla R. Barriers and solutions for timely initiation of antenatal care in Kigali Rwanda: Health facility professionals' perspective. Midwifery. 2013;30:96–102. https://doi.org/10.1016/j.midw.2013.1001.1016.

29. Aluisio A, Richardson BA, Bosire R, John-Stewart G, Mbori-Ngacha D, Farquhar C. Male antenatal attendance and HIV testing are associated with decreased infant HIV infection and increased HIV-free survival. J Acquir Immune Defic Syndr. 2011;56(1):76–82. https://doi.org/10.1097/QAI.1090b1013e3181fdb1094c1094.

30. Gross K, Schellenberg JA, Kessy F, Pfeiffer C, Obrist B. Antenatal care in practice: An exploratory study in antenatal care clinics in the Kilombero Valley, South-Eastern Tanzania. BMC Pregnancy Childbirth. 2011, 36;11. https://doi.org/10.1186/1471-2393-11-36.

31. Nyamtema AS, Jong AB, Urassa DP, Hagen JP, Roosmalen J. The quality of antenatal care in rural Tanzania: What is behind the number of visits? BMC Pregnancy Childbirth. 2012;12(70). https://doi.org/10.1186/1471-2393-12-70.

32. Mahiti GR, Mkoka DA, Kiwara AD, Mbekenga CK, Hurtig A, Goicolea I. Women's perceptions of antenatal, delivery, and postpartum services in rural Tanzania. Glob Health Action. 2015;8. https://doi.org/10.3402/gha.v3408.28567.

33. Mrisho M, Obrist B, Schellenberg JA, Haws RA, Mushi AK, Mshinda H, Tanner M, Schellenberg D. The use of antenatal and postnatal care: perspectives and experiences of women and health care providers in rural southern

Tanzania. BMC Pregnancy Childbirth. 2009;9(10). https://doi.org/10.1186/1471-2393-1189-1110.

34. McDonagh M: Is antenatal care effective in reducing maternal morbidity and mortality? Health Policy Plan 1996, 11(1):1–15.

35. Bergsjø P. What is the evidence for the role of antenatal care strategies in the reduction of maternal mortality and morbidity? Stud HSO   P. 2001:35–54.

36. Baker U, Okuga M, Waiswa P, Manzi F, Peterson S, Hanson C, Group TEs. Bottlenecks in the implementation of essential screening tests in antenatal care: Syphilis, HIV, and anemia testing in rural Tanzania and Uganda. Int J Gynecol Obstet. 2015;130:S43–50. https://doi.org/10.1016/j.ijgo.2015.1004.1017.

37. Paruzzolo S, Mehra R, Kes A, Ashbaugh C. Targeting poverty and gender inequality to improve maternal health. Washington DC: International Center for Research on Women; 2010.

38. Adjiwanou V, LeGrand T. Gender inequality and the use of maternal healthcare services in rural sub-Saharan Africa. Health Place. 2014;29:67–78. https://doi.org/10.1016/j.healthplace.2014.1006.1001.

10

Associations between social support, mental wellbeing, self-efficacy and technology use in first-time antenatal women: data from the BaBBLeS cohort study

Samuel Ginja[1], Jane Coad[2], Elizabeth Bailey[2], Sally Kendall[3], Trudy Goodenough[4], Samantha Nightingale[2], Jane Smiddy[5], Crispin Day[6], Toity Deave[4†] and Raghu Lingam[7*†]

Abstract

Background: Information and communication technologies are used increasingly to facilitate social networks and support women during the perinatal period. This paper presents data on how technology use affects the association between women's social support and, (i) mental wellbeing and, (ii) self-efficacy in the antenatal period.

Methods: Data were collected as part of an ongoing study - the BaBBLeS study - exploring the effect of a pregnancy and maternity software application (app) on maternal wellbeing and self-efficacy. Between September 2016 and February 2017, we aimed to recruit first-time pregnant women at 12–16 gestation weeks in five maternity sites across England and asked them to complete questionnaires. Outcomes included maternal mental wellbeing (Warwick-Edinburgh Mental Wellbeing Scale), and antenatal self-efficacy (antenatal version of the Tool to Measure Parenting Self-Efficacy). Other variables assessed were perceived social support (Multidimensional Scale of Perceived Social Support), general technology use (adapted from Media and Technology Usage and Attitudes Scale). Potential confounders were age, ethnicity, education, socioeconomic deprivation, employment, relationship status and recruitment site. Linear regression models were developed to analyse the relationship between social support and the outcomes.

Results: Participants ($n = 492$, median age = 28 years) were predominantly white British (64.6%). Half of them had a degree or higher degree (49.3%), most were married/living with a partner (83.6%) and employed (86.2%). Median (LQ-UQ) overall scores were 81.0 (74.0–84.0) for social support (range 12–84), 5.1 (4.7–5.4) for technology use (range 1–6), 54.0 (48.0–60.0) for mental well-being (range 14–70), and 319.0 (295.5–340) for self-efficacy (range 0–360). Social support was significantly associated with antenatal mental well-being adjusting for confounders [adj $R^2 = 0.13$, $p < .001$]. The addition of technology use did not alter this model [adj $R^2 = 0.13$, $p < .001$]. Social support was also significantly associated with self-efficacy after adjustment [adj $R^2 = 0.14$, $p < .001$]; technology had limited impact on this association [adj $R^2 = 0.13$, $p < .001$].

(Continued on next page)

* Correspondence: R.lingam@unsw.edu.au
†Toity Deave and Raghu Lingam contributed equally to this work.
Toity Deave and Raghu Lingam are both senior authors.
[7]Population Child Health Research Group, Women's and Children's Health, University of New South Wales, Sydney, Australia
Full list of author information is available at the end of the article

(Continued from previous page)

Conclusions: Social support is associated with mental well-being and self-efficacy in antenatal first-time mothers. This association was not significantly affected by general technology use as measured in our survey. Future work should investigate whether pregnancy-specific technologies yield greater potential to enhance the perceived social support, wellbeing and self-efficacy of antenatal women.

Keywords: Antenatal, Pregnancy, Wellbeing, Self-efficacy, Social support, Technology use

Background

Maternal mental health disorders during the antenatal and postnatal periods, most commonly depression and anxiety, are a significant public health problem. In the UK, around 12% of pregnant women experience depression and 13% experience anxiety, with many experiencing both. Rates of depression and anxiety increase to 15 to 20% of women in the first year after childbirth [1]. Worryingly, as many as half of all cases of perinatal depression and anxiety go undetected [2]. Evidence suggests that maternal depression continues to emerge many months after the point where routine depression screening currently occurs [3]. Maternal perinatal mental health disorders are associated with an increased risk of cognitive, emotional and behavioural difficulties in the child, which in turn can lead to adverse long-term life chances [4, 5]. It is estimated that perinatal mental health disorders cost the UK economy £8.1 billion per annum, 72% of these costs being related to adverse impacts on the child [6].

One major factor affecting perinatal mental health is social support. Although definitions of social support vary widely, this concept is often used to refer to the emotional and instrumental assistance received from various sources, with a focus on how the support is perceived by the recipient [7, 8]. A large body of research has demonstrated the link between maternal mental health and social networks, where the most supported mothers experience the best mental health outcomes [9–11]. For example, mothers are five times more likely to experience postpartum depression if they received no support or minimal support after the birth of the baby than women who received appropriate support [12]. Better levels of social support are thought to improve the mother's ability to cope with stressful life events and to interact with her child in more positive and stimulating ways. Possible reasons for this include easier access to information on developmentally appropriate methods of parenting and the fact that other people can act as buffers against maladaptive parenting and stressful life situations [13]. Despite the increased demands of motherhood, there is some evidence for a decline in social support perceived by new mothers, from pregnancy to postpartum [14]. Stronger social networks during pregnancy can protect against postpartum depression [15], which highlights the role of prevention programmes from an early stage.

With the increasing use of the internet and social media, transformation of the traditional family and austerity cuts to health and social care services [16], there is increasing interest in delivering information and supplement support to pregnant women through information and communication technologies. It has been suggested that the support that perinatal women receive through online technologies can be grouped as emotional support and instrumental support (both formal and informal), as well as community building and protection [17]. The internet is a major source of ante- and postnatal information with as many as three quarters of pregnant women using the internet for medical advice globally [18]. Use of technology has been identified as a way of increasing new mothers' confidence in mothering by enabling access to information and reassurance about their choices or concerns [19]. It has been reported that online support groups provide women experiencing postpartum depression with a safe place to connect with others and receive 'information, encouragement and hope' [20]. Blogging is thought to enhance the connection with extended family and friends, increasing social networks, which in turn has a positive impact on maternal well-being [21]. Another key technology are mobile apps, which should be linked to trustworthy websites, containing short answers to everyday concerns and information on local support services for pregnant and post-birth women [22]. Despite the potential benefits of existing technologies, there is still a lack of quantitative research that assesses the relationship between technology use and social support amongst women in the perinatal period.

The current paper assessed the association between social support and i) mental wellbeing and ii) self-efficacy in a large sample of UK, first-time antenatal women, and how general technology use affected these associations.

Methods

We used baseline data collected as part of the BaBBLeS study (Bumps and Babies Longitudinal Study), which aimed to assess the impact of a specific mobile software application (app) - Baby Buddy app [23] – on maternal self-efficacy and mental wellbeing at three-month post-partum [24]. In short, this cohort study was conducted in England (UK) to compare both of the above outcomes between first-time prospective mothers who used the Baby Buddy app and women who did not use it, ante- and postnatally, adjusting for key confounders [25]. The current article does not specifically look at the use of the Baby Buddy app but rather investigates the impact of general technology use on the association between social support, maternal mental wellbeing and self-efficacy.

First-time pregnant women aged 16 years or older were recruited in five maternity sites across England between September 2016 and February 2017. To ensure national geographical spread, maternity units were located in different areas of the country: West Midlands (site 1), London (site 2), Lancashire (site 3), East Midlands (site 4) and West Yorkshire (site 5). We aimed to recruit women and collect baseline data during the period of 12–16 weeks gestation.

The maternity services identified eligible women who were then invited to take part in the study in one of two ways. Women were either approached by research midwives when they attended a maternity appointment and were given a recruitment pack, or they were sent a recruitment pack through the post by their local maternity services. The recruitment pack contained information about the study, a consent form, contact sheet, a baseline questionnaire and reply envelope. Women were asked to complete the baseline questionnaire, consent form and contact sheet, and return them in the pre-paid envelope provided. Optionally, the survey (including consent form and contact details) could be completed online. The study questionnaire had been pilot tested and adapted for ease of use and meaning with nine mothers before administration.

The recruitment period lasted 5 months; if a questionnaire was not returned by 2 weeks after the initial questionnaire was sent, women were sent a reminder pack.

Questionnaire data were entered on an online survey platform [26], either directly by participants, or by the research team in the case of participants who had returned paper questionnaires. A 10% subsample of paper questionnaires was randomly chosen and double-data entered to ensure accuracy of data entry. The error rate was less than 2% which was deemed acceptable. This process was carried out in consultation with the local clinical trials unit.

Ethics

Study ethical approval was gained from NHS Research Ethics Committee (NRES) West Midlands-South Birmingham REC (16/WM/0029) and from the University of the West of England, Bristol Research Ethics Committee (HAS.16.08.001). Research & Development (R&D) departments within each of the study sites confirmed their capability and capacity to conduct the research.

Measures

The baseline questionnaire is presented in Additional file 1. Questions asked about perceived social support (exposure variable), maternal mental wellbeing and self-efficacy (outcome variables) and sociodemographic data and general technology use (potential confounders). Sociodemographic questions were asked to collect information on age, ethnicity, postcode (from which a socioeconomic deprivation score was derived), relationship status and employment. Recruitment site was determined based on the unique code that identified each questionnaire pack. Participants had the opportunity to write down any comments as free text.

Exposure variable

The primary exposure variable assessed in this study was perceived social support, measured using the Multidimensional Scale of Perceived Social Support (MSPSS) [27]. This scale consists of 12 statements about the support received from family (4 items), friends (4 items) and a significant other (4 items), e.g., 'My family really tries to help me' or, 'There is a special person in my life who cares about my feelings'. Participants rated their level of agreement with each statement on a seven-item Likert scale, from 1 (very strongly disagree) to 7 (very strongly agree) (range 1–7). Item scores were summed to provide total scores, both overall (range 12–84) and for each of the three subscales (range 4–28). Higher scores indicated perception of greater social support. The factorial validity and internal reliability of the MSPSS have been demonstrated in a number of studies, with alpha scores from 0.87 to 0.93 [27–29], including amongst pregnant women (alpha 0.92) [30].

Outcome variables

The two outcome variables in this study were maternal mental wellbeing and self-efficacy. Maternal mental well-being was assessed by the Warwick-Edinburgh Mental Well-Being Scale (WEMWBS) [31]. This scale comprises of 14 statements describing feelings (e.g., 'I have been feeling useful') and functional aspects (e.g., 'I've been dealing with problems well') over the previous 2 weeks. Items were scored from 1 (none of the time) to 5 (all of the time) and summed to provide an overall score between 14 and 70, where higher scores corresponded to higher levels of wellbeing. This scale has shown good content and criterion-related validity, as well as high test-retest reliability (0.83), in various groups and public health contexts, including parenting programmes [32].

Maternal self-efficacy was measured with a 36-item scale adapted for use in the antenatal period from the tool to measure Parenting Self-Efficacy (TOPSE) [33] to assess parents' beliefs about their ability to manage their child. This antenatal adaptation was carried out in consultation with the tool developer (SK, one of the co-authors of this paper). All TOPSE statements were reworded to the future tense, e.g., 'I am able to have fun with my baby' ➜ 'I will be able to have fun with my baby'. The scale is divided into six sections, each section containing six items and addressing a different domain of parenting, such as 'emotion and affection', or 'play and enjoyment'. Participants were requested to select how much they agreed with each item, from 0 (completely disagree) to 10 (completely agree) on a Likert scale. Five items were reverse-scored (items 6, 19, 20, 21 and 27). A total sum score was calculated from the 36 items, ranging from 0 to 360, where larger scores indicated greater self-efficacy. The postnatal scale has shown very high internal consistency (alpha 0.96) as well as good content and convergent validity [33, 34].

Potential confounders

Potential confounding variables taken into account in our analysis were women's age, ethnic group, socioeconomic deprivation, highest level of formal education, relationship status and employment. Many of these sociodemographic variables have been previously reported to be linked to social support; for example, experiencing lower levels of social support have been associated with giving birth at an earlier age [12, 35], being from an ethnic minority [36], lower educational attainment [37], lower socioeconomic status [38] and not having or not living with a partner [39]. Index of multiple deprivation (IMD) decile, a common indicator of socioeconomic deprivation in the UK, was obtained by searching participants' postcodes using a standard online tool [40]. The geographical site where participants were recruited was also included as a potential confounder. Questions and responses relating to sociodemographic information were identical to those from previous Census surveys [41].

We explored the impact of technology use on the association between social support and maternal wellbeing and self-efficacy. Technology use was assessed using the Media and Technology Usage and Attitudes Scale (MTUAS) which has shown high internal consistency, from 0.61 to 0.96 across all 15 subscales [42]. After discussion with the author, to avoid respondent fatigue, nine items were selected from the original scale, which described general aspects of technology use. Items assessed the frequency of text messaging, phone calls, smartphone use, internet searching and social media use. Smartphone use includes browsing the web and using apps of any type on a smartphone or tablet. Internet searching includes searching the web for news and information. General social media use includes checking page, posting photos or commenting on Facebook or other social networks. To make the scale simpler, the number of Likert scale points was reduced from 10 to 6; feedback from pilot respondents had suggested the appropriateness of these changes.

Participants indicated the frequency of each of these behaviours, e.g., 'Check your Facebook page or other social networks', from 1 (Never/Not applicable) to 6 (Several times a day). Average scores were calculated and ranged from 1 to 6, where 6 corresponded to the highest frequency of technology use.

The MTUAS scale was compared between pregnancy app users and non-pregnancy app users as a test of content validity. The premise underlying this content validity test was that pregnancy app users would show higher frequency of technology use than non-pregnancy app users; this analysis is presented here to increase understanding of the tools used. As hypothesised, participants who reported using pregnancy apps had significantly higher general technology use (mean = 5.12, SD = .03) compared to participants who reported not using pregnancy apps (mean = 4.94, SD = .07), t (487) = − 2.84, p = 0.005, supporting the content validity of the shorter MTUAS scale used.

Data analysis

All analysis was completed in Stata 14 [43]. Descriptive statistics were performed to characterise the sample, including median, lower quartile (LQ) and upper quartile (UQ). Categories were re-grouped to remove low number cells and improve the stability of the model for the analysis: ethnicity was divided into two groups 1) White British and 2) Other (other white European, Asian or Asian British, Black or Black British or a Mixed background); education level was split into 1) women with a degree or higher and 2) women without a degree; relationship status was divided into 1) being married or living with partner vs 2) being single, having a partner but not living together or other status; employment comprised of 1) being in paid employment (full-time, part-time, self-employment, or on leave from employment) and 2) not being in paid employment (studying, training, not employed). In the UK, the word 'degree' usually refers to an undergraduate academic degree but it is possible that it covers other qualifications in other countries. The variable for the evaluation site was retained without alterations as there was a reasonable number of participants recruited in all of the five sites. Age and IMD decile were used as continuous variables for analysis.

Linear regression models were developed to test the independent associations between each of the potential confounders and social support. The alpha level was set at 0.05. For this analysis we reported the F statistic and p value for each of the models overall. In addition, linear regression models were developed in three steps to assess: 1) the unadjusted association between social support and mental well-being, 2) this association adjusting for the potential confounders and, 3) the effect of technology use on the adjusted model. This three-step process was followed for both outcome variables, maternal well-being and self-efficacy. For this analysis, we reported the adjusted R-squared and significance level (alpha = 0.05) for all the models, as well as the regression coefficients and 95% confidence intervals independently for social support (models 1, 2 and 3) and for technology use (model 3).

There were only a small amount of missing data, therefore no imputation procedures were undertaken. Overall scores consisting of sums excluded participants with one or more items missing.

Results

A total of 492 participants returned a completed baseline questionnaire across all five maternity sites. Baseline characteristics of the study participants are presented in Table 1. On average (median), participants were 28 years old (LQ 24 – UQ 32; overall range 16 to 46), 13 weeks pregnant upon recruitment (LQ 12.4 – UQ 14.4; overall range 7 to 24) and were on the 4th IMD decile (LQ 2-UQ 6; overall range 1 (highest deprivation) to 10 (lowest

deprivation)). Approximately half of them had a degree or higher degree (49.3%); of the other half, 18.9% had professional qualifications. The vast majority were married or living with a partner (83.6%) and were in paid employment (86.2%). Most women identified themselves as white British (64.6%); the remaining were other white European (16.3%), Asian or Asian British (13.8%), black or black British (4.0%), mixed (0.6%) or other (0.6%).

Data on the exposure variable (perceived social support), outcome variables and technology use, are presented in Table 2. Analysis excluded participants with all of the MTUAS items missing ($n = 1$; 0.2%) or with one or more items missing on the WEMWBS ($n = 17$; 3.5%), antenatal TOPSE ($n = 44$; 8.9%) or MSPSS ($n = 8$; 1.6%). For all the scales used in this study, higher scores meant a higher level of the measured variable and no threshold has been established for 'high scores' and 'low scores'.

The median overall social support (MSPSS) score was 81.0 (IQR 10.0), with little variation between subscales.

Table 1 Sample characteristics ($N = 492$)

	n missing (%)	n (%)	Median (LQ - UQ)	Min	Max
Age (years)	19 (3.9%)		28 (24–32)	16	46
Gestation (weeks)	10 (2.0%)		13 (12.4–14.4)	7.7	24.9
IMD decile	15 (3.0%)		4 (2–6)	1	10
Geographical area	0 (0.0%)				
Site 1 (West Midlands)		171 (34.8%)			
Site 2 (London)		140 (28.5%)			
Site 3 (Lancashire)		61 (12.4%)			
Site 4 (East Midlands)		53 (10.8%)			
Site 5 (West Yorkshire)		67 (13.6%)			
Ethnicity	20 (4.1%)				
White British		305 (64.6%)			
Other		167 (35.4%)			
Education Level	11 (2.2%)				
Degree or higher		237 (49.3%)			
No degree		244 (50.7%)			
Relationship status	4 (0.8%)				
Married, or living with partner		408 (83.6%)			
Not married, or not living with partner		80 (16.4%)			
Employment	14 (2.8%)				
In paid employment		412 (86.2%)			
Not in paid employment		66 (13.8%)			

Age data approximated a normal distribution; data for weeks' gestation and IMD were highly skewed. Therefore, median and LQ-UQ are reported for all of the three variables

Ethnicity: 'Other' includes other white, Asian or Asian British, black or black British, mixed, and other

Education level: 'No degree' includes those who left school before completing GCSE's, completed GCSE's, hold A Levels or an apprenticeship, or professional qualifications

Relationship status: 'Not married, or not living with partner' includes single and other (e.g. widow)

Employment: 'In paid employment' includes full- and part-time employment, self-employed and on leave from employment; 'Not in paid employment' includes studying/training and not in paid employment

LQ lower quartile, UQ upper quartile; n (%) - denominator is n of participants with data

IMD Index of multiple deprivation, ranging from decile 1 (most deprived) to 10 (least deprived)

Table 2 Descriptive data on exposure variable, outcomes and technology use

	Scale score range	n responses missing (N = 492)	Median (LQ - UQ)
MSPSS overall	12–84		81.0 (74.0–84.0)
MSPSS Significant other	4–28		28.0 (28.0–28.0)
MSPSS Family	4–28	8 (1.6%)	28.0 (25.0–28.0)
MSPSS Friends	4–28		27.0 (24.0–28.0)
WEMWBS overall	14–70	17 (3.5%)	54.0 (48.0–60.0)
Antenatal TOPSE overall	0–360	44 (8.9%)	319.0 (295.5–340)
MTUAS overall	1–6		5.1 (4.7–5.4)
MTUAS Text messaging	1–6		6.0 (6.0–6.0)
MTUAS Phone calling	1–6	1 (0.2%)	6.0 (5.0–6.0)
MTUAS Smartphone use	1–6		6.0 (6.0–6.0)
MTUAS Internet searching	1–6		6.0 (5.0–6.0)
MTUAS General social media use	1–6		4.0 (3.3–5.0)
		n responses missing (N = 492)	n (%)
Uses mobile phone		1 (0.2%)	490 (99.8%)
Uses a tablet (e.g. iPad/Android)		4 (0.8%)	317 (65.0%)
Accesses the internet on phone/tablet		7 (1.4%)	485 (99.8%)
Accesses the internet at home		3 (0.6%)	481 (98.4%)
Uses pregnancy app(s)		3 (0.6%)	356 (72.8%)

MSPSS, WEMWBS and Antenatal TOPSE consist of sum scores. MTUAS consists of mean scores

All four scale variables were not normally distributed, therefore median and LQ-UQ are reported. However, error terms of the outcome variables were normally distributed

MSPSS Multidimensional Scale of Perceived Social Support, MTUAS Media and Technology Usage and Attitudes Scale, WEMWBS Warwick-Edinburgh Mental Wellbeing Scale, TOPSE Tool to Measure Parenting Self-Efficacy

Median overall scores were 54.0 (IQR = 12.0) for the WEMWBS, and 319.0 (IQR = 44.5) for the antenatal TOPSE. In the MTUAS scale, the average overall score was 5.1 (IQR 0.8), which suggests that technologies were used at least once a day (i.e. on the Likert scale, 5 corresponded to 'Once a day'). Text messaging, phone calls, smartphone use and internet searching had a median score of 6.0 (IQR varied between 0.0 and 1.0), i.e. 'Several times a day'. Less frequently, participants used social media - median 4.0 (IQR 1.7) - i.e. 'Several times a week'. Nearly all participants reported using a mobile phone (n = 490, 99.8%), accessed the internet on a mobile phone or tablet (n = 485, 99.8%) and accessed the internet at home (n = 481, 98.4%). Almost two thirds of women used a tablet (n = 317, 65.0%).

Potential confounders for inclusion in the final analysis, including technology use, were pre-specified based on existing literature. Their association with social support was tested through linear regression models (Table 3) prior to the main regression analysis. Social support was significantly associated with IMD decile, F $(1, 470)$ =4.10, p = .044, relationship status, F $(1, 483)$ = 17.09, $p < .001$ and with employment status, F $(1, 473)$ = 6.17, p = .013. An increase of one decile of IMD decile was associated with a 0.45 increase in social support; not being married or not living with a partner was associated

with a 5.51 decrease in social support; not being in paid employment was associated with a 3.64 decrease in social support. None of the other variables revealed significant associations with social support.

Further linear regression models were developed to examine the association between social support and each of the outcomes and to what extent technology use affected those associations. All the regression models showed that social support was significantly associated

Table 3 Associations between potential confounders and social support

Potential confounders	F (df)	p value
Age (n = 468)	F (1) = 0.21	.650
IMD decile (n = 470)	F (1) = 5.14	.024*
Ethnicity (n = 467)	F(1) = 0.06	.809
Education (n = 476)	F(1) = 0.91	.341
Relationship status (n = 483)	F(1) = 17.09	<.001**
Employment (n = 473)	F(1) = 6.17	.013*
Recruitment site (n = 484)	F(4) = 1.58	.178
Technology use (n = 483)	F(1) = 0.21	.648

F statistic is reported rather than the coefficient, due to the difficulty in interpreting the coefficients associated to the variable recruitment site which was the only true categorical variable

n number of observations; df Degrees of Freedom

*$p < .05$; **$p < .001$

with mental well-being (Table 4) and antenatal self-efficacy (Table 5) with and without adjustment for confounding factors (in all models $p < .001$). When potential confounders were taken into account in model 2, 13% of the variance in mental wellbeing was explained by the model. A 1 point increase on the social support scale was associated with a 0.30 point increase in mental well-being (95% CI 0.22 to 0.38) (Table 4). For antenatal self-efficacy, the model 2, 14% of the variance in antenatal self-efficacy was explained by the model. A 1 point increase in the social support scale was associated with a 1.04 increase in the antenatal self-efficacy scale (95% CI 0.70 to 1.39) (Table 5).

Technology use was not significantly associated with mental well-being (0.39, 95% CI -0.97 to 1.75) and had no impact on the adjusted model's goodness of fit (model 3, Table 4). In addition, there was no significant association between technology use and self-efficacy (0.92, 95% CI -4.71 to 6.54) and this variable decreased the model's goodness of fit by approximately 1% (model 3, Table 5).

Discussion

To the best of our knowledge, this is the first study to assess the impact of technology use on the association between social support and mental well-being amongst women in early pregnancy. Although the data clearly showed a positive association between social support and maternal well-being, our findings suggest that technology use had no impact on this association. Similarly, social support was positively associated with self-efficacy, which did not change significantly when technology use was taken into account.

Our findings add to the growing body of evidence for the positive association between social support and maternal mental health [9, 10], which has implications for early intervention. Social support may increase well-being both directly, when a person feels integrated in a large social network and indirectly, by acting as a buffer against potentially adverse effects of stressful events [44]. Our study, which used a measure of perceived social support in 'situations of need' or 'when things go wrong', provides empirical evidence for the buffering role of the support supplied by partner, family and friends. Consistent with this interpretation is the fact that social support was significantly

associated with having a partner and with being employed (presumably through interactions in the work place).

The negative association between socioeconomic deprivation and social support found in this study is in line with previous findings [38]. Others have also reported a significant association between social support and maternal age (negative, though not linear) [45], ethnic minority background (negative) [36] and education level (positive) [37] which we failed to observe. The characteristics of our sample may account for these differences. The proportion of participants with a degree or higher degree (49.3%) outnumbered that reported in a previous study [46] and the national average of 42% [47]. Deprivation scores were above what would be expected in the areas where the study was carried out [40]; the mean IMD decile across the five sites (i.e. Local Authority Districts) was 3.2, compared to a mean of 4.3 (SD 2.6) among study participants (higher IMD deciles indicate lower socioeconomic deprivation). This suggested a relatively higher mean socioeconomic status in our sample when compared to the population in those geographical areas from which the participants were recruited. This aspect, coupled with the sample being predominantly white British (reflective of the English population), may explain why levels of social support were above those reported previously [48, 49]: participants in these two studies were from black and minority ethnic groups, a factor that has been found to be linked to lower levels of social support [36].

The unemployment rate (13.8%) was above the national average for females (3.3%) [50]. A post-hoc comparison of mean IMD decile between employed (mean = 4.6, SD = 0.13) and non-employed women (mean = 2.77, SD = 0.24) shows that the latter experience higher levels of deprivation, rather than not working due to lack of need. This suggests that both the most affluent and, to a lesser extent, the least affluent were common in our study which could be related to a number of reasons. For analytical purposes, we grouped participants who reported not being in paid employment (10.5%) with those who were studying or in training (3.3%) resulting in a total of 13.8%. It is possible that some of those studying/ in training had a source of income (e.g. postgraduate

Table 4 Associations between mental well-being and both social support and technology use

Model	R^2 adjusted	Social support		Technology use	
		Regression coefficient (SE)	95% CI	Regression coefficient (SE)	95% CI
Model 1 (n = 470)	0.12***	0.31 (0.04) ***	0.24 to 0.39		
Model 2 (n = 411)	0.13***	0.30 (0.04) ***	0.22 to 0.38		
Model 3 (n = 410)	0.13***	0.30 (0.04) ***	0.21 to 0.38	0.39 (0.69)	- 0.97 to 1.75

Model 1: Mental well-being (outcome) and social support (exposure), unadjusted
Model 2: Same as Model 1 adjusting for confounders (age, ethnicity, education, relationship status, employment status, IMD decile and site)
Model 3: Same as Model 2 adjusting for technology use
***$p < .001$

Table 5 Associations between self-efficacy and both social support and technology use

Model	R^2 adjusted	Social support		Technology use	
		Regression coefficient (SE)	95% CI	Regression coefficient (SE)	95% CI
Model 1 ($n = 446$)	0.05***	0.76 (0.16) ***	0.45 to 1.06		
Model 2 ($n = 400$)	0.14***	1.04 (0.18) ***	0.70 to 1.39		
Model 3 ($n = 399$)	0.13***	1.03 (0.18) ***	0.68 to 1.38	0.92 (2.86)	-4.71 to 6.54

Model 1: Self-efficacy (outcome) and social support (exposure), unadjusted
Model 2: Same as Model 1 adjusting for confounders (age, ethnicity, education level, relationship status, employment status, IMD decile and site)
Model 3: Same as Model 2 adjusting for technology use
***$p < .001$

students on a scholarship). Self-selection, in that more highly educated women are more likely to agree taking part in research, could also have occurred [51]. At the same time, the fact that our study took place in some of the most deprived areas of the country could have led to the enrolment of a considerable number of women who were unemployed.

Measures used in this study have been widely used in antenatal research and allow comparisons between groups, or within groups across time points (no threshold of clinical significance exists to distinguish groups, e.g. high vs low wellbeing). Overall WEMWBS scores in our sample (median 54.0 (12.0)) were slightly above those from another study with prenatal women in the UK (mean 50.1 (7.9)) [52]. Besides chance, a possible explanation for this difference is the gestational stage of participants. In the latter study, women were in the third trimester of pregnancy whereas in ours participants were in their first trimester. The risk of poor mental health (i.e., lower wellbeing) has been found to increase with the greater demands of advancing pregnancy [53]. With regards to the antenatal TOPSE, comparisons are difficult because only postnatal TOPSE data have been published to date. Furthermore, previous assessments of antenatal self-efficacy involved instruments other than the TOPSE and focused on self-efficacy with respect to specific behaviours or tasks, such as breastfeeding [54] or childbirth [55].

Consistent with existing data [56–58], the use of technologies was widespread among participants, reiterating the presence of technology in modern society. However, an important finding of our study is that the associations between social support and both wellbeing and self-efficacy were not significantly affected by the level of technology use. This is somewhat unexpected as there is extensive use of self-care technologies in countries such as the UK or the US, including for the delivery of antenatal and postnatal services [59]. Agencies such as the National Institute for Health and Care Excellence (UK), in their guidance for the management of antenatal and postnatal mental health, include the use of technological devices namely phones and computers [1]. However, there seems to be a paucity of evidence about the impact

of technologies on maternal well-being. In keeping with research pointing to the potential negative effects of social media on young people's mental health [60], postnatal women ($n = 721$, mean age 30.4 years) who made social comparisons on social networking websites were found to be at increased risk of various detrimental outcomes, including perceptions of lower parental competence, lower social support and higher levels of depression [61]. On the other hand, another study with new mothers ($n = 157$, average age 27 years) reported that blogging, but not social networking, was associated with feelings of connection to extended family and friends which then predicted perceptions of social support and, in turn, maternal well-being [21]. According to the authors, these results could be related to the nature of activities involved in blogging and social networking: women were able to share successful parenting experiences on blogs, receive feedback and learn from others while reading blogs, whereas in social networks they could see what friends and family were doing but may not have received much support in return [21]. In fact, learning through others (vicarious experience) is known to enhance self-efficacy [62].

Altogether, these findings suggest that the impact of technology use on antenatal wellbeing is dependent on the type of activity. Our scale of general technology use, derived from a validated tool, focused on more general activities. It is also conceivable that some technologies and online activities yield greater benefits later in pregnancy or postnatally when demands increase. This question warrants further investigation.

Our study is one of the few quantitative studies to date investigating how technology use affects the wellbeing of women in the antenatal period. This topic is highly relevant if we consider the role increasingly played by technologies in the delivery of healthcare services, antenatal or otherwise. However, our study also had a number of limitations. The cross-sectional design of the study can only show if an association exists between variables, not a causal relationship. Degree holders were overrepresented in the sample which limits the generalisability of our findings. The conclusion that technology use has no impact on social support and well-being and self-efficacy requires caution because of the very high levels of general technology use observed in our sample. Ceiling effects have been noted in previous research that evaluated the impact of a school programme to increase technology use and skill, where baseline levels of some activities were already too high to allow room for improvement [63]. This may have happened in our case; a real lack of low technology users may have affected the power of the regression analysis. Although we provide some data supporting the validity of the adapted MTUAS scale, the changes made could also have altered the precision of the original scale.

Conclusion

Our findings indicate that the use of technologies, in its general form, has no or minimal influence on the association between social and mental well-being and self-efficacy during the early antenatal period. Future research, both quantitative and qualitative, should explore what aspects of technology use can facilitate social networks. Additional work is needed to investigate whether pregnancy-specific and technology-mediated activities, such as sharing pregnancy experiences online or using pregnancy apps, offer more potential to improve the lives of expectant mothers. This should include the development of health literacy skills where needed, such as information-seeking skills and internet access, which can impact positively on the psychological outcomes of perinatal women [64]. The next stage of this project is to evaluate and explore the impact of a pregnancy and parenthood-related technology on antenatal and early postnatal wellbeing and self-efficacy. Understanding the impact of such technologies, if any, is important if we are to develop more effective and cost-effective interventions to support and improve the lives of antenatal and postnatal women and, in turn, that of their children.

Acknowledgements
We would like to acknowledge that this work was funded by the charity Best Beginnings following a competitive tender process. Best Beginnings was awarded funding from the Big Lottery Fund to develop and promote their Baby Buddy app as a digital health innovation and to commission the academic evaluation of the app. This research was undertaken whilst the first (SG) and last author (RL) were based at the Institute of Health & Society, Newcastle University. We are grateful to the women who took part in the BaBBLeS study and all the midwives and other healthcare staff who were involved in the recruitment of participants. We are also indebted to a number of individuals who provided valuable technical and statistical support including Dr. Viviana Albani, Dr. Tomos Robinson, Professor Elaine McColl and Ms. Helen Mossop.

Funding
This study was funded by Best Beginnings through the Big Lottery Fund. The funder played no role in the collection, analysis, or interpretation of data, nor in the writing of this manuscript.

Authors' contributions
SG designed the baseline questionnaire, analysed the data and drafted this manuscript, under the supervision of RL, and with the input from all the other authors. JC, SK, CD, TG, EB, SN, JS and TD were in regular contact with recruitment sites to facilitate the process of data collection. TD, as chief investigator, drafted the research protocol and oversaw all aspects of the study design, data collection and analysis with input from the team. All authors read, commented on, and approved the manuscript. Both TD and RL were senior authors of this manuscript.

Competing interests
The authors declare that they have no competing interests.

Author details
[1]School of Psychology, Ulster University, Cromore Road, Coleraine, Co., Londonderry BT52 1SA, UK. [2]Centre for Innovative Research Across the Life Course (CIRAL), Faculty of Health & Life Sciences, Coventry University, Priory Street, Coventry CV1 5FB, UK. [3]Centre for Health Services Studies, University of Kent, Canterbury, Kent CT2 7NF, UK. [4]Centre for Child & Adolescent Health, University of the West of England Bristol, Oakfield House, Oakfield Grove, Clifton, Bristol BS8 2BN, UK. [5]Nursing, Midwifery and Health, Health and Life Sciences, Northumbria University, Coach Lane Campus, Benton, Newcastle upon Tyne NE7 7XA, UK. [6]Department of Psychology, Child & Adolescent Mental Health Service Research Unit, King's College London, Institute of Psychiatry, Psychology and Neuroscience, De Crespigny Park, London SE5 8AB, UK. [7]Population Child Health Research Group, Women's and Children's Health, University of New South Wales, Sydney, Australia.

References
1. NICE. Antenatal and postnatal mental health: clinical management and service guidance | guidance and guidelines. London: National Institute for Health and Care Excellence; 2014. https://www.nice.org.uk/guidance/cg192
2. National Maternity Review Team. Better Births. Improving Outcomes of Maternity Services in England. A Five Year Forward View for Maternity Care. 2016. https://www.england.nhs.uk/wp-content/uploads/2016/02/national-maternity-review-report.pdf
3. Kothari C, Wiley J, Moe A, Liepman MR, Tareen RS, Curtis A. Maternal depression is not just a problem early on. Public Health. 2016;137:154–61. https://doi.org/10.1016/J.PUHE.2016.01.003.
4. Deave T, Heron J, Evans J, Emond A. The impact of maternal depression in pregnancy on early child development. BJOG. 2008;115:1043–51. https://doi.org/10.1111/j.1471-0528.2008.01752.x.
5. Stein A, Pearson RM, Goodman SH, Rapa E, Rahman A, McCallum M, et al. Effects of perinatal mental disorders on the fetus and child. Lancet. 2014; 384:1800–19. https://doi.org/10.1016/S0140-6736(14)61277-0.
6. Bauer A, Parsonage M, Knapp M, Iemmi V, Adelaja B. The costs of perinatal mental health problems. London: Centre for Mental Health and London School of Economics; 2014.
7. Haber MG, Cohen JL, Lucas T, Baltes BB. The relationship between self-reported received and perceived social support: a meta-analytic review. Am J Community Psychol. 2007;39:133–44. https://doi.org/10.1007/s10464-007-9100-9.
8. Reblin M, Uchino BN. Social and emotional support and its implication for health. Curr Opin Psychiatry. 2008;21:201–5. https://doi.org/10.1097/YCO.0b013e3282f3ad89.
9. Halbreich U, Karkun S. Cross-cultural and social diversity of prevalence of postpartum depression and depressive symptoms. J Affect Disord. 2006;91: 97–111. https://doi.org/10.1016/J.JAD.2005.12.051.
10. Fisher J, de Mello MC, Patel V, Rahman A, Tran T, Holton S, et al. Prevalence and determinants of common perinatal mental disorders in women in low- and lower-middle-income countries: a systematic review. Bull World Health Organ. 2012;90:139–49. https://doi.org/10.1590/S0042-96862012000200014.
11. Leahy-Warren P, McCarthy G, Corcoran P. First-time mothers: social support, maternal parental self-efficacy and postnatal depression. J Clin Nurs. 2012; 21:388–97. https://doi.org/10.1111/j.1365-2702.2011.03701.x.
12. Kim TH, Connolly JA, Tamim H. The effect of social support around pregnancy on postpartum depression among Canadian teen mothers and adult mothers in the maternity experiences survey. BMC Pregnancy Childbirth. 2014;14:162. https://doi.org/10.1186/1471-2393-14-162.

13. Balaji AB, Claussen AH, Smith DC, Visser SN, Morales MJ, Perou R. Social support networks and maternal mental health and well-being. J Womens Health. 2007;16:1386–96. https://doi.org/10.1089/jwh.2007.CDC10.

14. Asselmann E, Wittchen H-U, Erler L, Martini J. Peripartum changes in social support among women with and without anxiety and depressive disorders prior to pregnancy: a prospective-longitudinal study. Arch Womens Ment Health. 2016;19:943–52. https://doi.org/10.1007/s00737-016-0608-6.

15. Morikawa M, Okada T, Ando M, Aleksic B, Kunimoto S, Nakamura Y, et al. Relationship between social support during pregnancy and postpartum depressive state: a prospective cohort study. Sci Rep. 2015; 5:10520. https://doi.org/10.1038/srep10520.

16. Karanikolos M, Mladovsky P, Cylus J, Thomson S, Basu S, Stuckler D, et al. Financial crisis, austerity, and health in Europe. Lancet. 2013;381:1323–31. https://doi.org/10.1016/S0140-6736(13)60102-6.

17. Drentea P, Moren-Cross JL. Social capital and social support on the web: the case of an internet mother site. Sociol Health Illn. 2005;27:920–43. https://doi.org/10.1111/j.1467-9566.2005.00464.x.

18. RCM. Internet advice for pregnant women. London: Royal College of Midwives; 2017. https://www.rcm.org.uk/news-views-and-analysis/news/internet-advice-for-pregnant-women

19. Gibson L, Hanson VL. Digital motherhood. Proceedings of the SIGCHI Conference on Human Factors in Computing Systems - CHI '13. New York: ACM Press; 2013. p. 313. https://doi.org/10.1145/2470654.2470700.

20. Evans M, Donelle L, Hume-Loveland L. Social support and online postpartum depression discussion groups: a content analysis. Patient Educ Couns. 2012;87:405–10. https://doi.org/10.1016/J.PEC.2011.09.011.

21. McDaniel BT, Coyne SM, Holmes EK. New mothers and media use: associations between blogging, social networking, and maternal well-being. Matern Child Health J. 2012;16:1509–17. https://doi.org/10.1007/s10995-011-0918-2.

22. Hearn L, Miller M, Fletcher A. Online healthy lifestyle support in the perinatal period: what do women want and do they use it? Aust J Prim Health. 2013;19:313. https://doi.org/10.1071/PY13039.

23. Best Beginnings. Best Beginnings. About Baby Buddy 2017. https://www.bestbeginnings.org.uk/about-baby-buddy. Accessed 17 Sept 2017.

24. Deave T, Coad J, Lingam R, Kendall S, Day C. Bumps and babies longitudinal study (BaBBLeS). Community Practitioners' and Health Visitors' Association Annual Conference. Telford: Telford International Centre; 2016.

25. Deave T, Kendal S, Lingam R, Day C, Goodenough T, Bailey E, et al. A study to evaluate the effectiveness of Best Beginnings' Baby Buddy phone app in England: a protocol paper. Prim Health Care Res Dev. 2018:1–6. https://doi.org/10.1017/S1463423618000294 Cambridge University Press.

26. Qualtrics. Qualtrics [Internet]. Provo, Utah, USA; 2005. https://www.qualtrics.com

27. Zimet GD, Dahlem NW, Zimet SG, Farley GK. The multidimensional scale of perceived social support. J Pers Assess. 1988;52:30–41. https://doi.org/10.1207/s15327752jpa5201_2·

28. Eker D, Arkar H. Perceived social support: psychometric properties of the MSPSS in normal and pathological groups in a developing country. Soc Psychiatry Psychiatr Epidemiol. 1995;30:121–6. https://doi.org/10.1007/BF00802040.

29. Canty-Mitchell J, Zimet GD. Psychometric properties of the multidimensional scale of perceived social support in urban adolescents. Am J Community Psychol. 2000;28:391–400. https://doi.org/10.1023/A:1005109522457.

30. Zimet GD, Powell SS, Farley GK, Werkman S, Berkoff KA. Psychometric characteristics of the multidimensional scale of perceived social support. J Pers Assess. 1990;55:610–7. https://doi.org/10.1080/00223891.1990.9674095.

31. Tennant R, Hiller L, Fishwick R, Platt S, Joseph S, Weich S, et al. The Warwick-Edinburgh mental well-being scale (WEMWBS): development and UK validation. Health Qual Life Outcomes. 2007;5:63. https://doi.org/10.1186/1477-7525-5-63.

32. Stewart-Brown S, Platt S, Tennant A, Maheswaran H, Parkinson J, Weich S, et al. The Warwick-Edinburgh mental well-being scale (WEMWBS): a valid and reliable tool for measuring mental well-being in diverse populations and projects. J Epidemiol Community Health. 2011;65:A38–9. https://doi.org/10.1136/jech.2011.143586.86.

33. Kendall S, Bloomfield L. Developing and validating a tool to measure parenting self-efficacy. J Adv Nurs. 2005;51:174–81. https://doi.org/10.1111/j.1365-2648.2005.03479.x.

34. Benzies K, Clarke D, Barker L, Mychasiuk R. UpStart parent survey: a new psychometrically valid tool for the evaluation of prevention-focused parenting programs. Matern Child Health J. 2013;17:1452–8. https://doi.org/10.1007/s10995-012-1152-2.

35. Elsenbruch S, Benson S, Rücke M, Rose M, Dudenhausen J, Pincus-Knackstedt MK, et al. Social support during pregnancy: effects on maternal depressive symptoms, smoking and pregnancy outcome. Hum Reprod. 2007;22:869–77. https://doi.org/10.1093/humrep/del432.

36. Shields MA, Price SW. Exploring the economic and social determinants of psychological well-being and perceived social support in England. J R Stat Soc Ser A. 2005;168:513–37. https://doi.org/10.1111/j.1467-985X.2005.00361.x.

37. Mangrio E, Hansen K, Lindström M, Köhler M, Rosvall M. Maternal educational level, parental preventive behavior, risk behavior, social support and medical care consumption in 8-month-old children in Malmö, Sweden. BMC Public Health. 2011;11:891. https://doi.org/10.1186/1471-2458-11-891.

38. Klebanov PK, Brooks-Gunn J, Duncan GJ. Does neighborhood and family poverty affect mothers' parenting, mental health, and social support? J Marriage Fam. 1994;56:441. https://doi.org/10.2307/353111.

39. Priscilla K. Coleman, Katherine Hildebrandt Karraker. Parenting Self-Efficacy among Mothers of School-Age Children: Conceptualization, Measurement, and Correlates. Family Relations 2000;49(1):13-24.

40. DCLG. English indices of deprivation 2015 - GOV.UK. London: Department for Communities and Local Government. http://imd-by-postcode.opendatacommunities.org/. Accessed 23 Oct 2018.

41. ONS. Finalising the 2011 questionnaire. Office for National Statistics. 2009. https://www.ons.gov.uk/census/2011census/howourcensusworks/howwe plannedthe2011census/questionnairedevelopment/finalisingthe2011 questionnaire. Accessed 23 Oct 2018.

42. Rosen LD, Whaling K, Carrier LM, Cheever NA, Rokkum J. The media and technology usage and attitudes scale: an empirical investigation. Comput Human Behav. 2013;29:2501–11 http://www.ncbi.nlm.nih.gov/pubmed/25722534.

43. StataCorp. Stata Statistical Software: Release 14. College Station: StataCorp LP; 2015.

44. Cohen S, Wills TA. Stress, social support, and the buffering hypothesis. Psychol Bull. 1985;98:310–57 Available: http://www.ncbi.nlm.nih.gov/pubmed/3901065.

45. Bornstein MH, Putnick DL, Suwalsky JTD, Gini M. Maternal chronological age, prenatal and perinatal history, social support, and parenting of infants. Child Dev. 2006;77:875–92. https://doi.org/10.1111/j.1467-8624.2006.00908.x.

46. Berridge K, Hackett A, Abayomi J, Maxwell S. The cost of infant feeding in Liverpool, England. Public Health Nutr. 2004;7:1039–46. https://doi.org/10.1079/PHN2004650.

47. ONS. Graduates in the UK labour market. London; 2017. https://www.ons.gov.uk/employmentandlabourmarket/peopleinwork/employmentandemployeetypes/articles/graduatesintheuklabourmarket/2017. Accessed 23 Oct 2018.

48. Akhtar A, Rahman A, Husain M, Chaudhry IB, Duddu V, Husain N. Multidimensional scale of perceived social support: psychometric properties in a south Asian population. J Obstet Gynaecol Res. 2010;36:845–51. https://doi.org/10.1111/j.1447-0756.2010.01204.x.

49. Husain N, Cruickshank K, Husain M, Khan S, Tomenson B, Rahman A. Social stress and depression during pregnancy and in the postnatal period in British Pakistani mothers: a cohort study. J Affect Disord. 2012;140:268–76. https://doi.org/10.1016/j.jad.2012.02.009.

50. ONS. LFS: Unemployment rate: UK: Female: Aged 25–49. London; 2018. https://www.ons.gov.uk/employmentandlabourmarket/peoplenotinwork/unemployment/timeseries/mgxd/lms. Accessed 23 Oct 2018.

51. Braig S, Grabher F, Ntomchukwu C, Reister F, Stalder T, Kirschbaum C, et al. The Association of Hair Cortisol with self-reported chronic psychosocial stress and symptoms of anxiety and depression in women shortly after delivery. Paediatr Perinat Epidemiol. 2016;30:97–104. https://doi.org/10.1111/ppe.12255.

52. Mannion A, Slade P. Psychotic-like experiences in pregnant and postpartum women without a history of psychosis. Schizophr Res. 2014;160:118–23. https://doi.org/10.1016/j.schres.2014.10.003.

53. Bennett HA, Einarson A, Taddio A, Koren G, Einarson TR. Prevalence of depression during pregnancy: systematic review. Obstet Gynecol. 2004;103: 698–709. https://doi.org/10.1097/01.AOG.0000116689.75396.5f.

54. Blyth R, Creedy DK, Dennis C-L, Moyle W, Pratt J, De Vries SM. Effect of maternal confidence on breastfeeding duration: an application of breastfeeding self-efficacy theory. Birth. 2002;29:278–84. https://doi.org/10.1046/j.1523-536X.2002.00202.x.

55. Beebe KR, Lee KA, Carrieri-Kohlman V, Humphreys J. The effects of childbirth self-efficacy and anxiety during pregnancy on prehospitalization labor. J Obstet Gynecol Neonatal Nurs. 2007;36:410–8. https://doi.org/10.1111/j.1552-6909.2007.00170.x.

56. Ofcom. The UK is now a smartphone society. Available: https://www.ofcom. org.uk/about-ofcom/latest/media/media-releases/2015/cmr-uk-2015. Accessed 20 Aug 2017.

57. Peragallo Urrutia R, Berger AA, Ivins AA, Beckham AJ, Thorp JM Jr, Nicholson WK. Internet use and access among pregnant women via computer and Mobile phone: implications for delivery of perinatal care. JMIR MHealth UHealth. 2015;3:e25. https://doi.org/10.2196/mhealth.3347.

58. Kennedy RAK, Mullaney L, Reynolds CME, Cawley S, McCartney DMA, Turner MJ. Preferences of women for web-based nutritional information in pregnancy. Public Health. 2017;143:71–7. https://doi.org/10.1016/j.puhe.2016.10.028.

59. Boulos MNK, Brewer AC, Karimkhani C, Buller DB, Dellavalle RP. Mobile medical and health apps: state of the art, concerns, regulatory control and certification. Online J Public Health Inform. 2014;5:229. https://doi. org/10.5210/ojphi.v5i3.4814.

60. Rosen LD, Whaling K, Rab S, Carrier LM, Cheever NA. Is Facebook creating "iDisorders"? The link between clinical symptoms of psychiatric disorders and technology use, attitudes and anxiety. Comput Human Behav. 2013;29: 1243–54. https://doi.org/10.1016/j.chb.2012.11.012.

61. Coyne SM, McDaniel BT, Stockdale LA. "Do you dare to compare?" associations between maternal social comparisons on social networking sites and parenting, mental health, and romantic relationship outcomes. Comput Human Behav. 2017;70:335–40. https://doi.org/10.1016/J.CHB.2016.12.081.

62. Bandura A. Self-efficacy mechanism in human agency. Am Psychol. 1982;37: 122–47. https://doi.org/10.1037/0003-066X.37.2.122.

63. Oliver KM, Corn JO. Student-reported differences in technology use and skills after the implementation of one-to-one computing. EMI Educ Media Int. 2008;45:215–29. https://doi.org/10.1080/09523980802284333.

64. Shieh C, Mays R, McDaniel A, Yu J. Health literacy and its association with the use of information sources and with barriers to information seeking in clinic-based pregnant women. Health Care Women Int. 2009;30:971–88. https://doi.org/10.1080/07399330903052152.

11

Association of intimate partner violence during pregnancy, prenatal depression, and adverse birth outcomes in Wuhan, China

Honghui Yu[1], Xueyan Jiang[2], Wei Bao[3], Guifeng Xu[3,4], Rong Yang[5] and Min Shen[2*]

Abstract

Background: Intimate partner violence (IPV) among pregnant women constitutes a global public health problem and a potential risk factor for adverse maternal and fetal outcomes. The present study aimed to examine the associations among IPV during pregnancy, prenatal depression, and adverse birth outcomes in Wuhan, China.

Methods: A cross-sectional study was performed from April 2013 to March 2014 in Wuhan, China. Sociodemographic characteristics, IPV during pregnancy, and depressive symptoms during pregnancy were assessed in the third trimester of pregnancy. Birth outcomes were collected after delivery using medical records. Chi-square tests and logistic regression analysis were used to examine the association between IPV and prenatal depression, as well as the association between IPV combined with prenatal depression and adverse birth outcomes.

Results: After adjustment for covariates, there was a statistically significant association between IPV during pregnancy and prenatal depression (adjusted odds ratio [aOR] = 2.50, 95% confidence interval [CI]: 1.60–3.90). IPV during pregnancy (aOR = 1.67, 95% CI: 1.08–2.56) and prenatal depression (aOR = 1.72, 95% CI: 1.11–2.68) were significantly associated with adverse birth outcomes. Women experiencing psychological abuse had a significantly higher odds of prenatal depression (aOR = 2.04, 95% CI: 1.19–3.49) and of adverse birth outcomes (aOR = 2.13, 95% CI: 1.08–2.58), compared with women who did not experience IPV and prenatal depression.

Conclusions: IPV during pregnancy and prenatal depression were significantly associated with adverse birth outcomes, after adjustment for socio-demographic and behavior factors. The findings suggest that early recognition of IPV and prenatal depression during antenatal care may protect pregnant women and improve birth outcomes.

Keywords: Intimate partner violence, Prenatal depression, Adverse birth outcome, Pregnancy

Background

Intimate partner violence (IPV) among pregnant women constitutes a global public health problem [1, 2] and is a potential risk factor for adverse maternal and fetal outcomes [3, 4]. IPV includes physical abuse, psychological abuse, sexual violence, and economic abuse in the home setting [5, 6]. A study conducted by World Health Organization [7] based on household data from the Demographic and Health Surveys (DHS) and the International Violence Against Women Survey (IVAWS) across 19 countries showed that the prevalence of physical IPV during pregnancy was 3.8~ 13.5% in Africa, 4.1~ 11.1% in Americas, 1.8~ 6.6% in Europe and 2.0–5.0% in Asia. Previous studies have suggested that IPV disproportionately affects low-income women, especially for pregnant women [8]. A previous survey showed that the prevalence of domestic violence among pregnant women was 15.9% in Japan [9], 6.5% in the United States [10], 7.7% in Spain [11], and 34.8% in northern European countries [12]; however, the prevalence rates were much higher in less developed countries such as Iran (72.8%) [13] and Nigeria (44.6%) [14]. In China, the prevalence rates of IPV among pregnant women have been reported as 18.8% in Hong Kong [15] and 11.3% in Changsha [16].

* Correspondence: shenmin@hust.edu.cn
[2]Department of Maternal and Child Health, School of Public Health, Tongji Medical College, Huazhong University of Science and Technology, Wuhan 430030, China
Full list of author information is available at the end of the article

IPV during pregnancy does not only affect women's health; it also has adverse health effects for newborns and affects their development in childhood [17–19]. Previous studies have demonstrated a relationship between abuse during pregnancy and both low birth weight (LBW) and preterm birth (PTB) [13, 18–20]. Many studies have shown that pregnancy constitutes a particularly critical period because of women's increased vulnerability and body changes, increased economic pressure, and less frequent sexual relations [18, 21, 22]. Pregnant women experiencing IPV also experience depression and anxiety. Studies have shown that women experiencing abuse during pregnancy are 2.5 times more likely to report depressive symptomatology, compared with their non-abused counterparts [23, 24]. These symptoms may be the direct consequence trauma or the indirect consequence of domestic violence [25–27].

In China, little is known about the experience of IPV among pregnant women or about its impacts on mental health and on children. Therefore, this study aimed to investigate the association between IPV during pregnancy and prenatal depression and the associations of these variables with adverse birth outcomes, adjusting for covariates.

Methods

This study was carried out in Qiaokou District Maternal and Child Health Hospital, Dongxihu District People's Hospital, and Tongji Hospital from April 1, 2013, to March 31, 2014, in Wuhan, China. The participants were pregnant women attending prenatal examinations or delivery at the selected hospitals during the study period. All participants were assessed in the third trimester of pregnancy or prior to delivery. This study was approved by the Ethics Board of Tongji Medical College, Huazhong University of Science and Technology. Written informed consent was obtained from the participants.

The Abuse Assessment Screen (AAS) was used to assess IPV during pregnancy [28]. Women reporting yes on any of the IPV items for the period of the current pregnancy were defined having been exposed to IPV. The Chinese version of AAS was first used in 1999 by Leung to screen for IPV among Chinese women [28]. The Chinese AAS has demonstrated a satisfactory level of measurement accuracy, with high specificity (≥ 89%) and positive predictive values (≥ 80%) and satisfactory-to-high negative predictive values (66–93%) [29]. IPV was defined as physical abuse, psychological abuse, sexual abuse, or economic abuse. Prenatal depression was measured using the Center for Epidemiologic Studies-Depression Scale (CES-D) [30]. The CES-D is a 20-item self-report scale designed to measure current levels of depressive symptoms and has been widely used in China. The

Cronbach's α of the CES-D overall has been shown to be 0.90, and it is 0.68–0.86 for each of the scale's factors [31]. CES-D scores range from 0 to 60, with higher scores signifying more severe symptoms of depression. The participants were considered likely to be depressed if their scores were ≥ 20.

Data were collected on the demographic characteristics of pregnant women and their partners, husbands' smoking and alcohol use behaviors, family status, and pregnancy-related complications. Information on birth outcomes and pregnancy-related complications was collected from medical records after delivery. Adverse birth outcomes included PTB, LBW, birth defects, asphyxia, and stillbirth. PTB was defined as birth prior to 37 weeks' gestation, following the definition of the World Health Organization [32]. Using the typical definition, stillbirth was defined as fetal death at or after 20 to 28 weeks of pregnancy [32]. LBW was defined using the World Health Organization's definition of an infant having a birth weight of 2499 g or less, regardless of gestational age. "Birth defect" is a phrase commonly used to describe congenital malformations (i.e., a congenital or physical anomaly that is recognizable at birth) [33]. Perinatal asphyxia is the medical condition resulting from a newborn infant being deprived of oxygen (hypoxia) for long enough to cause apparent harm. Miscarriage was defined as an early pregnancy loss, and live birth was defined as the baby being born alive, even if he/she died shortly afterward.

All statistical analyses were performed using SAS software, Version 9.4 (SAS Institute Inc., Cary, North Carolina). Descriptive statistics were used to calculate the prevalence of overall IPV and subtypes of IPV, including physical, psychological, and sexual abuse—categorical variables described by frequency distributions. Chi-square tests were used for bivariate analyses to assess differences in the prevalence rates of IPV. Continuity-adjusted chi-square analysis was applied when 25% of the cells had expected counts of less than five. Multivariable logistic regression was used to estimate the adjusted odds ratios (ORs) and 95% confidence intervals (CIs) for differences between the abused group and the non-abused group. All statistical tests were two-sided, and significance was determined using an alpha level of 0.05.

Results

A total of 900 pregnant women participated in the survey. Of these women, 797 returned questionnaires that were eligible for data analysis. The average maternal age was 27.4 ± 4.2 years. More than one-third of the participants had received a bachelor's degree or higher, and more than half had monthly household incomes of less than 6000 yuan (Table 1).

Table 1 Characteristics of pregnant women participated in the survey in Wuhan, China

Variables	IPV (%)	No IPV (%)	x^2 value	P value
Age (years)				
20–24	43 (20.00)	172 (80.00)	0.6547	0.8838
25–29	62 (17.42)	294 (82.58)		
30–34	33 (18.44)	146 (81.56)		
35+	8 (17.02)	39 (82.98)		
Maternal education level[**]				
Junior middle school or below	30 (24.59)	92 (75.41)	17.2640	0.0006
High school	52 (25.49)	152 (74.51)		
Vocational degree	25 (13.66)	158 (86.34)		
Bachelor degree or above	39 (13.54)	249 (86.46)		
Maternal occupation				
Employed	70 (14.68)	407 (85.32)	10.5410	0.0012
Unemployed	76 (23.75)	244 (76.25)		
Education level of husband				
Junior middle school or below	31 (27.68)	81 (72.32)	9.7016	0.0213
High school	39 (19.50)	161 (80.5)		
Vocational degree	30 (17.65)	140 (82.35)		
Bachelor degree or above	46 (14.60)	269 (85.4)		
Occupation of husbands				
Employed	126 (18.89)	541 (81.11)		
Unemployed	20 (15.38)	110 (84.62)		
Household income monthly (Yuan)				
> 3000	43 (25.6)	125 (74.4)	0.8937	0.3445
3000-	61 (19.55)	251 (80.45)		
6000-	28 (14.66)	163 (85.34)		
≥ 10,000	14 (11.11)	112 (88.89)		
Abortion history[**]				
Yes	66 (23.9)	210 (76.1)	8.8310	0.0030
No	80 (15.4)	441 (84.6)		
Parity[**]				
1	67 (14.5)	396 (85.5)	11.9798	0.0025
2	44 (21.9)	157 (78.1)		
≥ 3	35 (26.3)	98 (73.7)		
Husband's smoking behavior				
Yes	80 (19.4)	332 (80.6)	0.6882	0.4068
No	66 (17.1)	319 (82.9)		
Husband's drinking behavior				
Yes	113 (17.4)	537 (82.6)	2.0550	0.1517
No	33 (22.4)	114 (77.6)		
Pregnancy related complications				
Yes	31 (19.38)	129 (80.62)	0.1493	0.6992
No	115 (18.05)	522 (81.95)		
Adverse birth outcomes				
Yes	39 (26.53)	108 (73.47)	8.1744	0.0042

Table 1 Characteristics of pregnant women participated in the survey in Wuhan, China *(Continued)*

Variables	IPV (%)	No IPV (%)	χ^2 value	P value
No	107 (16.44)	544 (83.56)		
Prenatal depression				
Yes	43 (32.58)	89 (67.42)	21.4908	<.0001
No	103 (15.49)	562 (84.51)		
Total	146 (18.32)	651 (81.68)		

A total of 146 (18.32%) of the pregnant women reported that they had experienced IPV by their husbands during the pregnancy. The prevalence rates of psychological, physical, economic, and sexual abuse were 14.3%, 2.1%, 2.0%, and 0.3%, respectively. The overall prevalence rate of adverse birth outcomes was 18.44% (147/797). The prevalence rates of neonatal asphyxia, PTB, and LBW were 12.3%, 8.9%, and 5.3%, respectively. The women who had adverse birth outcomes had a higher rate of IPV during pregnancy than did women without adverse birth outcomes (26.53% vs. 16.44%, $P = 0.0044$). The IPV group had a higher prevalence rate of depression than did the non-IPV group (32.58% vs. 15.49%, $P < 0.001$) (Table 1).

Table 2 showed the differences of prevalence rates among IPV group and no IPV group. The results suggested that women experienced IPV had higher rates of prenatal depression than those no IPV ($P < 0.0001$). For subtype of IPV, women experienced psychological, psychological and physical abuse had significant higher prevalence rates of prenatal depression ($P < 0.01$).

In the multivariable logistic regression analysis, after adjusting for potential confounding factors, IPV was significantly associated with prenatal depression. Pregnant women who had experienced IPV were 2.50 times more likely to report prenatal depression (OR = 2.50, 95% CI:

1.60–3.90). In terms of the type of IPV, psychological abuse (OR = 2.04, 95% CI: 1.19–3.49), psychological and economic abuse (OR = 6.16, 95% CI: 1.48–25.58), and psychological and physical abuse (OR = 21.81, 95% CI: 5.23–91.04) were significantly associated with prenatal depression (Table 3).

After adjusting for confounding factors, both IPV and prenatal depression had a significant association with adverse birth outcomes; the adjusted ORs for these variables were 1.72 (OR = 1.72, 95% CI: 1.11–2.68) and 1.67 (OR = 1.67, 95% CI: 1.08–2.56), compared with women reporting no IPV and no prenatal depression, respectively (Table 4). Regarding IPV subtype, only psychological abuse had a significant association with adverse birth outcomes (OR = 2.13, 95% CI: 1.08–2.58).

Discussion

In this study, the prevalence of IPV among pregnant women in Wuhan, China, was 18.32%. We observed a significant and positive association between IPV and prenatal depression among pregnant women. Moreover, both maternal IPV and prenatal depression were associated with adverse birth outcomes. The prevalence rate was similar to a previous study's finding of an 18.8% prevalence of IPV among pregnant women in Hong Kong [15]. The prevalence rate was higher than a

Table 2 The differences of prevalence rates of depression among the IPV or the type of IPV group compared to no IPV group

IPV or subtype of IPV	Prenatal depression (%)	No prenatal depression (%)	χ^2 value	P value
Overall IPV			21.4908	<.0001
No	89 (13.67)	562 (86.33)		
Yes	43 (29.45)	103 (70.55)		
Psychological abuse			7.7637	0.0053
No	107 (15.22)	596 (84.78)		
Yes	25 (26.60)	69 (73.40)		
Psychological + physical abuse			17.1939[a]	<.0001
No	125 (15.88)	662 (84.12)		
Yes	7 (70.00)	3 (30.00)		
Psychological+ economic abuse			3.2836[a]	0.0700
No	128 (16.24)	660 (83.76)		
Yes	4 (44.44)	5 (55.56)		
Total	132 (16.60)	665 (83.40)		

[a]Continuity Adjusted Chi-Square was applied because 25% of the cells have expected counts less than 5

Table 3 Association between domestic violence during pregnancy and prenatal depression

Variables	Model 1*		Model 2*	
	OR (95% CI)	P value	OR (95% CI)	P value
Overall IPV	2.50 (1.60, 3.90)	<.0001	–	–
Subtypes				
Psychological abuse	–	–	2.04 (1.19, 3.49)	0.0092
Psychological+ economic abuse	–	–	6.16 (1.48, 25.58)	0.0123
Psychological+ physical abuse	–	–	21.81 (5.23, 91.04)	<.0001

Model 1: Adjusted for maternal age, maternal education, maternal occupation, husbands' education, husbands' occupation, husbands' drinking and smoking characteristics, pregnancy related complications and abortion history, overall domestic violence as an independent factor;
Model 2: Adjusted for maternal age, maternal education, maternal occupation, husbands' education, husbands' occupation, husbands' drinking and smoking characteristics, pregnancy related complications and abortion history, subtypes of domestic violence as independent factors

previous finding of 11.3% for overall prevalence of IPV among women during pregnancy in Changsha city [16]. Psychological abuse (14.6%) was the most common form of abuse, accounting for 64.38% of abuse experienced by the women in this study. This was followed by physical abuse (2.1%). This finding was consistent with a previous study in China, which found that psychological violence was the most common form of violence among pregnant Chinese women (59/96 = 61.5%) [16]. A previous study in Iran also found that psychological violence was the most common form of violence among pregnant women (51.3%) [34]. A study in Thailand reported that 54% of women had been exposed to emotional violence, 27% to physical violence, and 19% to sexual violence [35]. Further, a meta-analysis of 92 studies from 23 countries focusing on IPV among pregnant women reported the prevalence of domestic violence as 13.3% in developed countries, compared to 27.7% for developing countries ($P = 0.14$) [36].

We found that women who had experienced IPV during pregnancy had a higher prevalence of depressive symptoms than did those who had not experienced IPV (29.45% vs. 13.67%, $P < 0.0001$). After adjustment for women's and their husbands' demographic characteristics, smoking, and alcohol use, overall IPV was associated with an increased risk of prenatal depression (OR = 2.50, 95% CI: 1.60–3.90). Additionally, psychological abuse was significantly associated with prenatal depression (OR = 2.04, 95% CI: 1.19–3.49), and psychological abuse combined with economic abuse increased

the odds of developing prenatal depression by six times (OR = 6.16, 95% CI: 1.48–25.58) compared to those no IPV and prenatal depression. Our findings confirmed that IPV could lead to maternal depression and to a variety of adverse pregnancy outcomes.

Previous work has found strong associations between IPV and adverse outcomes, including LBW and PTB among women [37, 38]. In this study, we found that IPV during pregnancy was significantly associated with an increased odds of adverse birth outcomes (OR = 2.50, 95% CI: 1.60–3.90). This finding was consistent with previous studies. In Iran, a significant association was found between IPV and preterm labor (OR = 1.54, 95% CI: 1.16–2.03) [13]. In Vietnam, exposure to IPV was found to be associated with an increased risk of PTB (OR = 13.3, 95% CI: 2.5–69.9) and an increased risk of LBW (OR = 9.4, 95% CI: 2.0–44.3) among pregnant women [20]. Similar results were found in the United States, where IPV exposure was shown to increase the odds of the prematurity (OR = 1.45, 95% CI: 1.29–1.62), LBW (OR = 1.57, 95% CI: 1.25–1.97), and respiratory problems (OR = 1.17, 95% CI: 1.04–1.32) [4]. A recent study in India using adjusted regression models also revealed a significant association between IPV and both miscarriage (OR = 1.35, 95% CI: 1.11–1.65) and stillbirth (OR = 1.36, 95% CI: 1.02–1.82) [39].

We also found that women exposed to different types of IPV had different effects on prenatal depression and adverse birth outcome. Previous studies found that exposure to psychological and sexual violence may

Table 4 Association of domestic violence during pregnancy+ prenatal depression and adverse birth outcomes

Variables	Model 1*		Model 2*	
	OR (95% CI)	P	OR (95% CI)	P
Prenatal depression	1.72 (1.11, 2.68)	0.0161	1.76 (1.13, 2.73)	0.0124
Domestic violence	1.67 (1.08, 2.56)	0.0202	–	–
Only psychological abuse	–	–	2.13 (1.08, 2.58)	0.0026

Model 1: Adjusted for maternal age, maternal education, maternal occupation, husbands' education, husbands' occupation, husbands' drinking and smoking characteristics, pregnancy related complications and abortion history, prenatal depression and overall domestic violence as independent factors;
Model 2: Adjusted for maternal age, maternal education, maternal occupation, husbands' education, husbands' occupation, husbands' drinking and smoking characteristics, pregnancy related complications and abortion history, prenatal depression and subtypes of domestic violence as independent factors

influence the pregnancy through alterations in women's psychological wellbeing and lifestyle habits. Poor psychological wellbeing, in turn, may lead to hypertension or preeclampsia, which may be associated with insufficient weight gain and PTB [40, 41]. We also found significant associations between psychological abuse and prenatal depression (OR = 2.04, 95% CI: 1.19–3.49) and between psychological abuse and adverse birth outcomes (OR = 2.13, 95% CI: 1.08–2.58). In addition, women experiencing psychological abuse combined with subtype of physical IPV or economic IPV had higher odds ratios of adverse birth outcomes, compared with women who were not exposed to abuse. Taken together, our results show that IPV exposure, especially to psychological abuse, was significantly associated with prenatal depression and with adverse birth outcomes. These findings were consistent with a previously conducted prospective cohort study of IPV during pregnancy and adverse pregnancy outcomes in Vietnam [20].

The present study had several limitations. First, because the data on IPV and depression during pregnancy were collected in a cross-sectional study, we cannot establish the temporal relation between these two conditions. Second, we did not consider experiences of IPV or depressive symptoms prior to pregnancy that might be a potential factor of prenatal depression. The separate and combined associations of these conditions before and during pregnancy with birth outcomes warrant further investigation. Third, we should be careful to generalize the data to the completely pregnant population because the finding was obtained from a city of central China.

Conclusions

This study has shown that IPV and prenatal depression were common among pregnant women in Wuhan, China. IPV was significantly associated with prenatal depression, and both IPV and prenatal depressive symptoms were associated with risk increasing of adverse birth outcomes, which are deleterious to maternal and newborn outcomes. The findings suggested that screening for IPV and prenatal depressive symptoms during prenatal care is necessary and might be helpful in reducing adverse outcomes for both mothers and newborns.

Abbreviations
AAS: The Abuse Assessment Screen; ABO: Adverse birth outcomes; aOR: Adjusted odds ratio; CES-D: The Center for Epidemiologic Studies-Depression scale; CI: Confidence interval; IPV: Intimate partner violence; LBW: Low birth weight; PTB: Preterm birth; WHO: World Health Organization

Acknowledgments
We are extremely grateful to all the mothers who took part in the study, to the nurses for their help in recruiting them. We thank Jennifer Barrett, PhD, from Liwen Bianji, Edanz Editing China (www.liwenbianji.cn/ac), for editing the English text of a draft of this manuscript.

Funding
The fund for this research was obtained from the Natural and Science Foundation of Hubei Province (2013CFB125). However, it had no role in the design of the study, collection, analysis, interpretation of data, and in writing the manuscript.

Authors' contributions
Conceived and designed the study: MS. Supervised and performed the survey, involved in participant recruitment and interpreted the analysis: HHY and RY. Involved in Collecting, managing and analysis of the data: XYJ. Drafted the manuscript, revised the paper upon reviewers' comments and wrote the final manuscript: HHY and MS. Critical review and thoroughly edited the manuscript: WB and GFX. WB and GFX also supported the suggestion and explanation on the data analysis of the manuscript. All authors read and approved the final manuscript.

Consent for publication
Not applicable.

Competing interests
The authors declare that they have no competing interests.

Author details
[1]Department of Anesthesiology, Tongji Hospital affiliated Tongji Medical College, Huazhong University of Science and Technology, Wuhan 430030, China. [2]Department of Maternal and Child Health, School of Public Health, Tongji Medical College, Huazhong University of Science and Technology, Wuhan 430030, China. [3]Department of Epidemiology, College of Public Health, University of Iowa, Iowa City, IA 52242, USA. [4]Center for Disabilities and Development, University of Iowa Stead Family Children's Hospital, Iowa City, IA 52242, USA. [5]Wuhan Children's Hospital (Wuhan Maternal and Child Healthcare Hospital), Tongji Medical College, Huazhong University of Science & Technology, Wuhan 430015, China.

References
1. Tjaden P. TNE: nature and consequences of intimate partner violence: findings from the National Violence against Women Survey. Washington, DC: Department of Justice; 2000.
2. Petersen R, Gazmararian JA, Spitz AM, Rowley DL, Goodwin MM, Saltzman LE, Marks JS. Violence and adverse pregnancy outcomes: a review of the literature and directions for future research. Am J Prev Med. 1997;13(5):366–73.
3. Shah PS, Shah J. Knowledge synthesis group on determinants of preterm LBWB: maternal exposure to domestic violence and pregnancy and birth outcomes: a systematic review and meta-analyses. J Women's Health (Larchmt). 2010;19(11):2017–31.
4. Pavey AR, Gorman GH, Kuehn D, Stokes TA, Hisle-Gorman E. Intimate partner violence increases adverse outcomes at birth and in early infancy. J Pediatr. 2014;165(5):1034–9.
5. Committee on Health Care for Underserved W. ACOG Committee opinion no. 518: intimate partner violence. Obstet Gynecol. 2012;119:412–7.
6. Hinkle SN, Laughon SK, Catov JM, Olsen J, Bech BH. First trimester coffee and tea intake and risk of gestational diabetes mellitus: a study within a national birth cohort. BJOG. 2015;122(3):420–8.
7. Devries KM, Kishor S, Johnson H, Stockl H, Bacchus LJ, Garcia-Moreno C, Watts C. Intimate partner violence during pregnancy: analysis of prevalence data from 19 countries. Reprod Health Matters. 2010;18(36):158–70.
8. Alhusen JL, Bullock L, Sharps P, Schminkey D, Comstock E, Campbell J. Intimate partner violence during pregnancy and adverse neonatal outcomes in low-income women. J Women's Health (Larchmt). 2014; 23(11):920–6.
9. Kita S, Yaeko K, Porter SE. Prevalence and risk factors of intimate partner violence among pregnant women in Japan. Health Care Women Int. 2014; 35(4):442–57.

10. Beydoun HA, Tamim H, Lincoln AM, Dooley SD, Beydoun MA. Association of physical violence by an intimate partner around the time of pregnancy with inadequate gestational weight gain. Soc Sci Med. 2011;72(6):867–73.

11. Velasco C, Luna JD, Martin A, Caño A, Martin-de-las-Heras S. Intimate partner violence against Spanish pregnant women: application of two screening instruments to assess prevalence and associated factors. Acta Obstet Gynecol Scand. 2014;93(10):1050–8.

12. Lukasse M, Schroll AM, Ryding EL, Campbell J, Karro H, Kristjansdottir H, Laanpere M, Steingrimsdottir T, Tabor A, Temmerman M, et al. Prevalence of emotional, physical and sexual abuse among pregnant women in six European countries. Acta Obstet Gynecol Scand. 2014;93(7):669–77.

13. Hassan M, Kashanian M, Roohi M, Yousefi H. Maternal outcomes of intimate partner violence during pregnancy: study in Iran. Public Health. 2014;128(5):410–5.

14. Onoh R, Umeora O, Ezeonu P, Onyebuchi A, Lawani O, Agwu U. Prevalence, pattern and consequences of intimate partner violence during pregnancy at Abakaliki Southeast Nigeria. Ann Med Health Sci Res. 2014;3(4):484–91.

15. Chan KL, Brownridge DA, Tiwari A, Fong DY, Leung WC, Ho PC. Associating pregnancy with partner violence against Chinese women. J Int Viol. 2011;26(7):1478–500.

16. Zhang Y, Zou S, Cao Y, Zhang Y. Relationship between domestic violence and postnatal depression among pregnant Chinese women. Int J Gynecol Obstet. 2012;116(1):26–30.

17. Jasinski JL. Pregnancy and domestic violence a review of the literature. Trauma Violence Abuse. 2004;5(1):47–64.

18. Alhusen JL, Bullock L, Sharps P, Schminkey D, Comstock E, Campbell J. Intimate partner violence during pregnancy and adverse neonatal outcomes in low-income women. J Women's Health. 2014;23(11):920–6.

19. Donovan BM, Spracklen CN, Schweizer ML, Ryckman KK, Saftlas AF. Intimate partner violence during pregnancy and the risk for adverse infant outcomes: a systematic review and meta-analysis. BJOG. 2016;123(8):1289–99.

20. Hoang TN, Van TN, Gammeltoft T, D WM, Nguyen Thi Thuy H, Rasch V. Association between intimate partner violence during pregnancy and adverse pregnancy outcomes in Vietnam: a prospective cohort study. PLoS One. 2016;11(9):e0162844.

21. McFarlane J, Parker B, Soeken K, Bullock L. Assessing for abuse during pregnancy. Severity and frequency of injuries and associated entry into prenatal care. JAMA. 1992;267(23):3176–8.

22. Alhusen JL, Ray E, Sharps P, Bullock L. Intimate partner violence during pregnancy: maternal and neonatal outcomes. J Women's Health (Larchmt). 2015;24(1):100–6.

23. Connelly CD, Hazen AL, Baker-Ericzen MJ, Landsverk J, Horwitz SM. Is screening for depression in the perinatal period enough? The co-occurrence of depression, substance abuse, and intimate partner violence in culturally diverse pregnant women. J Women's Health (Larchmt). 2013;22(10):844–52.

24. Witt WP, Wisk LE, Cheng ER, Hampton JM, Creswell PD, Hagen EW, Spear HA, Maddox T, Deleire T. Poor prepregnancy and antepartum mental health predicts postpartum mental health problems among US women: a nationally representative population-based study. Womens Health Issues. 2011;21(4):304–13.

25. Audi CA, Segall-Correa AM, Santiago SM, Andrade Mda G, Perez-Escamila R. Violence against pregnant women: prevalence and associated factors. Rev Saude Publica. 2008;42(5):877–85.

26. Gazmararian JA, Lazorick S, Spitz AM, Ballard TJ, Saltzman LE, Marks JS. Prevalence of violence against pregnant women. JAMA. 1996;275(24):1915–20.

27. Shamu S, Abrahams N, Temmerman M, Musekiwa A, Zarowsky C. A systematic review of African studies on intimate partner violence against pregnant women: prevalence and risk factors. PLoS One. 2011;6(3):e17591.

28. Leung W, Leung T, Lam Y, Ho P. The prevalence of domestic violence against pregnant women in a Chinesecommunity: social issues in reproductive health. Int J Gynecol Obstet. 1999;66(1):23–30.

29. Zhang Y, Zou S, Cao Y, Zhang Y. Correlation of domestic violence and postnatal depression among pregnant women. Chin J Clin Psychol. 2012;20(4):506–9.

30. Radoff LS. The CES-D scale: a self-report depression scale for research in the general population. Appl Psychol Meas. 1977;1:385–401.

31. Zhang J, Wu Z, Fang G, et al. Development of the Chinese age norms of CES-D in urban area. Chin Ment Health J. 2010;24(2):139–43.

32. Lawn JE, Gravett MG, Nunes TM, Rubens CE, Stanton C, Group GR. Global report on preterm birth and stillbirth (1 of 7): definitions, description of the burden and opportunities to improve data. BMC Pregn Childbirth. 2010;10(Suppl 1):S1.

33. World Health Organization Congenital anomalies. http://www.who.int/mediacentre/. Accessed 20 Oct 2018.

34. Jamshidimanesh M, Soleymani M, Ebrahimi E, Hosseini F. Domestic violence against pregnant women in Iran. J Family Reprod Health. 2013;7(1):7–10.

35. Saito A, Creedy D, Cooke M, Chaboyer W. Effect of intimate partner violence on antenatal functional health status of childbearing women in northeastern Thailand. Health Care Women Int. 2013;34(9):757–74.

36. James L, Brody D, Hamilton Z. Risk factors for domestic violence during pregnancy: a meta-analytic review. Violence Vict. 2013;28(3):359–80.

37. Grote NK, Bridge JA, Gavin AR, Melville JL, Iyengar S, Katon WJ. A meta-analysis of depression during pregnancy and the risk of preterm birth, low birth weight, and intrauterine growth restriction. Arch Gen Psychiatry. 2010;67(10):1012–24.

38. Fonseca-Machado Mde O, Alves LC, Monteiro JC, Stefanello J, Nakano AM, Haas VJ, Gomes-Sponholz F. Depressive disorder in pregnant Latin women: does intimate partner violence matter? J Clin Nurs. 2015;24(9–10):1289–99.

39. Dhar D, McDougal L, Hay K, Atmavilas Y, Silverman J, Triplett D, Raj A. Associations between intimate partner violence and reproductive and maternal health outcomes in Bihar, India: a cross-sectional study. Reprod Health. 2018;15(1):109.

40. Zhang Y, Zou S, Zhang X, Zhang Y. Correlation of domestic violence during pregnancy with plasma amino-acid neurotransmitter, cortisol levels and catechol-o-methyltransferase Val(158)met polymorphism in neonates. Asia Pac Psychiatry. 2013;5(1):2–10.

41. Zhang Y, Zhang YL, Zou SH, Zhang XH, Cao YP, Yang SC. Correlation between domestic violence in pregnancy and the levels of plasma amino acids and cortisol in the neonates. Zhonghua Nei Ke Za Zhi. 2008;47(3):209–12.

12

The pregnancy experience of Korean mothers with a prenatal fetal diagnosis of congenital heart disease

Yu-Mi Im[1], Tae-Jin Yun[2], Il-Young Yoo[3], Sanghee Kim[4], Juhye Jin[5] and Sue Kim[4*] ⊙

Abstract

Background: Prenatal diagnosis of fetal congenital heart disease (CHD) is becoming widely available but there is a lack of understanding on such expectant mothers' experiences during pregnancy. This was the first study to investigate the pregnancy experience of Korean mothers with a prenatal fetal diagnosis of CHD.

Methods: In-depth interviews were conducted with 12 mothers regarding their child's prenatal diagnosis of CHD and the adaptive processes during pregnancy. The data were transcribed and analyzed according to the grounded theory framework.

Results: When the diagnosis of fetal CHD was suspected, mothers desperately sought accurate information regarding CHD while hoping in vain for a misdiagnosis. When the definitive diagnosis was made, most pregnant women experienced psychological trauma and pain, framed in the stigma and burden of having an imperfect child. Provision of accurate health advice and emotional support by a multidisciplinary counseling team was crucial at this phase, forming recognition that CHD could be treated. When fetal movements were felt, mothers came to acknowledge the fetus as an independent being, and made their best efforts to protect the fetus from harmful external influences using traditional *TaeKyo* mindset and practices, which in turn, were helpful in restructuring the meaning of the pregnancy.

Conclusions: Mothers went through a dynamic process of adapting to the unexpected diagnosis of CHD, which was closely linked to being able to believe that their child could be treated. Early counseling with precise information on CHD, continuous provision of clear explanations on prognosis, sufficient emotional support, and well-designed prenatal education programs are the keys to an optimal outcome.

Keywords: Congenital heart disease, Prenatal diagnosis, Pregnancy, Experience, Grounded theory

Background

The incidence of congenital heart disease (CHD) is estimated as 8.8 in 1000 liveborn infants [1]. Congenital malformations are one of the leading causes of infant death in the United States and other developed nations, and critical CHD is responsible for more deaths than is any other type of malformation [2].

Among prenatal examinations performed during pregnancy, fetal echocardiography can be performed at first trimester [3, 4]. The cardiac screening examination,

* Correspondence: suekim@yuhs.ac
[4]College of Nursing, Mo-Im Kim Nursing Research Institute, Yonsei University, 50 Yonsei-ro, Seodaemun-gu, Seoul 03722, Korea
Full list of author information is available at the end of the article

however, is performed optimally between 18 and 22 weeks' gestational age and many anatomical structures can still be visualized satisfactorily beyond 22 weeks [5]. If fetal CHD is suspected, pregnant women are transferred to a tertiary medical institution that can provide an accurate prenatal diagnosis, specialized birth plans, neonatal intensive care, and emergency cardiac surgeries to increase the viability of the fetus [6–8].

Prenatal diagnosis of congenital anomaly creates an idiosyncratic situation. For newborns who do not have additional risk factors and their families pursued treatment, prenatal diagnosis reduced the risk of death with planned cardiac surgery [9]. But pregnant women who become aware of fetal CHD experience deep grief, anger, loss of affection for the fetus, and worry owing to the lack of information regarding the disease as well as its uncertain future [10]. A substantial proportion of mothers have been reported to exhibit evidence for traumatic stress, with nearly 40% exceeding clinical cutoff values for posttraumatic stress disorder [11]. Moreover, the parents may blame each other or feel guilty, thus leading to discord between them [12].

During this difficult phase, pregnant women consult with a variety of healthcare professionals to obtain information regarding the disease. Counseling provided by healthcare professionals is remarkably influential in the decision-making process [13, 14] and the particular role of nurses, such as empathizing with the parents' emotions, coordinating with other healthcare professionals on behalf of parents, and supporting the parents' decisions has also been reported [15]. Fully understanding the experience of women with fetal CHD, the disease, and its treatment trajectory is required of health professionals to provide high-quality healthcare. However, there have been no such studies in Korea, despite increasing numbers of CDH diagnosed through prenatal screening. Thus, the purpose of this study was to explore the overall pregnancy experience of women starting from the time when they were told of definite diagnosis of fetal CHD, up to when they gave birth, exploring the context of accepting and deciding to continue with the pregnancy.

Methods

This study used grounded theory to explore and understand the pregnancy experience of mothers who had been told that their child has CHD. Since the primary purpose of grounded theory is to explore the dominant social processes that exist within human interactions [16], this method was considered most appropriate for our study. We attempted to assess how the mothers, as human beings, developed the meanings of each event and communicated with their inner selves in a variety of situations they encountered over the course of their pregnancy. These meanings were constructed through social experience and self-reflection, and by assigning such meanings to events the mothers could determine their responses [16].

Participants

Mothers with a prenatal fetal diagnosis of CHD diagnosed by a specialist, who were willing to talk about their pregnancy experience were invited to participate in this study. Mothers were recruited through purposeful and theoretical sampling [16]. Exclusion criteria were infants with conditions associated with genetic disorders, such as Down's syndrome, and if there were other congenital defects, such as cleft lip and palate.

The interval between birth and participating in the interviews did not exceed 6 months, in order to minimize the influence of parenting after birth on the mothers' recollection of the pregnancy experience. The timing of interviews was carefully selected to avoid adding stress/anxiety to participating mothers, which could influence their recall. The issue of time frame (intervals ranging from 1 to 6 months), from birth to time of interview, depended on when the participant wished to be interviewed. Many interviews ($n = 6$) were done in the out-patient department, following the infant's surgery, upon individual contact and setting a time. The remaining half ($n = 6$) were done in the hospital when the infant's condition was stable (e.g., the day before expected discharge). Of the total of 12 mothers who participated in in-depth interviews, five mothers participated within 3 months and seven mothers between 4 and 6 months postpartum. The gestational age of the fetus at prenatal screening differed between mothers, ranging from the 21st to 33rd week of pregnancy.

Data collection

In-depth interviews were undertaken from February to November 2013, following approval by the institutional review board of the tertiary level hospital from which mothers were recruited. Mothers provided written consent regarding voluntary participation and publishing the data in anonymous form. To collect enough vivid descriptions regarding the pregnancy experience, the main question was "Let's recall the day when you were told that your baby had congenital heart defects. How did you feel about that and what was your reaction?" Most interviews were conducted in locations where participants felt comfortable, such as in their homes, at a counseling office in the hospital, or at the bedside of the infants following cardiac surgery. The researcher met the participants in casual attire rather than a hospital uniform to facilitate a natural, comfortable ambiance. Each mother participated in one to four interviews, with most participating two to three times. The first interview lasted for 1–2 h on a face-to-face basis, and additional interviews lasted for 30–60 min, either in person or by telephone. The researcher also took field notes and compiled analytical memos following the interviews, as a means of clarifying salient issues and preparing for the next interview.

Data analysis

The data were analyzed based on the methodology proposed by Strauss and Corbin following open coding, axial coding, and selective coding, and we proceeded simultaneously with the process of data collection, abiding by the constant comparative method at the stage of coding mentioned above [17]. This iterative process made it possible to compare the concepts generated during the process of data collection with the pre-existing concepts and to discover their differences and similarities.

The interviews were recorded with consent having been obtained from the participants. Recorded interviews were transcribed by an assistant, and the researcher double-checked the recording to validate or modify the transcripts. All interviews were conducted and transcribed in Korean, and analysis was carried out in Korean, in order to recognize subtle nuances and cultural contexts. The themes that emerged from the study were translated into English at the final stage, and verified by the research team for accuracy and relevance.

Results

General characteristics of the participants
The general characteristics of the 12 mothers who participated in this study are presented in Table 1. The median age of the participants was 31.5 years. Half were stay-at-home mothers, and the remainder had professional occupations such as bankers, teachers or others. For most participants, this was their first pregnancy. The gestational age when a fetal diagnosis of CHD was made ranged from 21 to 33 weeks, with the first counseling being provided by the hospital's counseling team between 22 and 36 weeks.

Progression of pregnancy in mothers with prenatal diagnosis of CHD
The chronological process following initial suspicion and confirmation of fetal CHD progressed along four phases, depicted by wavy arrows that reflect mothers'

fluctuating state: "Shock and pain from frustration and despair," "Phase of worries," "Recognition of the baby as a living human being," and "Restructuring and endeavoring to protect the baby" (Fig. 1). Mothers initially experienced psychological trauma upon the prenatal diagnosis of CHD of their child, suffered from inner conflicts between maintaining and terminating the pregnancy, became determined to maintain the pregnancy after becoming aware of fetal movement, and finally restructured their pregnancy experience of conceiving a fetus with cardiac anomalies. However, not every study participant underwent all of these phases consecutively, and some of them bypassed the first or second phases.

Phase of shock and pain
Because mothers had never imagined that their child would have any problem, they were shocked when they first heard about CHD. Mothers asked themselves what they had done wrong before their pregnancy and why this was happening to them. They were unable to determine what their next step should be and were greatly concerned about the fact that they knew nothing anything about the defects. Some did not even want to accept this baffling situation.

Why did this happen to me? My husband and I have never seen people around us who had babies with congenital heart defects. We were really sorry that God gave us a critically ill baby.

Table 1 General characteristics of the participants

Participant	Age group	GA at diagnosis (weeks)	GA at fetal counseling (weeks)	Timing of first interview (months)	Employment status	Birth order	Diagnosis
1	30s	23	23	6	Yes	1st	TGA with VSD, PS
2	20s	25	32	3	No	1st	FSV (AVSD, DORV, PS, TAPVR, Rt isomerism)
3	30s	23	26	6	Yes	1st	Truncus arteriosus
4	30s	25	26	5	Yes	1st	FSV (TA)
5	40s	27	27	3	Yes	2nd	TGA with VSD, PDA
6	30s	23	23	6	No	1st	FSV (Rt. Isomerism, DORV, CAVSD, PS, TAPVR
7	30s	34	37	3	No	1st	HLHS
8	30s	22	22	6	No	1st	DORV, VSD, CoA
9	20s	21	25	1	No	1st	FSV (DORV, DIRV, PS, ASD, rudimentary LV)
10	20s	25	26	4	No	1st	TOF
11	30s	23	32	1	Yes	2nd	PA with VSD, MAPCA
12	30s	22	27	4	Yes	1st	DORV, ASD

GA gestational age, *TGA* transposition of the great arteries, *VSD* ventricular septal defect, *PS* pulmonary stenosis, *FSV* functional single ventricle, *AVSD* atrioventricular septal defect, *DORV* double outlet right ventricle, *TAPVR* total anomalous pulmonary venous return, *Rt* right, *TA* tricuspid atresia, *PDA* patent ductus arteriosus, *HLHS* hypoplastic left heart syndrome, *CoA* coarctation of the aorta, *DIRV* double inlet right ventricle, *ASD* atrial septal defect, *LV* left ventricle, *TOF* tetralogy of Fallot, *PA* pulmonary atresia, *MAPCA* major aorto-pulmonary collateral artery

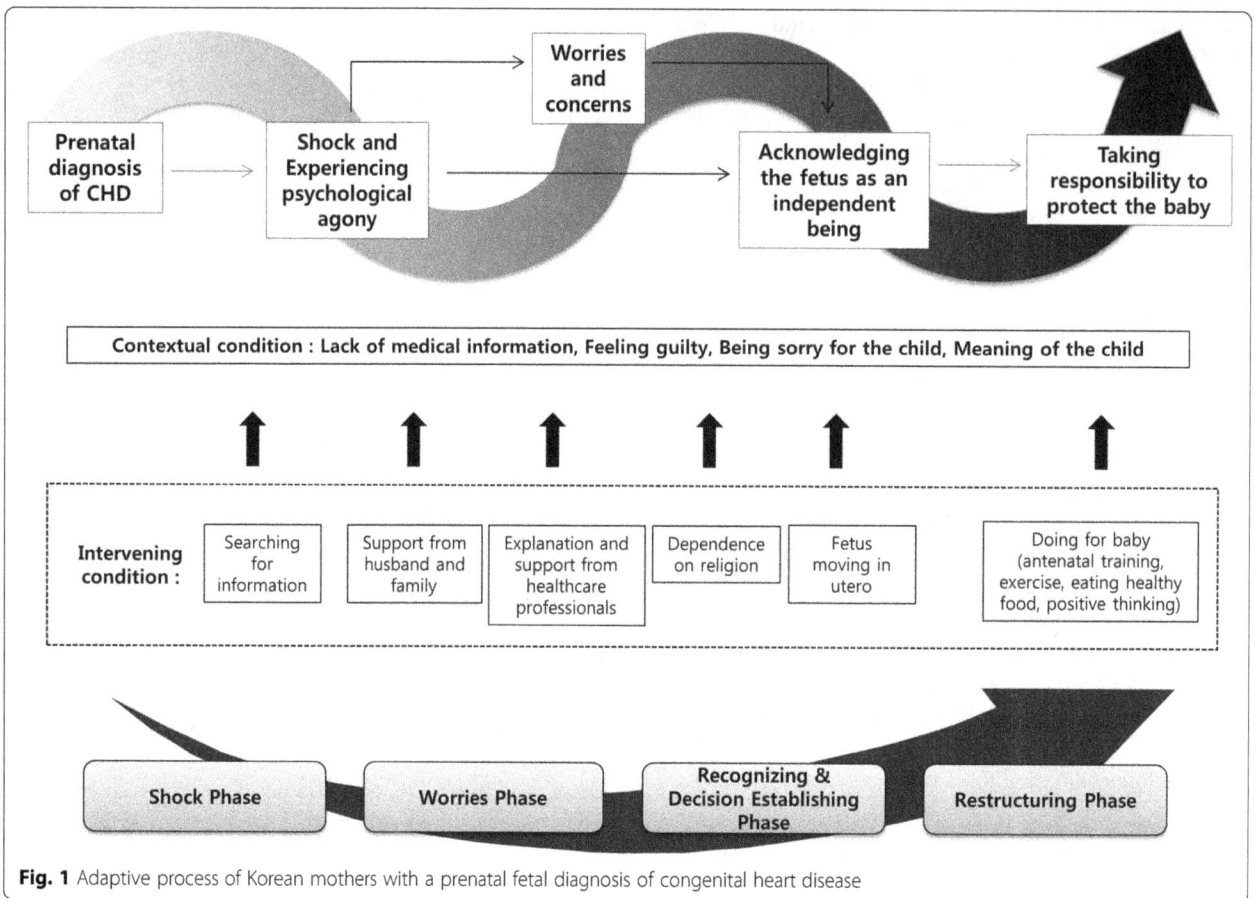

Fig. 1 Adaptive process of Korean mothers with a prenatal fetal diagnosis of congenital heart disease

I felt as if someone was hitting my head time and again, telling me that I would not be able to bear it. Actually, I thought to myself again and again that I could not accept this. Giving birth to a baby with an abnormal heart would never be a thing I could handle ... never ever!

In their search for as much information as possible about the cardiac anomalies, they often experienced difficulty in making sense of the information found online. Thus, the most prominent feelings reported by the pregnant mothers after the confirmation of fetal CHD were uncertainty, difficulty in accepting the diagnosis, psychological stress, depression, and loneliness. Two influential modes to help them overcome such difficulties at this phase were acquisition of precise information about the heart anomaly, and support from the husband and family members.

Phase of concern and worries
Although some mothers did not go through this phase, seven out of 12 participants entered the second stage of inner conflict immediately after being shocked by the recognition of fetal heart problems. They began to

agonize over whether or not they should maintain the pregnancy, as it conflicted with their cultural sense of duty to produce a healthy child. Termination of the pregnancy was occasionally proposed by the husband or other family members, framed in the stigma and burden of raising an imperfect child, which added to their distress and worries.

While I saw my baby as merely being sick, my mom thought the baby was completely 'abnormal,' like an alien. I could understand my mom because she is an old woman, not knowing about state-of-the-art medical technology. I thought my sister would see this matter differently. However, I was freaked out when my sister cautiously asked me whether I might consider therapeutic abortion. She said 'You'll be able to be pregnant easily next time, so why do you want to deliver an imperfect baby?'

Considering the baby, I felt I should go ahead with maintaining the pregnancy. Considering the rest of my life, however, I shouldn't. My thoughts were wandering from this side to that side like a pendulum. Thinking of my husband was the most painful part of my dilemma. When we got married, I promised I'd bear him a pretty and healthy baby ... I could have quietly given up the baby without him knowing at all. Actually, I knew several hospitals which could have done the job for me, but...

Some mothers immediately showed a determined attitude toward maintaining their pregnancy. For instance, women who became pregnant after failing several artificial fertilization procedures or having experienced miscarriages said they did not for a moment consider giving up the baby. Another participant stated that she did not consider an abortion because the fetus was a blessed gift from God, no matter how sick. Being able to have strong confidence in postnatal medical care and seeking assurance in religious beliefs were noted as influential ways to overcome the difficulties in this phase.

Recognition of the child as a living human being

Korean culture typically counts the baby's time spent in utero and the baby becomes 1 years-old at birth [18]. Such assumption of the fetus's being is tied to the practice of encouraging early prenatal interactions with the fetus, referred to as *TaeKyo*, a traditional concept thought to contribute to fetal development by focusing the pregnant mother's mind and behaviors throughout the pregnancy [19]. Although *TaeKyo* was not a focus in the initial phases of shock and worry, feeling fetal movements (quickening) brought the actual recognition of the fetus as a living human being. This propelled the mothers to more easily accept the baby and this phase was characterized by a shift to determined attitude to maintain the pregnancy. The most important intervention to overcome difficulties at this stage was the feeling of being connected with the baby through fetal movements.

It was a marvelous experience. I suddenly realized that something alive was in me. When I saw the ultrasound image of the baby's face, this realization became even more vivid and made me extremely happy.

The baby was most actively moving when I was driving. I used to talk to her 'Stop it!' If she was not moving, then I tapped my belly and talked to her again, 'Hey, what are you doing? Are you sleeping?' As a matter of fact, I became nervous when she was not moving, thinking that something might go wrong. This 'hide-and-seek' game continued till the day she was born. I felt happy when she was kicking my belly. I felt as if she was sending me a signal that 'Mommy, I'm here, and I will be OK later on after I'm born!

Restructuring the pregnancy experience

At this phase mothers began to actively engage in a *TaeKyo* mindset, i.e., maintaining a peaceful, optimistic, and affirmative attitude, and began to ease away from the difficulties they had been through and form a different idea regarding the meaning of conceiving a child with CHD. In this phase mothers actively took on responsibility to protect the fetus via specific *TaeKyo* practices, such as eating nutritious foods and working out regularly in hopes of optimizing the postnatal condition of their child. As such, actively enacting *TaeKyo* mindset and practices was a way to restructure and solidify the meaning of their pregnancy and overcome prior difficulties.

Yoga was one of the things I started to do after I decided to hang on to my baby. They taught me how to do abdominal breathing, and I felt as if my baby's heart and lung function improved as I breathed using my abdominal muscles. I don't know the scientific basis of this, but I just wanted to help my baby overcome the difficult surgeries after birth using his strong heart and lungs.

On prenatal counseling, I learned that the birth weight needs to be good enough for my baby to safely undergo the planned surgical procedures. The counselor told me I should eat meat, fruits, vegetables, and other nutritious foods as much as I could. I didn't like to eat meat before pregnancy, and I didn't even get to eat any meat after conception due to morning sickness. However, I began to eat meat every day, hoping that the birth weight would be greater than 3 kilograms. It was the only thing I could actually do for my baby.

Discussion

This was the first study to explore the experience of Korean women with a prenatal fetal diagnosis of CHD, starting from time of confirmed diagnosis to their adaptive process over time. Mothers within 6 months of delivery were invited to participate as we felt that including longer postnatal periods could incur greater recollection bias. The primary author's clinical experience with such mothers provided assurance that this time frame (3–6 months) allows for basic adjustment of the mother-infant while still being a valid time point for thinking back on their pregnancy. The pregnancy experiences of mothers is this study can be understood as the process of transition, from initial shock and agony to endeavoring to protect their child. It was obvious that they initially had a difficult time and experienced pain and shock. However, as the mothers finally acknowledged the fetus as an independent being, they began to do their utmost to protect their fetus from any harmful influences that might prompt the termination of the pregnancy.

When the mothers were told that their child had CHD, the majority were initially in shock, hoped in vain for a misdiagnosis, and attempted to gain information regarding the CHD. These findings were consistent with previous reports from Western countries that pregnant women who discover congenital deformities in their unborn child experience shock regardless of the severity or curability of the malformation [20, 21]. In a study investigating the experience of expectant mothers discovering fetal congenital deformities, it was difficult even for mothers who were professional nurses to accept the unexpected diagnosis [10].

Our study confirmed the strong influence of spousal and family members' attitude early on at diagnosis. We found this especially in relation to culturally engrained beliefs about gendered duties and social norms about the potential responsibility of the mother. This is parallel to studies in Asia that have noted that if a baby is born prematurely or with a low birth-weight, the mother may even be blamed by family or relatives for not observing the cultural practices appropriately, thus causing physical harm to the fetus [22]. Blame and stigma in Confucian-based cultures such as Korea should be considered and healthcare professionals can actively involve husbands and family members to understand CHD first-hand, and engage them to support the expectant mother.

Fetal movements, which can strengthen the bond between mother and child [23], were especially influential in facilitating the process of acceptance, and can be used by healthcare professionals as a point of reference when interacting with mothers of fetal CHD. Cultural practices of *TaeKyo* were tangible ways to solidify restructuring of the meaning of the pregnancy, likely related to its self-regulatory nature [24]. In addition to encouraging psychological and emotional preparations for becoming a mother, *TaeKyo* also has positive influence on maternal identity after childbirth [19]. *TaeKyo* reflects the responsibility of not only the expectant mother but also of the family and surrounding community [18], and can be a way to strengthen maternal-fetal attachment and self-efficacy in dealing with high risk pregnancy situations [24]. Healthcare professionals working with Korean mothers can encourage the cultural code of *TaeKyo* not only in its behavioral aspect aiming to maximize healthy fetal development, but also as a way to encourage development of a new view of the pregnancy as well as maternal identity.

In the initial phase of learning of the diagnosis, quick referral to a specialist and timely counseling is most important, supplemented by regular contacts with healthcare

professionals. In the early phase, healthcare professionals can actively provide mothers and family members with accurate knowledge of the pathophysiology of CHD to enable informed decision-making regarding maintaining the pregnancy. Seeking information is a common way to cope with a stressful event, and previous studies have consistently described the significance of as much information as possible at the point of diagnosis [14, 25, 26]. When having confidence that CHD is curable, expectant mothers were able to accept the diagnosis and began to do whatever they could to protect the "baby while in my body". In line with reports that mothers with fetal congenital anomaly needed more information throughout their pregnancy than their counterparts with a healthy pregnancy [20], during the course of pregnancy, our participants continuously searched for useful information and also sought information regarding the postnatal treatment process. However, the sources were often cases posted on online communities and it is imperative that maternal and neonatal professionals be a direct source of information through regular counseling. Emergency phone numbers may also be provided to allow mothers consistent access to information and support during pregnancy and after birth. The rapport established during pregnancy can continue to grow after childbirth and can have further positive impact on the continual process of their infant's treatments.

Nearly all the infants in this study had serious conditions of CHD. Yet as the purpose of this study was to explore the general pregnancy experience of mothers with prenatal diagnosis of fetal CHD, we did not analyze whether disease severity might have exerted an influence. We found that most mothers interviewed did not seem to fully grasp the implications of severity, but struggled with the diagnosis itself, which essentially prompted this exploratory study. Future studies could further determine whether the pregnancy process is different according to the severity of heart disease or whether it may differ depending on timing of diagnosis or counseling period.

Conclusions

Childbirth is considered as one of the most important life events not only for a mother, but a family as a whole. This research found that pregnant Korean women who learned that their fetus had CHD through prenatal screening experienced pain and shock, worry, recognition of the fetus as a human being, and, finally, restructuring of the pregnancy experience. Interventions by the healthcare professionals in this field need to be specific for each phase of transition. As better understanding is gained of the specific psychological transition undergone by these pregnant women, more appropriate and timely intervention may be enabled. At the initial point of encounter, healthcare providers can seek establishing a secure rapport with the mother, her spouse, and the immediate family. Clinical implications for healthcare providers also include the provision of clear information that is built up and repeated throughout the pregnancy so that expectant mothers can have factual and well-grounded understanding that CHD is treatable, thus avoiding an overly pessimistic view of the future. While the findings of this study may be more applicable to first time pregnancies, creating well-designed education programs and/or support groups for these mothers may be helpful measures that provide continuity and support. As spirituality and religiosity was an important aspect for this sample of Korean mothers, modes of spiritual expression may also be encouraged, and support from their faith community may provide additional benefit for these women.

Acknowledgements
The authors wish to thank the participants of this study, who shared their stories and lives with us.

Funding
Not applicable.

Authors' contributions
Yu-Mi Im and Sue Kim were responsible for designing the study, data collection and analysis, and overall write up of the manuscript. Tae-Jin Yun contributed to acquisition of the data and critically reviewing and revising the manuscript. Il-Young Yoo, Sanghee Kim, and Juhye Jin were involved in analysis and interpretation of the data and critically reviewing and revising the manuscript. All authors have agreed to be accountable for all aspects of the work in ensuring that questions related to the accuracy or integrity of any part of the work are appropriately investigated and resolved.

Competing interests
The authors declare that they have no competing interests.

Author details
[1]Department of Nursing, Seoul Women's College of Nursing, Seoul, South Korea. [2]Division of Pediatric Cardiac Surgery, Asan Medical Center, University of Ulsan College of Medicine, Seoul, South Korea. [3]College of Nursing, Yonsei University, Seoul, South Korea. [4]College of Nursing, Mo-Im Kim Nursing Research Institute, Yonsei University, 50 Yonsei-ro, Seodaemun-gu, Seoul 03722, Korea. [5]Department of Nursing, College of Health and Life Science, Korea National University of Transportation, Jeungpyeong-gun, South Korea.

References

1. McElhinney DB, Wernovsky G. Outcomes of neonates with congenital heart disease. Curr Opin Pediatr. 2001;13(2):104–10.

2. Mahle WT, Newburger JW, Matherne GP, Smith FC, Hoke TR, Koppel R, et al. Role of pulse oximetry in examining newborns for congenital heart disease: a scientific statement from the AHA and AAP. Pediatrics. 2009;124(2):823–36.

3. Vayna AM, Veduta A, Duta S, Panaitescu AM, Stoica S, Buinoiu N, et al. Diagnosis of fetal structural anomalies at 11 to 14 weeks. J Ultrasound Med. 2018;24 [Epub ahead of print].

4. Hutchinson D, McBrien A, Howley L, Yamamoto Y, Sekar P, Motan T, et al. First-trimester fetal echocardiography: identification of cardiac structures for screening from 6 to 13 Weeks' gestational age. J Am Soc Echocardiogr. 2017;30(8):763–72.

5. International Society of Ultrasound in Obstetrics and Gynecology, Carvalho JS, Allan LD, Chaoui R, Copel JA, GR DV, et al. ISUOG Practice Guidelines (updated): sonographic screening examination of the fetal heart. Ultrasound Obstet Gynecol. 2013;41(3):348–59.

6. Verheijen PM, Lisowski LA, Stoutenbeek P, Hitchcock JF, Brenner JI, Copel JA, et al. Prenatal diagnosis of congenital heart disease affects preoperative acidosis in the newborn patient. J Thorac Cardiovasc Surg. 2001;121(4):798–803.

7. Tworetzky W, McElhinney DB, Reddy VM, Brook MM, Hanley FL, Silverman NH. Improved surgical outcome after fetal diagnosis of hypoplastic left heart syndrome. Circulation. 2001;103(9):1269–73.

8. Blyth M, Howe D, Gnanapragasam J, Wellesley D. The hidden mortality of transposition of the great arteries and survival advantage provided by prenatal diagnosis. BJOG. 2008;115(9):1096–100.

9. Holland BJ, Myers JA, Woods CR Jr. Prenatal diagnosis of critical congenital heart disease reduces risk of death from cardiovascular compromise prior to planned neonatal cardiac surgery: a meta-analysis. Ultrasound Obstet Gynecol. 2015;45(6):631–8.

10. Upham M, Medoff-Cooper B. What are the responses & needs of mothers of infants diagnosed with congenital heart disease? MCN Am J Matern Child Nurs. 2005;30(1):24–9.

11. Rychik J, Donaghue DD, Levy S, Fajardo C, Combs J, Zhang X, et al. Maternal psychological stress after prenatal diagnosis of congenital heart disease. J Pediatr. 2013;162(2):302–7 e1.

12. Chenni N, Lacroze V, Pouet C, Fraisse A, Kreitmann B, Gamerre M, et al. Fetal heart disease and interruption of pregnancy: factors influencing the parental decision-making process. Prenat Diagn. 2012;32(2):168–72.

13. Menahem S, Grimwade J. Prenatal counselling - helping couples make decisions following the diagnosis of severe heart disease. Early Hum Dev. 2005;81(7):601–7.

14. Lalor JG, Devane D, Begley CM. Unexpected diagnosis of fetal abnormality: women's encounters with caregivers. Birth. 2007;34(1):80–8.

15. Rempel GR, Cender LM, Lynam MJ, Sandor GG, Farquharson D. Parents' perspectives on decision making after antenatal diagnosis of congenital heart disease. J Obstet Gynecol Neonatal Nurs. 2004;33(1):64–70.

16. Blumer H. The methodological position of Symbolic Interactionism, in Symbolic Interactionism: Perspective and Method. Berkeley: University of California Press; 1969. p. 1–60.

17. Strauss A, Corbin J. Basics of qualitative research: techniques and procedures for developing grounded theory. 2nd ed. London: Sage; 1998.

18. Kim Y. Conceptualizing prenatal care: recent research and the application of TaeKyo, Korean traditional beliefs and practices. Health Care Women Int. 2015;36(1):26–40.

19. Chae HJ, Song JE, Kim S. Predictors of maternal identity of Korean primiparas. J Korean Acad Nurs. 2011;41(6):733–41.

20. Askelsdottir B, Conroy S, Rempel G. From diagnosis to birth: parents' experience when expecting a child with congenital anomaly. Adv Neonatal Care. 2008;8(6):348–54.

21. Maijala H, Astedt-Kurki P, Paavilainen E, Väisänen L. Interaction between caregivers and families expecting a malformed child. J Adv Nurs. 2003; 42(1):37–46.

22. Choi H, Van Riper M. Adaptation in families of children with Down syndrome in east Asian countries: an integrative review. J Adv Nurs. 2016. https://doi.org/10.1111/jan.13235 [Epub ahead of print].

23. Cranley MS. Development of a tool for the measurement of maternal attachment during pregnancy. Nurs Res. 1981;30(5):281–4.
24. Seo JY, Kim W, Dickerson SS. Korean immigrant women's lived experience of childbirth in the United States. J Obstet Gynecol Neonatal Nurs. 2014; 43(3):305–17.
25. Garvin BJ, Kim CJ. Measurement of preference for information in U.S. and Korean cardiac catheterization patients. Res Nurs Health. 2000;23(4):310–8.
26. Grandjean H, Larroque D, Levi S. The performance of routine ultrasonographic screening of pregnancies in the Eurofetus study. Am J Obstet Gynecol. 1999;181(2):446–54.

13

Determinants of client satisfaction to skilled antenatal care services at Southwest of Ethiopia

Serawit Lakew[1*], Alaso Ankala[2] and Fozia Jemal[3]

Abstract

Background: Patient satisfaction to Antenatal care services has traditionally been linked to the quality of services given and the extent to which specific needs are met. Even though data in this area was limited in Ethiopia, improving quality of care was one of the strategies in health sector development program IV. This study, therefore, attempted to assess client satisfaction to skilled antenatal care services in the study area.

Methods and materials: A cross-sectional facility based survey was conducted among women who were attending antenatal care clinic, using quantitative method triangulated with qualitative data collection. Participants were selected using systematic sampling method according to the flow pregnant women to the antenatal care clinics. The study was carried out in all functional public health centers in the district. During the survey, 405 women were interviewed. A logistic regression model was applied to control for confounders.

Results: Out of the total respondents, overall satisfied to skilled antenatal care services were about 277(68%). The most common specific component of antenatal care that had good-satisfaction by the respondents was "Privacy" at examination (81.7%). Most satisfied health education session was "Diet and nutrition" session (82.2%). Absence of sonar test, no doctor and long waiting time were commonest causes of dissatisfaction. Respondents who have ≥ 2 previous antenatal care visit were 3 times more likely (AOR = 2.93; 95% CI, 1.21, 7.12) to have satisfaction to antenatal care services as compared to those with ≤ 1 visit. Women whose current visit fourth were 9 times more likely (AOR = 9.02, 95% CI; 1.76, 46.1) to be satisfied for antenatal services than those who were in the first visit. Women with family monthly income of $US 25–100 per month were 60% (AOR = 0.4, 95% CI; 0.2, 0.8) less likely to have satisfaction by skilled antenatal care services than those who had monthly household income below $US 25.

Conclusion and recommendation: Women who reported good-satisfaction to overall skilled antenatal care services were highest as compared to previous Ethiopian study findings. Demographic, economic, obstetric and distance factors were independent predictors of satisfaction to skilled antenatal care services. Non natives must be encouraged to seek satisfying services.

Keywords: Satisfaction, Skilled antenatal care, Women, Southwest of Ethiopia

* Correspondence: lserawit@yahoo.com
[1]Department of Nursing and Midwifery, Arbaminch University, Arba Minch, Ethiopia
Full list of author information is available at the end of the article

Background

Pregnancy is a very important event from both social and medical point of view. ANC is an opportunity to advice the women on how to prepare for complications and promote the benefit of skilled attendance at birth [1].

W.H.O recommends that pregnant women should feel welcome at clinics for ANC in that it should be user-friendly. Examinations and tests should be carried at times that suit the woman. The teamwork between professionals and the pregnant woman is decisive for the safety of the woman and her fetus [2]. Every woman has the right to obtain recommended services of ANC from a skilled attendant at her pregnancy. A skilled attendant is not only trained to attend to normal pregnancies but also to recognize and manage complications and make referrals to hospital if more advanced care is needed. Women in rural areas were most at risk of giving birth and ANC services in the absence of skilled attendant [3, 4].

Ratings of women satisfaction for ANC indicated higher across developing countries and vary from country to country [5–9]. Studies found that overall satisfaction was highest in Cameroon and Egypt. In Cameroon, it was about 96.9% satisfied [10]. In Egypt, more than 90% reported satisfied for waiting time in lab results, Staff help, trust the doctor followed by cleanness of the center, privacy, most of accessibility items, and most of physician performance items. Least satisfied (below 30%) for location of the center, health education program, and explanation of the problems by physicians [11].

In Riyadh, about 87.7% pregnant women attending ANC felt unhappy because they had to wait up to 1 hour before being seen by the physician. About 63.1% were satisfied with information regarding their treatment. Around 18.9% thought that information was not enough and 17.25% reported they did not receive any information about their treatment [12].

In Kenya, about 96% of women who attended FI ANC clinics and 97% who attended NI ANC clinics were either "satisfied" or "very satisfied" with their clinic visit. A 'very poor' grade of satisfaction was considered to be a weak area of antenatal services. The dissatisfaction expressed mainly related to the process of imparting health education (such as: commitment, availability of time and language barrier) and not to the availability of health education material [13].

In Nigeria, most respondents were satisfied by the services given at the clinic (81.1%). Sitting arrangement was most satisfied (97.9%). Toilet and bathroom facilities were least satisfied (39.3 and 38.1% respectively). About 91.6% respondents reported "diet and nutrition" more satisfied during the interactive session than others. Prevention of cervical cancer was least discussed topic (65.7%) [14]. Obafemi Awolowo University study findings added that about 55% of women attending ANC clinic were satisfied with the quality of health talk. Around 72.6% were satisfied by the opinion that the services of the hospital were good and met their needs. About 53.7% agreed with the competency of the hospital staff. About 39.1% agreed with timely response of the staff and 20.5% on the opinion that the staffs were friendly and polite [15].

In various African country, Continued utilization of ANC services in the future pregnancy was directly linked to the satisfaction of the clients ($p < 0.05$) [14]. Significant satisfaction was also observed for being attending in public centers over private in Cameroon and those who served in Mendera Kochi and Higher Two Centers over others at Jimma town of Ethiopia [10, 16]. Those who have no formal education, attended primary education, monthly income < 500 birr and between 750 and 1000 birr, planned pregnancy and no history of stillbirth had significant associations for satisfied ANC services over their counter parts at $p < 0.05$ [16].

In Cameroon, significant association was observed for good satisfaction at their first pregnancy, the sitting area comfort, and competence of staff as compared to its counterparts [10]. Pakistan qualitative discussants reported, distant location of facilities, lack of functional equipment, medicines and supplies as perceived poor satisfaction [17]. Previous Ethiopian studies focused on the relationship between women's satisfaction and the provision and utilization of health care services [18]. No data could have been found on specific component of services satisfaction in Ethiopia in general and the study area in particular. This study, therefore, attempted to place its contribution through its findings.

Conceptual frame work

As indicated by Fig. 1, this conceptual frame work was adopted from one systematic review on women satisfaction to maternity care services in developing world, since it matches with this local system [9]. ANC services satisfaction was one component with background characteristics, provider factors, obstetrics factors and amenities were independent predictors. The frame work was adjusted to local system for to make it more convenient (Fig. 1).

Methods

Study design and setting

Health facility based cross-sectional study was conducted from Jan 1 to March 12, 2016. Health Facility includes Hospitals, Health Centers, Health Posts and Private Clinics. Arba Minch Zuria was one of the districts in the southwest of Ethiopia. It was located in the Great Rift Valley. As per the report of district health department statistics office, it had 30 kebeles (kebele is the lowest administrative state in Ethiopia) and a total population of 202,495 of whom 100,842 are men and 101,653

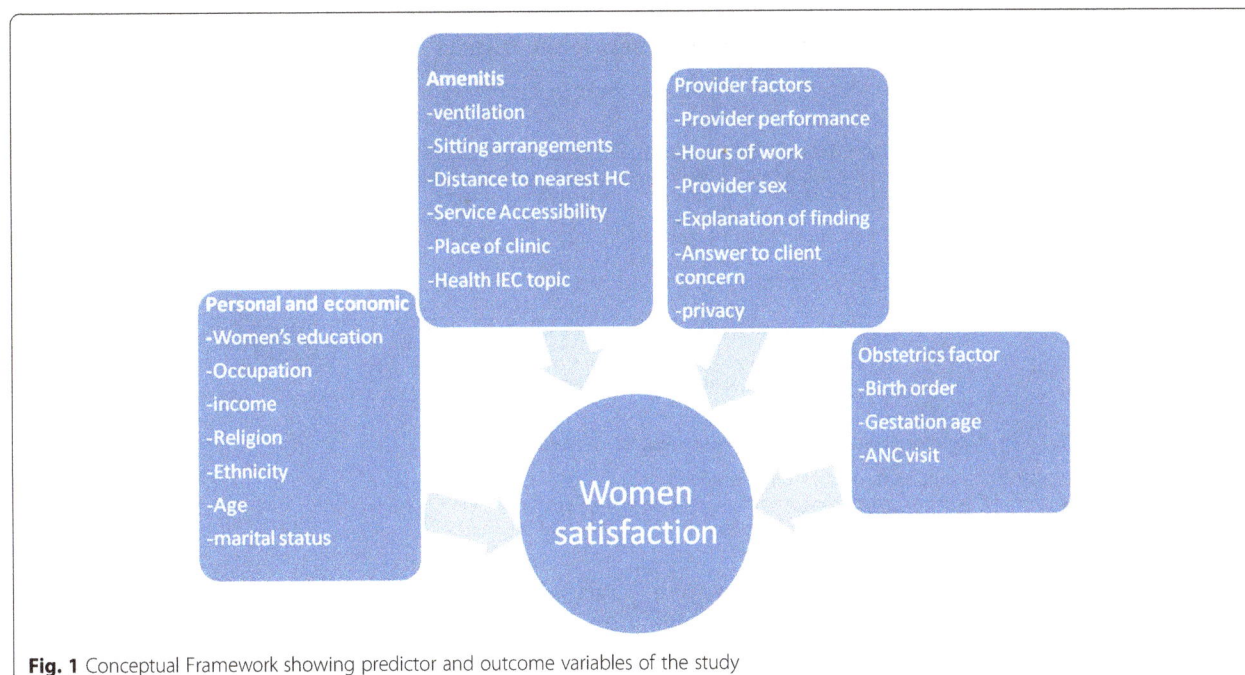

Fig. 1 Conceptual Framework showing predictor and outcome variables of the study

women. The district was located some 454kms south-west of Addis Ababa. The district had no any functional hospitals. But, it had five functional health centers and about thirty health posts (staffed by Health Extension Workers who are non-skilled providers) and private clinics together [19, 20]. The private clinics in the study region had no routine ANC services, since it had service fee and costly. Routine ANC services exist only in government health centers because services were free. In the district, skilled providers exist in the public health centers and private clinics only. Health Centers, therefore, were selected as study unit.

Sample size and sampling procedure

Sample size was determined by using single population proportion (SPP) formula based on the assumptions of 95% confidence level, 60.4% p-value (previous Rural Ethiopian study) and a 10% contingency. Accordingly, the total sample size was 405 women participant. Systematic sampling technique was used to select the study subjects. Number of Participants in each health centers was estimated based on three steps. First, total catchment population to each health centers were obtained from district health offices, department of statistics. Next, estimated proportion (N) of pregnancy in the catchment population of each health centers (using 4.5% of the whole population [21]) was obtained. Finally, the number of attendance for ANC (using 34% [22]) within the total estimated pregnancy was calculated in each health center. Respondents (n) who were registered for antenatal care during data collection at post-procedure

period were interviewed by systematic sampling technique until the required sample size was achieved in each health center. The Kth value was calculated based on number of registered for ANC of the day divided by expected sample a day (in each health center). From the first K^{th} values, one woman was selected by lottery method. The consecutive woman was selected by every k^{th} value. Also consider that ANC registration was performing in the morning for rural Ethiopian Health facility as tradition (Fig. 2).

For qualitative method, a convenience sampling technique was used to select pregnant women participant for the FGD by taking health center as homogeneity criteria. Accordingly, 10 FGDs were purposively selected with 2 FGDs in each of five active health centers. Selected respondents were not participant on quantitative. FGDs were conducted on two occasions with different days after the end of quantitative interview. It was accomplished by same data collectors under supervision.

Questionnaire development and measurement

Questionnaire was adapted from previous similar studies in the abroad [11] and adjusted in the local system. The questions and statements were grouped and arranged according to the particular that they can address. After extensive revision, the final version of the English questionnaire was developed. An individual who were expert for English and Amharic languages translated the English version into Amharic and the vice versa. For quantitative method: data were collected using face-to-face client interview questionnaires (by exit

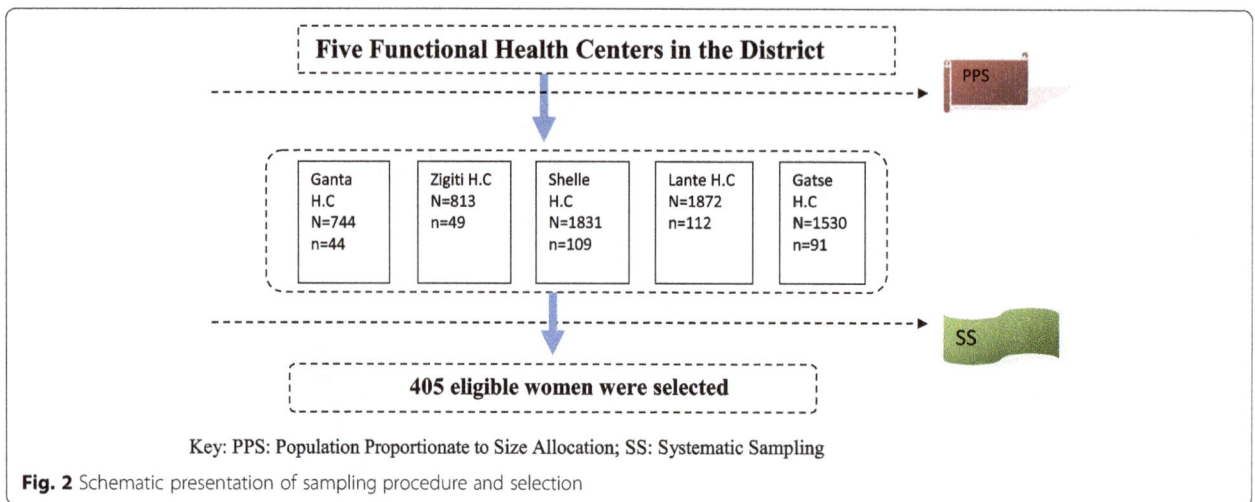

Fig. 2 Schematic presentation of sampling procedure and selection

interview). Having skilled Antenatal Care services were those participant who had ANC by skilled Health personnel, such as Nurse, Midwife, Health Officer and/ or Doctor at Health Facility. Having good satisfaction to Skilled Antenatal Care services were those women who answered 'good' to satisfaction questions in general and the vice versa for poor satisfaction. Predictor variables included in the data collection tool were demographic and Socio-economic variables; obstetrics variables; provider and staff variables; and amenities. For qualitative method: Focus group interview guideline was used to guide and probe the FGDs. The FGD interview guideline includes probing questions on areas of care clients satisfied and areas of care clients not satisfied. About 6–12 volunteered discussants were selected for each FGD session from each health centers. Every participant had given chance to talk as per the need to talk.

Statistical analysis

For quantitative method, after data collection each questionnaire was manually checked for completeness and then coded. After this validation, data were entered using EPI INFO version 3.5.2 and exported to SPSS statistical software package windows version 20 for analysis. Descriptive and summary statistics were used to describe the study population by variables of interest based on conceptual framework and for outliers. The degree of association between independent and dependent variables were described using crude and adjusted odds ratio. Bivariate analysis was applied to examine the association between each of the independent variables and satisfaction of ANC services. Multivariate statistical method used in the analysis was logistic regression model to control confounders. For qualitative methods, FGD data transcribed into English language verbatim, read critically and essential themes were identified. Ideas related to

various themes were color coded and then organized into concepts and presented using narratives. The result was presented in tri-angulations with the quantitative data using subjects verbatim as illustrations.

Data quality control

Data Collection tool was adopted and pretested [11]. Three days Training was given to data collectors and supervisors. Every day, completed questionnaires were reviewed and checked for completeness and relevance by the supervisors. All the necessary feedback was offered to data collectors in the next morning before the actual procedure. Data checked for completeness, coded, entered into computer, cleaned, and frequency checked for outliers and missing values before analysis.

Ethical issues

Ethical clearance was obtained from Arba Minch College of Health Sciences Research and Publication core process (RPCP) and Southern National regional state Health Bureau. The study was commenced after letter of cooperation written to each catchment health facility administrators from Zonal administrators (ZHB). Informed written consent was secured to all study subjects. Each respondent was informed for the objective of the study and assurance of confidentiality, risks and benefits. List of Colleges Ethics committee includes: Alemayehu Bekele Kassahun, Addisu Alemayehu Gube, Tarekegn Tadesse Hunede, and Bereket Workalemahu Ayele.

Results

Socio-demographic and personal characteristics

Of the total 405 sample, the response rate was 100%. Of the age distribution of the women, about 315 (77.8%) of the participant were the dominant group of 20–34 years. The mean age of the participant was 27.6 years ± 5.6 SD.

Concerning woman education, more than half 203 (50.1%) had reported no history of formal education. Gamo ethnic group were the dominant 346 (85.4%) over others among the attendee participated. Except the few, most of women arrived the health facility traveling ≥ 1 km from their home, around 323 (79.8%) (Table 1).

Table 1 Independent variables used in the analysis categories and percentage distribution, Arba Minch Zuria district, Southwest Ethiopia, March 2016

Variable	Status of Satisfaction, (n = 405)	
	Good satisfaction, n (%)	Poor satisfaction, n (%)
Age		
< 20 yrs	26(6.4)	16(4.0)
20-34 yrs	212(52.3)	103(25.4)
≥ 35 yrs	39(9.6)	9(2.2)
Woman education		
No education	153(37.8)	50(12.3)
primary	81(20.0)	56(13.8)
Secondary+	43(10.6)	22(5.4)
Distance to the nearest HC		
< 1 km	42(10.4)	40(9.9)
≥ 1 km	235(58.0)	88(21.7)
Ethnicity		
Gamo	255(63.0)	91(22.5)
Welayta	16(4.0)	24(5.9)
Others[a]	6(1.5)	13(3.2)
Birth order (n = 318)[d]		
1	48(15.1)	32(10.1)
2–3	106(33.3)	47(14.8)
4–5	49(15.4)	14(4.4)
6+	19(6.0)	3(0.9)
Previous ANC visit		
< 2 visit	195(48.1)	110(27.2)
≥ 2 visit	82(20.2)	18(4.4)
Marital Status		
Married	274(67.7)	118(29.1)
Others[b]	3(0.7)	10(2.5)
Religion		
Orthodox	123(30.4)	67(16.5)
Protestant	129(31.9)	58(14.3)
Others[c]	25(6.2)	3(0.7)
Family Monthly Income (n = 360)[d] (in $US)		
< 25	85(23.6)	23(6.4)
25–50	105(29.2)	65(18.1)
> 50	53(14.7)	29(8.1)

N.B: [a] include Zayse and Amhara, [b] widowed, divorced & single, [c] Muslim, catholic, traditional, [d] had missing values

Regarding respondents religion, Ethiopian Orthodox and Protestant Christianity religion followers alone account for 377 (93.1%) of the respondents. This showed the two religion dominance in the study region. Birth order of majority of woman was between 2 to 5 among the study participants, about 67.9%. When observing income, net monthly income of the women as family income grouping was higher in middle income categories ($US 25–50), accounting 218 (53.8%) of respondents. The median monthly income of the family was $US 37.5 (Table 1).

Satisfaction by components of skilled ANC services

Overall satisfaction was classified as poor or good satisfaction. Most women were satisfied with the services offered, about 277(68%). Satisfaction among components of services range from 24 to 82% satisfied. More importantly, satisfaction status was specifically described based on main components of services for Skilled Antenatal Care. Regarding accessibility for services, more women satisfied for staff hours of work 247 (61%) and sitting arrangements 289 (71.4%). Half and more of the women were satisfied by cleanness of the Center 241 (59.5%) and Toilet facility 226 (55.8%) (Table 2 and Fig. 3).

Provider "examination time" client satisfied was far large 309 (76.3%) among others within "performance of provider" responses category as women report suggested and relatively lower responses observed in "explanation of results of investigation", about 241 (59.5%). Major 'poor satisfaction' response in this category was 'location of the center' among others, about 211 (52.1%). Regarding privacy, poor-satisfaction report was 74 (18.3%), which is the lowest of all and the vice versa was the highest (Table 2).

Only about a third of the women had good satisfaction to explanation of the problem, explanation of rationale of the investigation on provider performance component, and delivering of the information in staff performance component, about (33.1, 31.6, and 33.6%), respectively (Table 2).

Majority of FGD respondents also reported that most providers had no respect for working hour's punctuality. For that reason our waiting time was beyond expected time to wait. Most of wasting time occurs on either exit time end or entrance beginning. Once they start the procedure, time utilization was effective. One 21 years old lady said, now I decided to visit the facility not based on government working hours, but providers working hours.

Describing satisfaction by health education and communication session in the ANC clinic

The health education and communication session on women satisfaction during ANC visit observed that overall health education program was not-satisfied by the majorities, about 245 (60.5%) of the

Table 2 Percent distribution of level of women Satisfaction to different components of ANC services, Arba Minch Zuria district, Southwest Ethiopia, March 2016 (*n* = 405)

Aspects of Care	Status of Satisfaction			
	Good Satisfied		Poor satisfied	
	Number	%	Number	%
Overall satisfaction to ANC services	277	68.4	128	31.6
Amenities				
Location of the center	194	47.9%	211	52.1%
Hours of work	247	61%	158	39%
Ventilation	196	48.4%	219	51.6%
Sitting arrangement	289	71.4%	116	28.6%
Cleanness of the center	241	59.5%	164	40.5%
Cleanness of the Toilet	226	55.8%	179	44.2%
Performance of provider				
Answering questions	290	71.6%	115	28.4%
Taking history	255	63%	150	37%
Explanation of problem	271	66.9%	134	33.1%
Trusting the doctor	289	71.4%	116	28.7%
Examination time	309	76.3%	96	23.7%
Explanation of rational for investigation	277	68.4%	128	31.6%
Explanation of results of Investigation	241	59.5%	164	40.5%
Performance of staff				
Delivering of information	269	66.4%	136	33.6%
Maintaining Privacy	331	81.7%	74	18.3%

respondents. When specifically observing, cervical cancer prevention IEC session was not satisfied by nearly half of women, about 206 (50.9%). The 'no-satisfaction' respondents report were highest for STI prevention, about 268 (66.1%), malaria prevention 214 (52.9%), Physical exercise 212 (52.4%), and Breast self examinations 302 (74.6%) (Table 3).

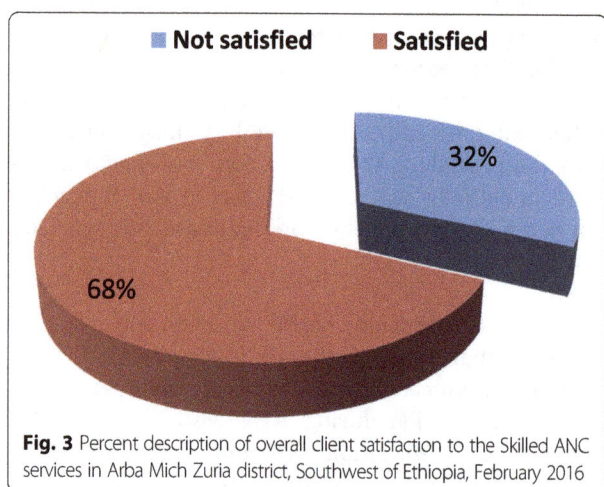

Fig. 3 Percent description of overall client satisfaction to the Skilled ANC services in Arba Mich Zuria district, Southwest of Ethiopia, February 2016

Highest client 'Good satisfaction' reports were observed as compared to "poor satisfaction" on some specific sessions. These included personal hygiene 284 (70.1%), tooth care 214 (52.8%), diet and nutrition 333 (82.2%), clothing 277 (68.4%), fetal movement monitoring 256 (63.2%), allowable medication 276 (68.1%), importance of breast feeding 247 (61%), basics of newborn care 211 (52.1%), follow-up for appointment 303 (74.8%), signs of labor 288 (71.1%), danger signs 286 (70.6%), and family planning and child spacing sessions 300 (74.1%) (Table 3). Majority discussants of focus group reported the major Health Education areas focused by the providers were diet at pregnancy and personal hygiene and its importance. We were happy with the sessions given. We identified healthier dietary selection for a pregnant woman. Providers also encouraged us to increase daily consumption of meal in that we have to have at least an additional two meal plan per a day over the routine. A single 34 years old respondent added "a provider told me to continue with the food that I was using even before pregnancy. Such as: vegetable diets, cereals and legumes that I get it from my farm land. Provider also addressed to balance my diet plan with my current weight and weight gain throughout the progress of pregnancy".

Table 3 Percent distribution of women satisfaction to health education and communication session on ANC clinic, Arba Minch Zuria district, Southwest Ethiopia, March 2016 ($n = 405$)

Health Education Topics	Status of Satisfaction			
	Good Satisfied		Poor satisfied	
	Number	%	Number	%
Overall Health education program	160	39.5%	245	60.5%
Prevention of Cervical Cancer	96	23.7%	309	76.3%
STI's prevention	137	33.8%	268	66.1%
Malaria prevention	191	47.2%	214	52.9%
Physical exercise	193	47.7%	212	52.4%
Personal hygiene	284	70.1%	121	29.8%
Teeth care	214	52.8%	191	47.2%
Diet and nutrition	333	82.2%	72	17.8%
Clothing	277	68.4%	128	31.6%
Fetal movement monitoring	256	63.2%	149	36.8%
Allowable medication	276	68.1%	129	31.9%
Breast feeding importance	247	61%	158	39%
Basics of newborn care	211	52.1%	194	47.9%
Follow-up appointment	303	74.8%	102	25.2%
Breast Self examination	103	25.4%	302	74.6%
Signs of labor	288	71.1%	117	28.8%
Danger signs of pregnancy	286	70.6%	119	29.4%
Family planning and child spacing	300	74.1%	105	25.9%

Describing satisfaction by number of current visit and gestational age

As observed, 'women satisfied' was increasing with frequently visiting for this pregnancy. Women satisfied were observed among the fourth and more visits of the respondents (88.6% Vs 66.7, 65.1, and 68.2%). Regarding gestational age, similar phenomena were observed in that in all trimester most women reported "good satisfaction" over that of "poor satisfaction". But, first trimester satisfaction and dissatisfaction was nearly closer each other (58.3 and 41.7% Vs 67.7 and 32.3%; 69.5 and 30.5%) as compared to second and third trimester. Third and second trimester satisfaction was huge over first, about (69.5 and 67.7% Vs 58.3%), respectively. The average gestational age at first visit of this pregnancy visit was 21.1 weeks $\pm$ 7.2 SD (Figs. 4 and 5).

Perceived main causes of dissatisfaction to skilled ANC services

A total of about 128 (32%) respondents had reported for having no satisfaction to Skilled Antenatal Care services in the facility of study district. Among this, reports of no sonar test (27.3%), unavailability of gynecologists (25%) and long waiting time in the clinic (20.3%) took the largest part. Even though they were lower 'no good laboratory services', 'not explaining about the clinic', 'overcrowding', and 'poor education session' reports also took proportions as the causes of dissatisfaction for overall Skilled Antenatal Care services (Fig. 6). In addition to this some of the discussants forwarded 'up on shortage of some medical instruments, providers usually used to refer us to the distant located hospital. Because of this, most of women did not go because of transportation and accommodation cost problem that we encounter at urban hospital and also hospital service was inconvenient than that of rural Health Centers'. A single 28 years old woman among the discussants of Gatse Health Center said 'I was not happy on the centers timely examination. There is long waiting and now I waited for long time'.

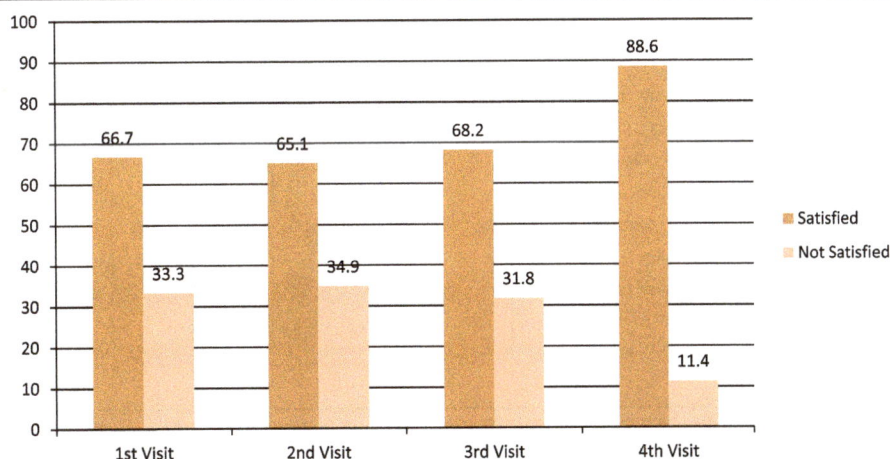

Fig. 4 Percent description of women current ANC visit by satisfaction status to ANC services, Arba Minch Zuria district, Southwest Ethiopia, March 2016 ($n = 405$)

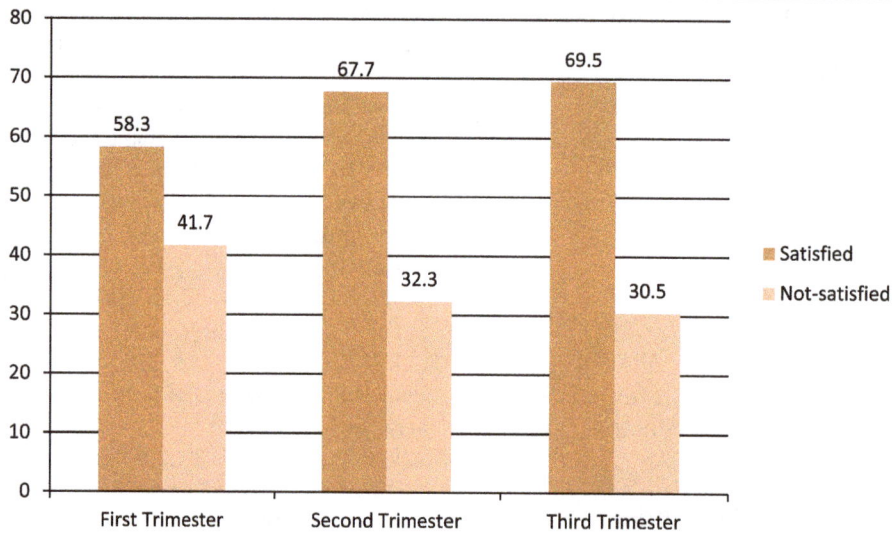

Fig. 5 Percent description of women gestational age of current pregnancy visit by satisfaction status to ANC services, Arba Minch Zuria district, Southwest Ethiopia, March 2016 ($n = 405$)

Factors associated with satisfaction to skilled ANC services

Bivariate and multivariable logistic regression analysis was used to calculate odds ratios and corresponding 95% confidence intervals for the predictors of satisfaction to Skilled Antenatal Care services. Concerning predictors of satisfaction in the bivariate analysis, having satisfaction to Skilled Antenatal Care services was associated with having birth order, distance to the nearest health center, previous ANC visit, family monthly income, marital status, ethnicity, and current visit type (Table 4).

When adjusted for other confounders in multivariable logistic regression analyses, only six variables, distance to the nearest health center, previous ANC visit, family monthly income, marital status, ethnicity, and current visit type were the potent predictors of women satisfaction to Skilled Antenatal Care services. Woman who arrived from 1 km or more distance to the center were 2.27 times more likely (AOR = 2.27; 95% CI, 1.27, 4.06) to have satisfied to Skilled Antenatal Care than those who are from below 1 km distance (Table 4).

Respondents who had 2 or more previous ANC visits were three times (AOR = 2.93; 95% CI, 1.21, 7.12) more likely to be satisfied to ANC services as compared to those with less or equal to one visit. Those women with family monthly income of $US 25–100 per month were

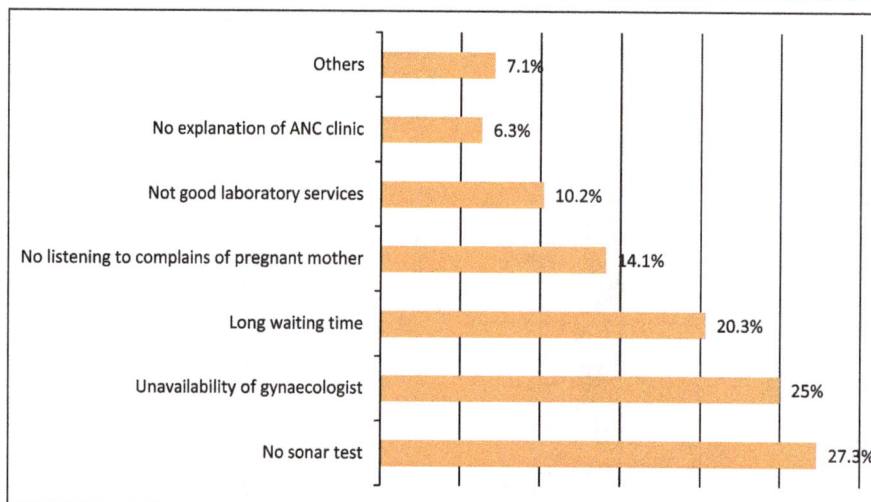

N.B. others include: Poor health education session and crowding clinic in the morning

Fig. 6 Percent distribution of women by main causes of dissatisfaction to skilled ANC services, Arba Minch Zuria district, Southwest Ethiopia, March 2016 ($n = 128$)

Table 4 Adjusted and unadjusted odds ratio of logistic regression model showing effects of predictor variables on the likely hood of client satisfaction for skilled ANC services, Arba Minch Zuria District, South West Ethiopia, March 2016

Predictor variables		Had satisfaction							
		Yes n = 277, 68.4%	No n = 128, 31.6%	COR	95% CI		AOR	95% CI	
					lower	upper		lower	upper
Birth Order (n = 318)	1	15.1%	10.1%	1.0+			1.0+		
	2–3	33.3%	14.8%	1.5	0.85	2.64	1.14	0.58	2.26
	4–5	15.4%	4.4%	2.33*	1.11	4.91	1.55	0.66	3.63
	6+	6%	0.9%	4.22*	1.15	15.4	3.45	0.38	31.4
Distance to the nearest HC[a]	< 1 km	9.9%	10.4%	1.0+			1.0+		
	≥ 1 km	21.7%	58%	2.54*	1.55	4.18	2.27**	1.27	4.06
Previous ANC visit	≤ 1	48.1%	27.2%	1.0+			1.0+		
	≥ 2	4.4%	20.2%	2.57*	1.47	4.5	2.93**	1.21	7.12
Family monthly income ($US)	< 25	23.6%	6.4%	1.0+			1.0+		
	25–50	29.2%	18.1%	0.44*	0.25	0.76	0.4**	0.2	0.8
	> 50	14.7%	8.1%	0.49*	0.26	0.94	0.67	0.27	1.67
Marital Status	Married	67.7%	29.1%	7.74*	2.09	28.6	8.17**	1.43	46.5
	Others[b]	0.7%	2.5%	1.0+			1.0+		
Ethnicity	Gamo	63%	22.5%	1.0+			1.0+		
	Welayta	4%	5.9%	0.24*	0.12	0.47	0.26**	0.13	0.54
	Others[c]	1.5%	3.2%	0.16*	0.06	0.45	0.2**	0.07	0.61
Current Visit	First	25.2%	12.6%	1.0+			1.0+		
	Second	20.7%	11.1%	0.93	0.57	1.53	1.09	0.57	2.08
	Third	14.8%	6.%	1.07	0.61	1.88	1.23	0.55	2.73
	Fourth and more	7.7%	1%	3.87*	1.3	11.57	9.02**	1.76	46.1

N.B: **Statistically Significant Association (p < 0.05), *significant by binary analysis, [1.0+] Reference category, [a]Health Center, [b]Singe, divorced, widowed, [c]Zeyse, Amhara

60% (AOR = 0.4, 95% CI; 0.2, 0.8) less likely to be satisfied by Skilled Antenatal Care services than those who had monthly household income below $US 25 (Table 4).

Compared to unmarried/divorced/widowed, married women were 8.17 times (AOR = 8.17, 95% CI; 1.43, 46.5) more likely to be satisfied to Skilled Antenatal Care. Non-native (Amhara, Zayse) ethnic groups were 80% (AOR = 0.2, 95% CI; 0.07, 0.61) decreased to have satisfied as compared to the native (Gamo) ethnic groups. And, women who come for fourth ANC visit were 9 times (AOR = 9.02, 95% CI; 1.76, 46.1) more likely to be satisfied than those who were in the first visit (Table 4).

Discussion

This health institution based cross-sectional study was attempted to assess the satisfaction status of women to Skilled Antenatal Care services in the district of Arba Minch Zuria, Southwest of Ethiopia. Findings of this study showed Skilled Antenatal Care services satisfaction were associated with demographic, economic, obstetric and accessibility factors of the respondents.

Accordingly, high number of respondents had reported they had good-satisfaction to the services. Many studies suggested that satisfaction of clients to ANC services varied from country to country [5–8]. This was inconsistent and higher finding as compared to Oman and previous Ethiopian (68% Vs 59% & 60%) [13, 16] and lower than Nigerian, Kenyan and Cameroons (68% Vs 81.1, 95, 96.4%) [10, 14, 23]. The highest finding could be an indication in Ethiopia for the ever-growing health sector development program for quality services so that it could be contributed to this comparative greater satisfaction. Conversely, the lower finding could be related to still the existence of comparative quality shortages in the study area of Ethiopia.

Satisfaction regarding location of the center, health education program and provider explanation of the problems on women ranges from about one-third to two-third, such as 39.5 to 66.9%. This was higher than Peruvian, Pakistan, European, and two African findings (39.5 to 66.9% Vs < 30%) [5–8, 17]. This higher finding of Ethiopia could be related to minimum surface area of the center due to few departments and buildings. This could give the center location closer to the roadside. Ethiopian provider usually had few minutes session for health education and explanation of the problem to the client. Greater satisfaction in this regard could be due to this short duration in the absence of intervention or treatment process that satisfies most of busy Ethiopian women to go to their home for home based work.

This study showed more than half women had satisfaction by 'hours of work' (61%). It was lower finding as compared to African Egyptian study finding (61% Vs 77.9%) [11]. This difference could be due to minimal working hours passed on work by providers in the facility of Ethiopia as per 24 h a day and 7 days a week. Shortage of skilled provider was also another issue to be considered in Ethiopia. Existence of these two facts alone were reported by Ethiopian HSDP-IV of 2012 report [24]. This comparative lower finding was also strengthened by majority of discussants that "………every health professionals within the department on which they were in-charge had not found at government work hours that as we know, we mean at early 2:30 to 3:00hrs morning and 8:00 hrs to 8:30 hrs afternoon. Some exist in the facility compound, but not availed in the department on time. Some others totally not availed, but come late. Others, but not all, exit the facility early, before exit time (exit time: 6:30 morning or 11:30 after noon). It is most disappointing to all of us………….thanks to opportunity to talk".

In this study, good satisfaction to sitting arrangements, ventilation and cleanness of the toilet reported were nearly ¾th (71.4%), below half (48.4%), and more than half (55.8%) of the respondents, respectively. These were still lower from the highest findings of Nigeria (71.4, 48.4, 59.5% Vs 97.5, 84.1, 60.7%) [14]. This could show still insufficient arrangements for the three variables here in Ethiopia in the extent of its proper functioning to until it brings highest good satisfaction as compared to Nigeria's center with-in the continent of Africa.

Regarding performance of the provider and staff, all the findings of 'good satisfaction' in the current study were more than average as reported, such as: answering questions (71.6%), taking history (63%), trusting the provider (71.4%), examination time (76.3%), explanation of rational for investigation (68.4%), explanation of results of Investigations (59.5%) delivering information (66.4%) and maintaining privacy (81.7%). All of the mentioned components of services were comparatively lower from the Shawa Village Egyptian finding [11]. The probable explanation in this regard could be shortage of professional ethics, availability of non-women friendly services, and performance negligence's by professionals were dominating here in Ethiopian as compared to outside higher satisfaction countries. As it is mentioned in various studies (such as: Bangladesh and India) [25–27], high satisfaction was also related to Maintenance of privacy via a separate room or screen for examination.

This study assessed 'poor- satisfaction' health education and communication sessions as components of services. These included: Prevention of Cervical cancer, STI's prevention, Malaria prevention, Physical exercise, and Breast Self examination. On the other hand, more than average women reported for each of major HE sessions as 'good-satisfaction' included: Personal hygiene, Teeth care, Diet and nutrition, Clothing, Fetal movement monitoring, Allowable medications, Breast feeding, Basics of newborn care, Follow-up appointment, Signs of labor, Danger signs of pregnancy, and Family planning and child spacing. The poor satisfaction was contrary to Nigerian finding [14]. This could be due to not addressing these specific tasks on HE session here in Ethiopia by majorities of providers as contrasted by Nigeria. The good satisfaction components was in-line with Nigerian and Cameroon findings [10, 14]. The positive relationship could be due to increasing health sector development program for education session development here and there.

More than average women reported for each of major HE sessions as 'good-satisfaction' included: Personal hygiene, Teeth care, Diet and nutrition, Clothing, Fetal movement monitoring, Allowable medications, Breast feeding, Basics of newborn care, Follow-up appointment, Signs of labor, Danger signs of pregnancy, and family planning and child spacing. This was in-line with Nigerian and Cameroon findings [10, 14]. This positive relation could be due to increasing health sector development program for education session development here and there. Focus group discussants also supported positive finding in that "…….ohhh, it was good and interesting. Health education session focusing on personal hygiene, diet and nutrition, and communicable disease prevention were clear to all of us. After education we have got special things to ourselves and our life. Our child can be protected from future infections, especially diarrhea and vomiting problems. One 38yrs old woman said: Now I will breast feed only for six months exclusively. Vaccinating baby is beneficial to me and to him".

Causes of dissatisfaction as client reported in the facility were: absence of sonar test, no doctor and long waiting time in the clinic. Other studies (Ghana, Nigeria and Ethiopia) also supported this as causes of dissatisfaction with services [16, 28, 29]. But, in this study, sonar test was the pioneer that reported by the majority of respondents as compared to other findings.

This study observed that having satisfied to Skilled Antenatal Care services was statistically significantly associated (AOR = 2.27; 95% CI, 1.27, 4.06) with distance ≥ 1 km that women traveled to arrive to the nearest Health Center. This was inconsistent with Pakistan qualitative finding [17] as far distance was one of the factors for dissatisfaction. This difference could be due to reduced expectations of women from outside village that she could get adequate services of her need. As suggested by developing countries study, women with low expectations with more services could result in good satisfaction of services and the vice versa [9].

Women Satisfied to SANC services was significantly associated (AOR = 2.93; 95% CI, 1.21, 7.12) with frequent (> 1times) previous ANC visits that women had. This was directly linked to Ibadan, Nigerian finding [14] and Riyadh [12] in which patient satisfaction was significantly higher among women in the highest visit groups. The positive association in this regard could be due to developing awareness on its importance by repeated visiting, increasing client need and effective response to this need by the health care workers here and there. Moreover, satisfied woman are more likely to increase the compliance with ANC visits [30]. Therefore, majority of subsequently visiting women could probably be satisfied groups in the current study and others.

In this study, having satisfied to Skilled Antenatal Care services was significantly associated (AOR = 0.4, 95% CI; 0.2, 0.8) with respondents who had monthly family income of $U.S 25–50/month. This was in line with previous home study [16] in that better satisfaction observed in lower income groups. Outside home, Malaysia, it was also positively linked as having no cost or low spending money for the ANC services had better services satisfaction [30]. The synonymous finding could probably indicate that low costly services are more satisfying to the poor ANC clients here and there.

Women in married marital status were significantly associated (AOR = 8.17, 95% CI; 1.43, 46.5) for having satisfied to Skilled Antenatal Care services. No other studies before could have observed this association directly. In this study, we could explain that this significant association could probably be related to existence of high number of married women among the study participants. This was because, married marital status and ANC service utilization had significant association in Ethiopia [31, 32].

This study revealed that having satisfied to Skilled Antenatal Care services were statistically significantly associated with being from Welayta (AOR = 0.26, 95% CI; 0.13, 0.54) and other (other includes: Amhara and Zayse) ethnic group (AOR = 0.2, 95% CI; 0.07, 0.61) respondents. This ethnic association with maternal Skilled Antenatal Care services satisfaction was also linked by Kenyan, Sri Lanka and Nigerian studies [33–35]. This particular ethnic discrimination could probably be related with non-native ethnic group's perception as being discriminated for services quality. This was because there was no one from minor ethnic group reported for ethnic related discrimination in FGDs. Concerned bodies needed to make specific interventions to poorly satisfied ethnic groups and further study is required.

This study shows that respondents who were in the fourth ANC visit were significantly associated (AOR = 9.02, 95% CI; 1.76, 46.1) for good-satisfaction to Skilled Antenatal Care services. This was supported by finding of Riyadh [12]. High good-satisfaction with highest visit gives the women opportunity to ask her concerns and this could increase her good feeling towards the services. Besides this, high number visit could possibly enhance positive relationship between providers and client, making maximum good feelings or satisfaction towards the women. This probable explanations were also supported by Tanzanian finding [36]. As satisfaction can be one of the effect for quality, perceived good quality services was also associated to that of subsequent ANC visit by a woman, as one home study suggested [37].

Strengths of the study

Being facility based is an advantage for better representing of the study district on the outcome variable as compared to being community based house to house survey. This was because it included respondents in the most recent service use. So, recall bias was highly minimized. Being triangulated design was also the strength. Moreover, being professional data collectors (nurse) used was an advantage for effective collection of obstetrics related information from the respondent's as it is difficult for non-health professionals.

Limitations of the study

Design related cause-effect relationship for all significant associations may not be established. Being facility based interviews could be disadvantageous in that it inhibits criticism of medical care by some of respondents even if it had weighted advantage over recall bias minimizations. The woman could depend on a single satisfying service for decisions of overall satisfaction, even though her self-report was the primary option for capturing customer satisfaction data. Social desirability bias could have affected the quality of data collected because study subjects might get difficulty to answer dissatisfaction in the presence of an interviewer. This bias was minimized via interviewing in a separate room by non-staff members' enumerator without wearing gown. Being non-scale based satisfaction measurement data collection tool could be the disadvantage for better observation of concentrated area in a scale of satisfaction. Moreover, women who were on a first visit could not be able to judge quality of some components of services accurately. This bias was reduced by clarification of components of services and allowing her to observe some amenities back again during the interview. Selection of questions and indicators could also have lead to a skewed interpretation.

Conclusion and recommendations

Women who reported having good-satisfaction to overall Skilled Antenatal Care services were highest. The most common specific component of ANC that had good-satisfaction by the respondents was maintaining "Privacy" during examination (81.7%). The most common health education topic during ANC services which was satisfied by the respondents was "Diet and nutrition" (82.2%). Absence of sonar test, no doctor, and long waiting time in the center were commonest causes of dissatisfaction by client report. Woman birth order, distance to the nearest health center, previous ANC visit, family monthly income, marital status, ethnicity, and current ANC visit type were independent predictors of satisfaction to Skilled Antenatal Care services. Providers must re-plan and improve their performances in the district for another highest satisfaction in the future. Especial attention must be given to those ethnics other than Gamo in the district regarding overall ANC services, since dissatisfaction was highest among them. Policy makers and other stake holders should give attention to increase ANC visit coverage in the country by developing strategies with the aim of maximum satisfaction to Skilled Antenatal Care services. Government officials should be engaged in development of middle income economy for women through women economy development strategy and intervention throughout the country. Early ANC visitors should also be given attention by providers to increase chance for return visit through maximizing client satisfaction in every component of services.

Abbreviations

ANC: Antenatal Care; FGD: Focus Group Discussion; HE: Health Education; IEC: Information, Education and Communication

Acknowledgements

Our special gratitude and appreciation goes to Arba Minch Health Sciences college research and publication core process for budgeting this research project. We were also grateful to Arba Minch Zuria administrators, Regional Health Bureau, data collectors, respondents and supervisors for their unreserved effort to the success of this work.

Funding

This study was undertaken by the grant from Arbaminch College of Health Sciences Office of Research and Publication Core Process. Funding includes for Data collection, entry and writing-up. Publication fee had not been funded from the college.

Authors' contributions

SL: Developed design and Conceptualization, performed statistical analysis and sequence alignment, and drafted the manuscript. AA: Participated on Design development, performed statistical analysis, participated drafting the manuscript. FJ: Coordinated the study, developed design, statistical analysis and participated manuscript draft development. All these authors read and approved the final manuscript.

Competing interests

We declare that we authors do not have any competing interests.

Author details

[1]Department of Nursing and Midwifery, Arbaminch University, Arba Minch, Ethiopia. [2]Department of Nursing and Midwifery, Arba Minch College of Health Sciences, Arba Minch, Ethiopia. [3]Department of Obstetrics and Gynecology, Tikur Anbesa Specialized Hospital, Addis Ababa University, Addis Ababa, Ethiopia.

References

1. Ethiopian Updated management protocol on selected obstetrics topics, Federal Democratic Republic of Ethiopia Ministry of Health.pdf. January 2010.
2. Holan S, Mathiesen M, Petersen K. A national clinical guideline for antenatal care. Oslo: Short version, Directorate for Health and Social Affairs; 2005.
3. Mafubelu D, Islam M. WHO, dept of making pregnancy safer annual report of 2006, P 6 of 56; 2007.
4. United Nations, author. The millenium development goals report. 2012.
5. Seclen-Palacin JA, Benavides B, Jacoby E, Velasquez A, Watanabe E. Is there a link between continuous quality improvement programs and health service users' satisfaction with prenatal care? An experience in Peruvian hospitals. Rev Panam Salud Public. 2004;16:149–57.
6. Luyben AG, Fleming VE. Women's needs from antenatal care in three European countries. Midwifery. 2005;21:212–23.
7. Bronfman-Pertzovsky MN, Lopez-Moreno S, Magis-Rodriguez C, Moreno-Altamirano A, Rutstein S. Prenatal care at the first level of care: characteristics of providers that affect users' satisfaction. Salud Publica Mex. 2003;45:445–54.
8. Uzochukwu BS, Onwujekwe OE, Akpala CO. Community satisfaction with the quality of maternal and child health services in Southeast Nigeria. East Afr Med J. 2004;81:293–9.
9. Srivastava A, Avan BI, Rajbangshi P, Bhattacharyya S. Determinants of women's satisfaction with maternal health care: a review of literature from developing countries. BMC Pregnancy Childbirth. 2015;15(97):p1–12.
10. Edie GEHE, Obinchemti TE, Tamufor EN, Njie MM, Njamen TN, Achidi EA. Perceptions of antenatal care services by pregnant women attending government health centres in the Buea Health District, Cameroon: a cross sectional study. Pan Afr Med J. 2015;21(45):1937–8688.
11. Montasser NAE-H, Helal RM, Megahed WM, Amin SK, Saad AM, Ibrahim TR, et al. Egyptian Women's satisfaction and perception of antenatal care. Int J Trop Dis Health. 2012;2(2):145–56.
12. Kamil A, Khorshid E. Maternal perceptions of antenatal care provision at a tertiary level hospital, Riyadh. Oman Med J. 2013;28(1):33–5.
13. Ghobashi M, Khandekar R. Satisfaction among expectant mothers with antenatal Care Services in the Musandam Region of Oman. Sultan Qaboos Univ Med J. 2008;8(3):325–32.
14. Nwaeze IL, Enabor OO, Oluwasola TAO, Aimakhu CO. PERCEPTION AND SATISFACTION WITH QUALITY OF ANTENATAL CARE SERVICES AMONG PREGNANT WOMEN AT THE UNIVERSITY COLLEGE HOSPITAL, IBADAN, NIGERIA. Ann Ib Postgrad Med. 2013;11(1):22–8.
15. Esimai O, Omoniyi-Esan G. Wait time and service satisfaction at antenatal clinic, Obafemi Awolowo University Ile-Ife. East Afr J Public Health. 2009;6(3):309–11.
16. Chemir F, Alemseged F, Workneh D. Satisfaction with focused antenatal care service and associated factors among pregnant women attending focused antenatal care at health centers in Jimma town, Jimma zone, South West Ethiopia; a facility based cross-sectional study triangulated with qualitative study. BMC Res Notes http://wwwbiomedcentralcom/1756-0500/7/164. 2014;7:164.
17. Majrooh MA, Hasnain S, Akram J, Siddiqui A, Memon ZA. Coverage and Quality of Antenatal Care Provided at Primary Health Care Facilities in the 'Punjab' Province of 'Pakistan'. PLoS One. 2014;9(11):e113390. https://doi.org/10.1371/journal.pone.0113390.
18. Biro MA, Waldenstrom U, Brown S. Satisfaction with team midwifery Care for low- and High-Risk Women: a randomized controlled trial. Birth. 2003;30:1–10.
19. SNNPR, Gamo Gofa Zone, Arba Minch Zuria Woreda Health Office Report, 2013.
20. Ethiopian Housing and population Census of 2007 : Southern Peoples, Nations and Nationalities Region of Ethiopia. https://en.wikipedia.org/wiki/Southern_Nations,_Nationalities,_and_Peoples%27_Region.retrived.

21. Addisse M. Ethiopia public health training initiative, the Carter Center, the Ethiopia Ministry of Health, and the Ethiopia ministry of education, University of Gondar; 2003.

22. Central Statistical Agency [Ethiopia] and ICF International, Ethiopia Demographic and Health Survey (EDHS) 2011. Central Statistical Agency and ICF International, Addis Ababa, Ethiopia and Calverton, Maryland, USA. 2012.

23. Baotran N, Craig CR, Rachel SM, Elizabeth BA, Maricianah O, Katie D, et al. PATIENT SATISFACTION WITH INTEGRATED HIV AND ANTENATAL CARE SERVICES IN RURAL KENYA. AIDS Care. 2012;24(11):1442–7.

24. Ethiopia Health Sector Development Programme (HSDP) IV of 2010. MOH, Ethiopia. VERSION 19. ethiopia_hsdp_iv_final_draft_2010_-2015.pdf.

25. Aldana JM, Piechulek H, Al-Sabir A. Client satisfaction and quality of health care in rural Bangladesh. Bull World Health Organ. 2001;79:512–7.

26. George A. Quality of reproductive care in private hospitals in Andhra Pradesh. Women's perception. Econ Polit Wkly. 2002;37:1686–92.

27. Das P, Basu M, Tikadar T, Biswas GC, Mirdha P, Pal R. Client satisfaction on maternal and child health services in rural Bengal. Indian J Community Med. 2010;35:478–81.

28. Fawole AO, Okunlola MA, Adekunle AO. Client's perceptions of the quality of antenatal care. J Nat Med Assoc. 2008;100:1052–8.

29. D'Ambruoso L, Abbey M, Hussein J. Please understand when I cry out in pain: women's accounts of maternity services during labour and delivery in Ghana. BMC Public Health. 2005;5:140.

30. Rahman MM, Ngadan DP, Arif MT. Factors affecting satisfaction on antenatal care services in Sarawak, Malaysia, evidence from a cross sectional study. Springerplus. 2016;5:725.

31. Mekonnen Y, Mekonnen A. Utilization of maternal health Care Services in Ethiopia. Calverton, Maryland: ORC Macro; 2002.

32. Kwast BE, Liff JM. Factors associated with maternal mortality in Addis Ababa, Ethiopia. Int J Epidemiol. 1998;17(1):115–21.

33. Senarath U, Fernando DN, Rodrigo I. Factors determining client satisfaction with hospital-based perinatal care in Sri Lanka. Tropical Med Int Health. 2006;11:1442–51.

34. Oladapo OT, Osiberu MO. Do sociodemographic characteristics of pregnant women determine their perception of antenatal care quality? Matern Child Health J. 2009;13:505–11.

35. Bazant ES, Koenig MA. Women's satisfaction with delivery care in Nairobi's informal settlements. Int J Qual Health Care. 2009;21:79–86.

36. Gupta S, Yamada G, Mpembeni R, Frumence G, Callaghan-Koru JA, et al. Factors Associated with Four or More Antenatal Care Visits and Its Decline among Pregnant Women in Tanzania between 1999 and 2010. PLoS ONE. 2014;9(7):e101893. https://doi.org/10.1371/journal.pone.0101893.

37. Fesseha G, Alemayehu M, Etana B, Haileslassie K, Zemene A. Perceived quality of antenatal care service by pregnant women in public and private health facilities in Northern Ethiopia. Am J Health Res. 2014;2(4):146–51.

14

Improving women's knowledge about prenatal screening in the era of non-invasive prenatal testing for Down syndrome – development and acceptability of a low literacy decision aid

Sian Karen Smith[1]*[iD], Antonia Cai[1], Michelle Wong[1], Mariana S. Sousa[1,2,3], Michelle Peate[4], Alec Welsh[5,6], Bettina Meiser[1], Rajneesh Kaur[1], Jane Halliday[7,8], Sharon Lewis[7], Lyndal Trevena[9], Tatiane Yanes[10], Kristine Barlow-Stewart[11] and Margot Barclay[12,13]

Abstract

Background: Access to information about prenatal screening is important particularly in light of new techniques such as non-invasive prenatal testing (NIPT). This study aimed to develop and examine the acceptability of a low literacy decision aid (DA) about Down syndrome screening among pregnant women with varying education levels and GPs.

Methods: We developed a DA booklet providing information about first-trimester combined testing, maternal serum screening, and NIPT. GPs and women participated in a telephone interview to examine the acceptability of the DA and measure screening knowledge before and after reading the DA. The knowledge measure was designed to assess whether women had understood the gist of the information presented in the decision aid. It comprised conceptual questions (e.g. screening tells you the chance of having a baby with Down syndrome) and numeric questions (e.g. the accuracy of different screening tests).

Results: Twenty-nine women and 18 GPs participated. Regardless of education level, most women found the booklet 'very' clearly presented ($n = 22$, 76%), and 'very' informative ($n = 23$, 80%). Overall, women's conceptual and numeric knowledge improved after exposure to the DA, from 4% having adequate knowledge to 69%. Women's knowledge of NIPT also improved after receiving the decision aid, irrespective of education. Most GPs found it 'very' clearly presented ($n = 13$, 72%), and that it would 'very much' facilitate decision-making ($n = 16$, 89%).

Conclusions: The DA was found to be acceptable to women as well as GPs. A comprehensive evaluation of the efficacy of the decision aid compared to standard information is an important next step. Strategies are needed on how to implement the tool in practice.

Keywords: Decision aid, Informed decision-making, Prenatal screening, Prenatal testing, Trisomy 21, Down syndrome, Non-invasive prenatal testing (NIPT), Low literacy

* Correspondence: sian.smith@unsw.edu.au
[1]Psychosocial Research Group, Lowy Research Centre, C25, Prince of Wales Clinical School, Faculty of Medicine, UNSW Sydney, Corner High and Botany St, Kensington, Sydney New South Wales 2033, Australia
Full list of author information is available at the end of the article

Introduction

Screening in early pregnancy for foetal abnormalities is an established part of routine care in Western countries [1]. Some countries, such as the UK and the Netherlands offer prenatal screening as part of their national screening programmes and costs are reimbursed [2, 3]. Other countries have not implemented screening programmes, but have policies in place to ensure women are made aware that screening tests are available [4]. Irrespective of a women's age or family history, a nuchal translucency ultrasound, with or without a maternal serum test is generally available to women in early pregnancy to assess a woman's risk of carrying a foetus with chromosomal abnormalities. The most common chromosome condition is Down syndrome which can lead to varying degrees of physical, behavioural, and cognitive problems. If an increased risk is identified, invasive diagnostic tests such as amniocentesis and chorionic villus sampling are available. Women could then be faced with the decision of terminating the pregnancy or preparing for the birth of a child with special needs [5, 6].

Following the discovery of cell-free foetal DNA in the mother's blood, non-invasive prenatal testing (NIPT) is steadily becoming available to screen for Down syndrome in early pregnancy [7, 8]. NIPT is more accurate than conventional screening with a higher detection rate (99% versus ~ 80–90%, respectively) [9, 10], and eliminates the risk of miscarriage associated with invasive tests [11]. Accuracy, safety, and peace of mind are often cited as the perceived benefits of NIPT by women and health care professionals [12, 13]. NIPT has largely been driven by the commercial sector [14]. However, several European countries have evaluated the impact of integrating NIPT into existing prenatal screening programmes [15–17]. In Australia, the context for current study, women have to fund NIPT themselves as it is not available on Medicare or reimbursed through private insurance [18]. Existing Australian clinical guidelines state that all pregnant women should be offered NIPT as an option, and that health care professionals should be informed about NIPT and how it fits into current screening and diagnostic pathways [19]. As such, different approaches have been adopted in different practices, and information provision is likely to vary.

Access to decision support information in early pregnancy is essential for making informed decisions, particularly in light of the availability of NIPT and the perception that it is "just a blood test" [20, 21]. The hallmarks of such decisions are possessing good knowledge of the consequences of participating in, or declining screening, being able to deliberate the options and outcomes, and making a choice consistent with their attitudes [22].

Decision aids (DAs) are tools designed to help people to make informed health decisions by explicitly stating the decision, providing information about the potential benefits and risks, and by clarifying values [23]. In prenatal care, DAs increase knowledge, lower decisional conflict and reduce anxiety [24]. An environmental scan of publicly available prenatal testing DAs – a process whereby internal and external data sources were searched, namely the DA Library Inventory, correspondence with research networks, and electronic databases – found that none of the 20 DAs identified fulfilled the International Patient Decision Aid minimum standards [25]. Only a few DAs included values clarification exercises, and most were developed prior to the availability of NIPT, with the exception of a web-based multimedia decision aid [26]. In addition, prenatal screening DAs rarely acknowledge the involvement of health care professionals in decision-making. Yet, health care professionals play an important role in supporting informed reproductive choices. [27]. In Australia, General Practitioners (GPs) or primary care physicians, are well positioned to provide decision support information about prenatal screening as they are typically the first health professional that women meet in the early stages of pregnancy when screening decisions are made.

A key challenge when designing health information is making sure that it is accessible and understood to people with different education and literacy skills [28]. Even women with higher levels of education may not be familiar with the various screening tests and struggle to understand information if it not communicated clearly [29]. In Australia, low health literacy is common, and up to 60% of the general population experience difficulties accessing and understanding information [30]. While there are prenatal screening decision aids [26, 31], few have been specifically developed using low literacy design principles to help expectant couples better understand information on equitable basis regardless of their education and literacy level [32].

To address the gaps highlighted above, this descriptive study aimed to: (1) develop a low literacy DA about prenatal screening for Down syndrome including NIPT, to complement counselling by a GP or other antenatal health care professional, (2) examine the acceptability and comprehensibility of the DA among GPs and among women with different education levels, and elicit suggestions for improvement, and (3) measure women's screening knowledge about the different screening tests available (including NIPT) before and after receiving the decision aid.

Method

Development of the low literacy DA

The DA was developed by a multidisciplinary steering committee (all authors) of health professionals and researchers with expertise in epidemiology, genetics education, genetic counselling, psychology, DA development, and maternal foetal medicine. Existing Australian prenatal screening resources and the International Patient Decision Aid Standards (IPDAS) informed the content [33–35]. The DA was designed as a written booklet because our previous work found that women preferred paper-based information [36]. It is intended to complement rather than replace information or counselling by a GP or other health care professional.

Various low-literacy design strategies were applied, including; plain language; colour coding; glossary of medical terms; visual illustrations; simple medical diagrams; and providing contextual information before factual information [37–40]. The first draft of the DA was piloted with the target group, namely six pregnant women (mean age 31 years) with lower and higher education attending a hospital-based ultrasound clinic - 3 women with higher school certificate, and 3 had completed a university degree. The DA was then further refined based on their suggestions (e.g. using brighter colours and presenting culturally sensitive illustrations). Table 1 presents the DA content, including a 100-dot

diagram (Fig. 1) and a worksheet (Fig. 2). The final version can be found – http://www.psychosocialresearch-groupunsw.org/decision-aids.html.

Acceptability of the DA

GP recruitment and procedure

GPs were invited to provide feedback on the DA and assist in recruiting eligible women. Invitation letters were sent to 320 GPs working in antenatal shared care listed on a hospital database in South Western Sydney, New South Wales (NSW), Australia. South Western Sydney is a metropolitan part of Sydney, with a higher proportion of lower socioeconomic groups compared to other areas of Sydney [41]. In Australia, antenatal shared care is an arrangement where pregnancy care is shared between the GP and the hospital or other birth setting. GPs who offer shared care must have extra training and qualifications [42]. NSW does not have a state-wide prenatal screening programme and often women have to pay for screening tests privately. NSW Health policy states that women should be made aware of screening and be supported in making an informed decision [43].

Interested GPs returned an expression of interest form and were visited by researchers (AC and SS), who explained the recruitment process, obtained written informed consent, and provided information packs (recruitment sheet, participant information sheet and

Table 1 Decision aid content

Component/feature	Description
General description	• Paper-based, 36-page, A5 booklet.
	• Written and quantitative information about prenatal screening (including NIPT) and diagnostic testing for Down syndrome.
Theoretical Framework	• Systemic functional linguistics were used to structure the information (Clerehan, Buchbinder et al. 2005).
Visual, format and design aspects	• Plain language, headings, bullet points, and white space were used.
	• Colour coding was consistently used to distinguish between screening and diagnostic tests.
	• A timeline was included to outline the timing of the different screening tests. Visual illustrations were used throughout the booklet to support key concepts and break up the text.
	• The image on the front cover was designed to set the scene for the booklet – a women contemplating the options.
	• Medical diagrams were presented of diagnostic testing.
Key factual content	• The difference between screening and diagnostic tests.
	• The chromosome conditions screened for.
	• The different types of screening tests (first-trimester, second-trimester and NIPT).
	• Accuracy of screening testing in detecting Down syndrome.
	• Diagnostic testing.
	• Options available after a diagnosis of Down syndrome.
	• Personal worksheet to help women/ couples decide about prenatal screening (Fig. 2).
Presentation of quantitative information	• Systematic 100-dot diagrams (see Fig. 1) used to convey sensitivity (rate at which women carrying babies with Down syndrome are detected) of the Combined First Trimester screening, Second Trimester Maternal Serum Screening and Non-Invasive Prenatal testing.

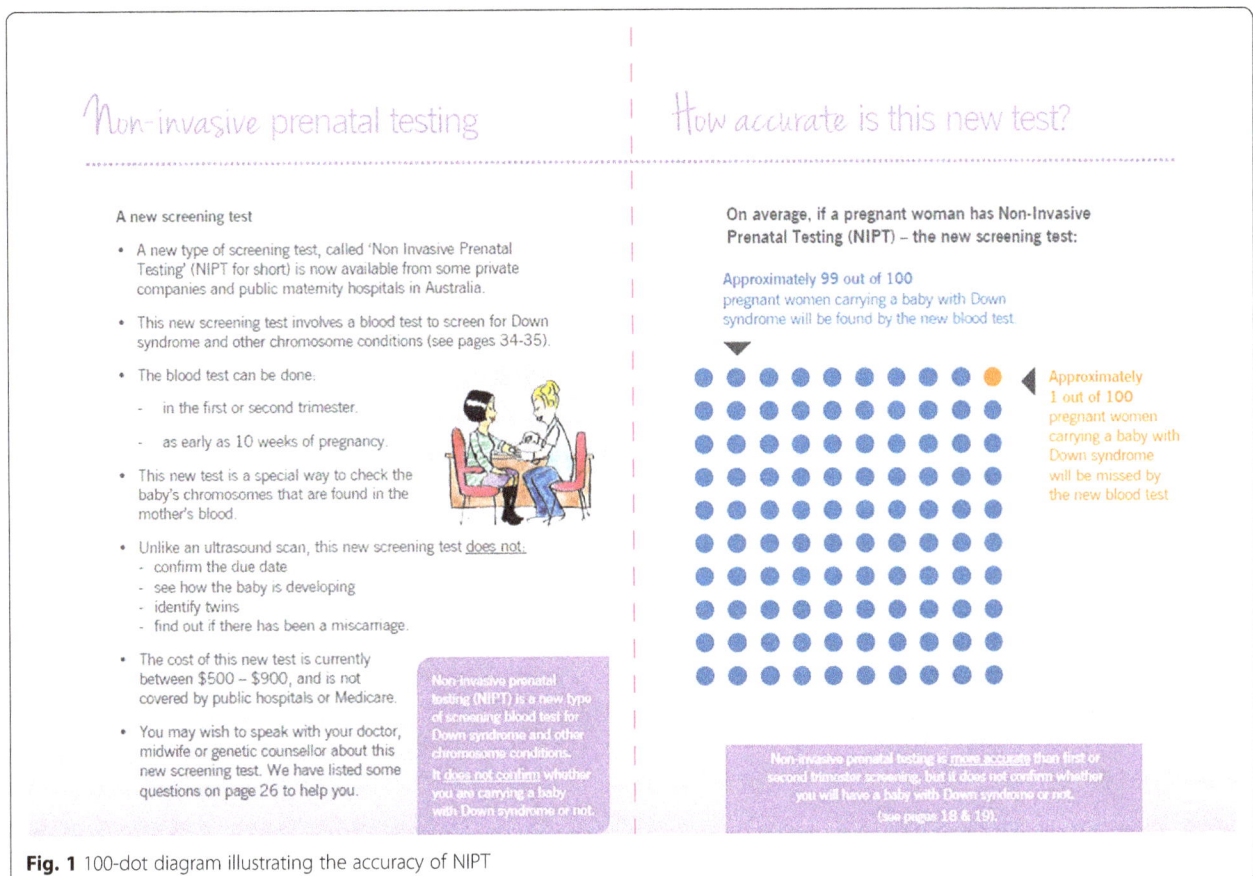

Fig. 1 100-dot diagram illustrating the accuracy of NIPT

DA). GPs were asked to invite all eligible women, until the target sample size of 30 was reached. In our previous decision aid work, a sample size of 30 has been found to be suitable for obtaining feedback on the acceptability and comprehensibility of DAs [44, 45]. We also telephoned GPs individually about once a month to thank them for their commitment to the study, and to identify barriers to recruitment and discuss ways to boost recruitment.

GPs took part in a 30-min telephone interview using closed/structured and open-ended questions to obtain feedback on the DA. The current study reports the responses to the structured questions; the qualitative data will be reported in a separate paper. For participation, GPs received continuing professional development points from the Royal Australian College of General Practitioners.

Recruitment of pregnant women and procedure

Eligible women were invited by their GP and given an information sheet. Women were eligible if they were aged 16 years or older, were able to speak English and equal to or less than 13 weeks and 2 days of gestation. This cut-off time was chosen because in Australia combined first trimester screening is carried out between 9

weeks and 13 weeks (plus 6 days). This cut-off point enabled us to recruit women slightly later on in gestation to widen the recruitment window [46]. Women who expressed an interest were contacted by researchers (AC & TY) to determine eligibility, obtain verbal consent, and measure knowledge prior to receiving the DA. Eligible and consenting participants were mailed a copy of the DA and telephoned approximately 2 weeks later to collect socio-demographic information, elicit DA feedback, and measure knowledge. To increase recruitment, we offered women reimbursement for their time (a gift voucher), and sent a monthly newsletter to GPs to update and remind them to recruit potential participants.

Participants were recruited between 2014 and 2015. Ethics approval was obtained from the South Eastern and South Western Sydney Local Health District Human Research Ethics Committees (ref number: 12/219).

Measures
GP measures
Socio-demographic data were collected from GPs. Closed questions (using Likert rating scales) adapted from our previous research were used to examine perceptions of its length, balance, clarity, and usefulness

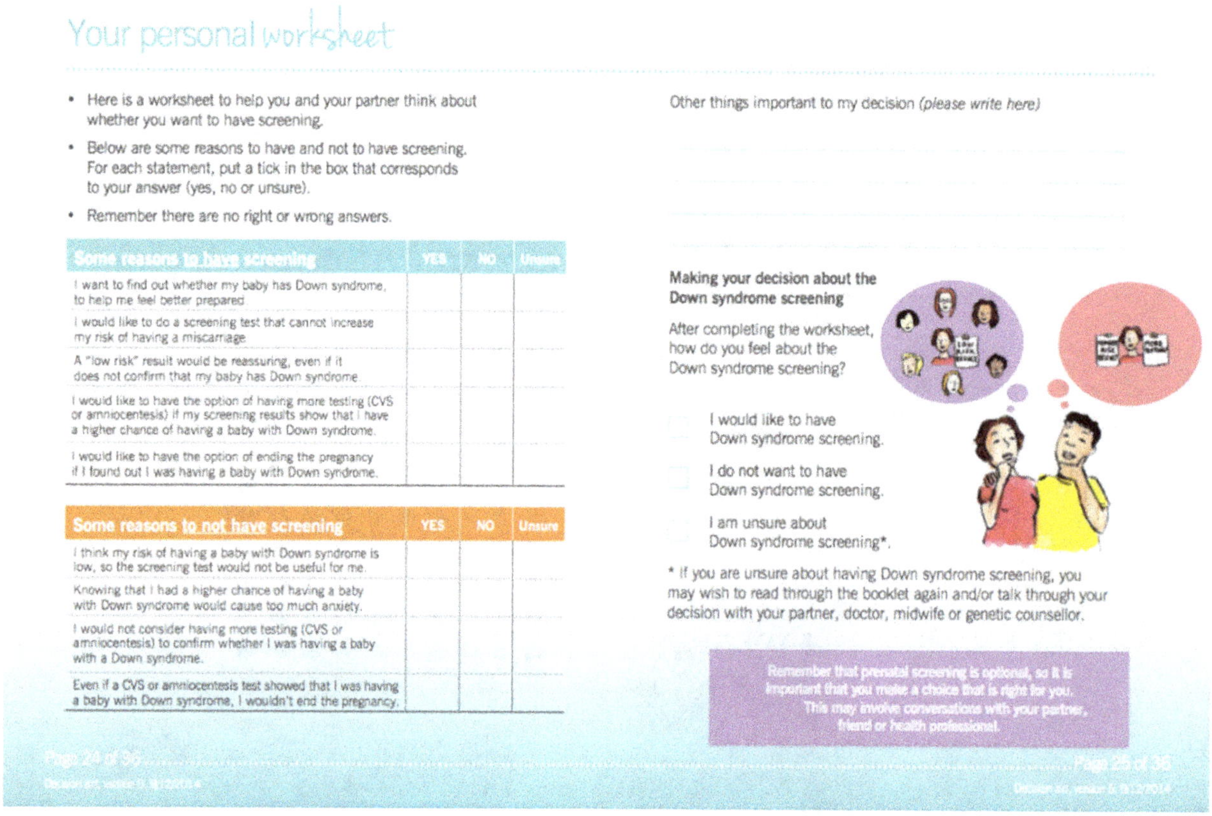

Your personal worksheet

- Here is a worksheet to help you and your partner think about whether you want to have screening.
- Below are some reasons to have and not to have screening. For each statement, put a tick in the box that corresponds to your answer (yes, no or unsure).
- Remember there are no right or wrong answers.

Some reasons to have screening	YES	NO	Unsure
I want to find out whether my baby has Down syndrome, to help me feel better prepared			
I would like to do a screening test that cannot increase my risk of having a miscarriage			
A "low risk" result would be reassuring, even if it does not confirm that my baby has Down syndrome			
I would like to have the option of having more testing (CVS or amniocentesis) if my screening results show that I have a higher chance of having a baby with Down syndrome.			
I would like to have the option of ending the pregnancy if I found out I was having a baby with Down syndrome.			

Some reasons to not have screening	YES	NO	Unsure
I think my risk of having a baby with Down syndrome is low, so the screening test would not be useful for me.			
Knowing that I had a higher chance of having a baby with Down syndrome would cause too much anxiety.			
I would not consider having more testing (CVS or amniocentesis) to confirm whether I was having a baby with a Down syndrome.			
Even if a CVS or amniocentesis test showed that I was having a baby with Down syndrome, I wouldn't end the pregnancy.			

Other things important to my decision *(please write here)*

Making your decision about the Down syndrome screening

After completing the worksheet, how do you feel about the Down syndrome screening?

- I would like to have Down syndrome screening.
- I do not want to have Down syndrome screening.
- I am unsure about Down syndrome screening*.

* If you are unsure about having Down syndrome screening, you may wish to read through the booklet again and/or talk through your decision with your partner, doctor, midwife or genetic counsellor.

Remember that prenatal screening is optional, so it is important that you make a choice that is right for you. This may involve conversations with your partner, friend or health professional.

Page 24 of 36 ... Page 25 of 36

Fig. 2 Personal worksheet included in the DA

[47]. Some open-ended questions were asked to elicit feedback on how to improve the DA.

Women measures: Socio-demographic and obstetric variables

Data on age, marital status, educational level, country of birth, years lived in Australia, first language, employment status, occupation, previous pregnancy outcomes and screening experience were collected.

DA acceptability and comprehensibility

Closed questions using Likert rating scales examined the acceptability of the DA in terms of its length, balance, clarity, and amount of information. Comments on the illustrations, colour coding, diagrams, and worksheet were elicited using open-ended questions, and participants were asked to offer suggestions on how to improve the DA.

Knowledge

Knowledge is a key component of informed decision-making. Prenatal screening knowledge was measured to identify the extent to which women's knowledge changed before and after exposure to the DA, and examine whether the resource would help inform women's decision-making during pregnancy. The knowledge questions and marking scheme were informed by Fuzzy Trace Theory, a dual-process theory which proposes two ways in which people process and store information in their memory: (i) processing and remembering the bottom-line meaning ('gist'), and (ii) processing and recalling information precise details ('verbatim') [48]. When making decisions, studies have shown that gist information processing tends to be superior to verbatim processing in improving the quality of the decision, possibly because it relies less on remembering the exact details [49] As such, our knowledge measure was designed to assess whether women understood the 'gist' of the information, including their (i) conceptual knowledge of screening for Down syndrome (e.g. screening tells you the chance of having a baby with Down syndrome) and, (ii) numeric knowledge (e.g. the accuracy of different screening tests). Nineteen items with true/false response options, adapted from previous questions developed by [50] and our previous work [51]. Existing knowledge measures did not include questions about NIPT so we developed our own items. A scoring scheme was developed providing a maximum score of 22 (16 for conceptual knowledge and 6 for numeric knowledge) (Additional file 1 knowledge scoring scheme and questions). It was decided a priori that a score of 75% or above (score ≥ 17 out of 22) would be considered 'adequate knowledge'. Although the 75% knowledge threshold might be considered high, it enabled us to identify whether the conceptual and numeric knowledge scales were responsive to exposure to the DA. Thus, to achieve 'adequate knowledge', participants needed to answer a combination of conceptual and numeric questions correctly.

Data analysis

Data were analysed using SPSS 24.0 (Statistical Program for the Social Sciences. Basic descriptive statistics, including means, medians, percentages, ranges and standard deviations were calculated to describe the samples in terms of socio-demographic characteristics.

Results

GP sample characteristics

Twenty-two GPs returned an expression of interest form and 18 GPs consented. The mean age of the GPs was 45 years (range 28–66 years), 72% were female, 50% were born in Australia, and 40% had more than 20 years' experience (Table 2).

Women sample characteristics

All of the GPs managed to invite at least one woman to participate. A total of 59 pregnant women were initially invited to take part. Of these, 22 did not meet the eligibility criteria and 8 were not interested. A total of 29 eligible women agreed to participate.

The mean age of the women was 32 years (range 25–40 years) (Table 3). Seventeen of the 29 women (59%) had a university education, 7 (24%) had a trade or technical qualification, and 5 (17%) had completed high (secondary) school education (aged between 15 and 16 years) or had achieved a Higher School Certificate. The Higher School Certificate (HSC) is the qualification awarded to senior high school students in Years 11 and 12 (aged between 16 to 18 years) who successfully complete high school. Participants were divided into two groups – (i) Higher education ($n = 17$, 59%) – undergraduate or postgraduate degree and, (ii) Lower education ($n = 12$, 41%) – completed secondary/ high school education or had successfully completed a Higher School Certificate, or trade/technical/ vocational qualifications.

Acceptability of the DA

GPs

Most GPs felt that the information was 'very' clear ($n = 13$, 72%), 'very' easy to read ($n = 13$, 72%), 'very' useful ($n = 16$, 89%), and 'very' appealing ($n = 14$,

Table 2 GP Characteristics ($n = 18$)[a]

Characteristics	N (%)
Age (years)	
Mean	45
Range	28–66
Gender	
Male	5 (28)
Female	13 (72)
Country of birth	
Australia	9 (50)
South-East Asia	5 (33)
Africa	3 (16)
UK	1 (6)
Primary language	
English	11 (61)
Other	7 (39)
Years of experience as a GP	
Less than a year	3 (20)
1–5 years	1 (7)
6–10 years	2 (13)
11–20 years	3 (20)
21–30 years	5 (33)
31+ years	1 (7)
Employment status	
Full-time	13 (72)
Part-time	5 (28)
Current role in general practice	
Registrar/in training	4 (22)
Contractor/sessional	7 (39)
Retainer/salaried	3 (17)
Partner/principal	4 (22)

[a]Some percentages do not add up to 100% due to rounding

78%) (Table 4). All GPs described the DA as 'very' informative ($n = 18$, 100%). The majority of GPs felt that the DA presented a balanced view of prenatal screening ($n = 16$, 89%), and would 'very much' assist women/couples in helping them to better understand about screening ($n = 15$, 83%) and facilitate their decision-making ($n = 16$, 89%).

Most felt the DA would make it 'somewhat' or 'much' easier to communicate to women about screening ($n = 16$, 88%). Just over half of GPs ($n = 10$, 56%) thought it would be 'very' feasible to implement the DA into practice, whereas the remaining GPs felt it would be 'somewhat' more challenging ($n = 8$, 44%). Half of the GPs described the information in the DA as just the right amount ($n = 9$, 50%), and the other half thought it would be 'too much' for women ($n = 9$, 50%).

Table 3 Characteristics of the women ($n = 29$)[a]

Characteristics	N (%)
Socio-demographic characteristics	
Age (years)	
Mean	32
Range	25–40
Marital Status	
Married	24 (83)
Living with partner	4 (14)
Not living with partner	1 (3)
Educational level	
Year 10 or below[b]	3 (10)
Year 12 Higher School Certificate (HSC)[c]	2 (7)
Trade or technical certificate	7 (24)
Bachelors/Undergraduate degree	10 (35)
Postgraduate degree	7 (24)
Country of birth	
Australia	22 (76)
Other	7 (24)
Language/s spoken at home	
English only	19 (66)
Bilingual	10 (34)
Current employment status	
Full-time employed	14 (48)
Part-time employed	7 (24)
Self-employed	3 (10)
Homemaker	4 (14)
Student	1 (3)
Has private health insurance	
Yes	22 (76)
No	6 (21)
Obstetric variables	
First pregnancy	
Yes	13 (45)
No	16 (55)
Previous pregnancy outcomes	
Previously experienced a miscarriage	7 (24)
Previously experienced a termination of pregnancy	2 (7)
Previous screening tests	
Yes	9 (31)
No	5 (17)
Unsure	3 (10)
Previous diagnostic tests	
No	16 (55)
Unsure	1 (3)

[a]Some percentages do not add up to 100% due to rounding
[b]In Australia, Year 10 is the 10th full year of compulsory secondary (or high school) education with students aged between 15 and 16 years. By the end of Year 10, all qualifying students complete secondary (high) school
[c]Senior secondary (high) school education runs from Year 11 and Year 12 with students aged between 16 to 18 years. The Higher School Certificate (HSC) is the qualification awarded to senior secondary school students who successfully complete senior high school

Table 4 GP responses regarding the acceptability of the DA ($n = 18$)

Questions and responses options	N (%)
How clear was the information?	
Very	13 (72)
Somewhat	5 (28)
How informative was the DA?	
Very	18 (100)
How easy to read was the DA	
Very	13 (72)
Somewhat	3 (17)
Not at all	2 (11)
How useful was the DA?	
Very	16 (89)
Somewhat	2 (11)
How appealing was the DA?	
Very	14 (78)
Somewhat	4 (22)
How would you describe the amount of information?	
Just right	9 (50)
Too much	9 (50)
How balanced did you find the information?	
Completely balanced	16 (89)
Encouraging prenatal screening	2 (11)
Will the DA make it easier for you to communicate with patients?	
Very much	8 (44)
Somewhat	8 (44)
Not at all	2 (11)
Do you think the DA will assist women/couples in helping them to understand about prenatal screening?	
Very much	15 (83)
Somewhat	3 (17)
Do you think the DA will assist women/couples in making decisions?	
Very much	16 (89)
Somewhat	2 (11)
How feasible would it be to implement the DA into routine practice?	
Very	10 (56)
Somewhat	5 (28)
Not very	3 (16)

Women

Overall, women reacted positively towards the DA (Table 5). The majority of participants reported reading all the information ($n = 25$, 86%), and that it took them less than 30 min to read ($n = 23$, 79%). Around half of the women reported that 'all' or 'most' of the information was new to them ($n = 15$, 51%). Most women felt the DA presented a balanced view of screening ($n = 21$, 72%),

Table 5 Women's responses regarding the acceptability of the decision aid by higher and lower education groups[a]

Questions and response options	Higher education (n = 17) N (%)	Lower education (n = 12) N (%)	Total women (n = 29) N (%)
How much of the DA did you read?			
I read all of it	14 (82)	11 (92)	25 (86)
I read part of it	0 (0)	1 (8)	1 (3)
My GP went through it with me	1 (6)	1 (8)	2 (7)
How long did it take you to read it?			
Less than thirty minutes	14 (82)	9 (75)	23 (79)
More than thirty minutes	3 (18)	3 (25)	6 (21)
What about the amount of information?			
Not enough	3 (18)	2 (18)	5 (18)
Just right	12 (71)	8 (73)	20 (71)
Too much	2 (12)	1 (9)	3 (11)
How balanced was the information?			
Encouraging prenatal screening	6 (35)	2 (17)	8 (28)
Completely balanced	11 (65)	10 (83)	21 (72)
Order of topics presented			
I liked the order	13 (89)	11 (92)	24 (89)
I'm not sure	2 (13)	1 (8)	3 (11)
How much of the information was new?			
All or most	10 (59)	5 (41)	15 (51)
Some	7 (41)	6 (50)	13 (45)
None	0 (100)	1 (8)	1 (3)
Did you show the booklet to anyone?			
Yes	11 (65)	7 (58)	18 (62)
No	6 (35)	5 (42)	11 (38)
Who did you show the booklet to?			
Husband/partner	9 (53)	6 (50)	15 (52)
Friend who is pregnant	0 (0)	1 (8)	1 (3)
GP + husband/partner	2 (12)	0 (0)	1 (7)
Would you recommend the DA?			
Yes I would	14 (82)	9 (75)	23 (79)
I'm not sure	2 (12)	2 (17)	4 (14)
No	1 (6)	1 (8)	2 (7)
How worried you felt after reading the DA?			
Not at all	8 (47)	7 (58)	15 (52)
A little bit	5 (29)	5 (42)	10 (35)
Somewhat	4 (24)	0 (0)	4 (14)
Did you use the worksheet?			
Yes	5 (29)	5 (42)	10 (34)
No	12 (71)	7 (58)	19 (66)
Please indicate if you thought the booklet was...			
Clearly presented	12 (71)	10 (83)	22 (76)
Informative	13 (77)	10 (83)	23 (80)
Easy to read	13 (77)	11 (92)	24 (83)

Table 5 Women's responses regarding the acceptability of the decision aid by higher and lower education groups[a] *(Continued)*

Questions and response options	Higher education (*n* = 17)	Lower education (*n* = 12)	Total women (*n* = 29)
	N (%)	N (%)	N (%)
Useful	14 (82)	10 (83)	24 (83)
Appealing to look at	10 (59)	9 (75)	19 (66)
How helpful was the DA in terms of…			
Increasing understanding of options	15 (88)	10 (83)	25 (86)
Clarifying the benefits of each option	9 (53)	9 (75)	18 (62)
Clarifying the risks of each option	12 (71)	8 (67)	20 (69)
Clarifying your decision-making	8 (47)	8 (67)	16 (55)
Helping you reach a decision	8 (47)	6 (50)	14 (48)

[a]Some percentages do not add up to 100% due to rounding

although a slightly higher proportion of women with higher education thought it was encouraging screening (*n* = 6, 35%) compared to those with lower education (*n* = 2, 17%). Most women thought the amount of information was 'just right' (*n* = 20, 71%), with only a few finding it to be 'too much' information (*n* = 3, 11%).

Most women found the booklet 'very' clearly presented (*n* = 22, 76%), 'very' informative (n = 23, 80%), 'very' easy to read (*n* = 24, 83%), and 'very' useful (n = 24, 83%) (Table 5). Slightly fewer women described the DA as 'very visually appealing to look at' (*n* = 19, 66%). The majority of women felt the booklet was 'very' helpful in increasing their understanding of the options (n = 25, 86%). Around half of the women reported it being 'very' helpful in clarifying their decision-making (*n* = 16, 55%) and reaching a decision (*n* = 14, 48%). Just over a third of women reported completing the personal worksheet (*n* = 10, 34%).

Women's responses to the open-ended questions

All of the women found the font size appropriate. The colours were described as 'bright', and 'consistent'. The illustrations and diagrams were generally well received; being described as 'appropriate', and 'a good mix of cultures'. However, a few women did not like the illustrations and found them 'condescending' and too 'upbeat' considering the serious nature of the topic.

The summary sheet, timeline, worksheet and glossary of medical words were described as 'useful', and helping to 'put it into perspective'. The 100 dot-diagrams (Fig. 1) received mixed responses – some described them as 'a clever visual representation', whereas others thought they were 'difficult to grasp' in terms of what they were representing (i.e. pregnant women carrying a baby with Down syndrome).

Women's screening knowledge – Conceptual and numeric

Overall, there was a difference in women's knowledge before and after exposure to the DA, with mean scores increasing from 12.7 (out of 22) to 18.3 (Table 6).

Conceptual knowledge scores improved from 12.0 to 14.4 (out of 16), and numeric knowledge scores increased from 0.7 to 3.9 (out of 6). Women's knowledge about NIPT also improved from 2.1 to 4.1 (out of 5) after receiving the decision aid. Both education groups showed improvements, and a slightly higher proportion of women with higher education had increased knowledge compared to women with lower education (77% versus 58%, respectively).

Key revisions to the DA based on participant feedback

Both women and GPs had useful suggestions on how to improve the booklet. The following revisions were made in accordance with their feedback. We included a summary page comparing the accuracy and potential risks (i.e. miscarriage) of the different types of screening and diagnostic tests so the reader had all the information in one to which they could refer to in their decision-making. Both women and GPs wanted more practical information on where NIPT could be done and who to ask about it; we included a list of questions about NIPT that women could ask their GP, or other antenatal health professional. Some women were interested to know where they could find more information on the practicalities or impact of raising a child with Down syndrome. As such, in our revisions, we provided details of several resources produced by Down syndrome Australia. Some GPs felt the booklet should explain that screening requires medical referral, and clarify that screening identifies other chromosomal conditions. Throughout the booklet, we made some wording changes in accordance with Down syndrome Australia protocol on how to communicate with the public about Down syndrome. For example, we replaced the term 'risk' with 'chance', and 'problem' or 'disease' with 'condition'. Based on GP feedback, we described diagnostic tests as 'definite' tests and replaced 'detecting Down syndrome' with 'identifying Down syndrome'. We also reworded the 100-dot diagrams to clarify that the

Table 6 Women's conceptual and numeric screening knowledge before and after receiving the decision aid by education group

	Higher education (n = 17)	Lower education (n = 12)	Total women (n = 29)
Pre Knowledge Scores, Mean (SD)[a]			
Conceptual (maximum score 16)	12.1 (1.7)	11.9 (2.2)	12 (1.9)
Numeric (maximum score 6)	0.9 (1.4)	0.3 (0.7)	0.7 (1.2)
NIPT knowledge (maximum score 5)	2.1 (1.2)	2.2 (0.6)	2.1 (1.0)
Total knowledge score (max score n)	13.1 (2.3)	12. 2 (1.8)	12.7 (2.1)
Adequate knowledge[b] (total score ≥ 17 out of 22), n (%)	1(6)	0 (0)	1(4)
Post Knowledge Scores, Mean (SD)			
Conceptual (maximum score 16)	14.7 (1.4)	14.1 (1.5)	14.4 (1.4)
Numeric (maximum score 6)	4.2 (2.4)	3.4 (2.4)	3.9 (2.4)
NIPT knowledge (maximum score 5)	4.3 (1.0)	3.8 (1.1)	4.1 (1.09)
Total knowledge score (max score 22)	18.9 (3.2)	17.5 (3.4)	18.3 (3.3)
Adequate knowledge (total score ≥ 17 out of 22), n (%)	13 (77)	7 (58)	20 (69)

[a]Data missing for 1 participant
[b]Participants were classified as having 'adequate' or 'inadequate' knowledge using the midpoint of the scale. It was decided a priori that a pass mark of 75% or above (score ≥17 out of 22) would be considered 'adequate knowledge'

diagrams represented 100 pregnant women carrying a baby with Down syndrome.

Discussion

This article describes the development and acceptability of a low literacy DA about Down syndrome screening. The DA was well received by women with different education levels and GPs. Women's knowledge of the different types of screening tests, including NIPT, increased after exposure to the DA. Most women felt the information was very clearly presented, easy to read, informative, and rated the amount of information and length favourably. The DA was considered to be relevant, with most reporting they would recommend it to others. Similarly, most GPs reported the DA as clear, and that it would assist women in decision-making.

Although conceptual and numeric knowledge increased for both higher and lower education groups, a slightly higher proportion of women with higher education were found to have adequate knowledge compared to those with lower education. Although this is a small sample, it nonetheless echoes previous work showing that women from lower education groups experience greater difficulties making an informed decision [32]. Similarly, women with higher education have shown to benefit more from decision aids than those with lower education, possibly because they are more familiar with the engaging in decision-making and critically appraising health information [33, 47, 52].

Both women and GPs reviewed the DA positively, and there were few discrepancies in their views towards it. However, they did differ with regard to the amount of information, with half of the GPs thinking there was too much information, yet most women thinking it was just

about right. Women expressed the need for more experiential information about living with a child who has Down syndrome. The final version includes website links with information about this. It is not uncommon for health professionals to underestimate how much information patients want to receive, possibly through fear of overloading patients, or underestimating their understanding [53].

Not all GPs agreed that the DA would be easy to implement and some felt it would not necessarily facilitate communication. The challenges of implementing DAs in clinical practice are widely reported [54–56]. Although DAs have proven to be effective, they are not commonly used in practice because of communication, cultural, ideological, organisational, and practical barriers [57]. Lepine et al. (2016) identified a number of factors influencing whether health professionals would use a prenatal screening DA, ranging from whether the tool was positively appraised, considered relevant, or being readily accessible to having enough time and colleagues endorsing the tool [58].

Our results showed that around two-thirds of women reported not using the values clarification worksheet. Perhaps the information on its own without a values clarification exercise might be enough to improve knowledge and enhance decision-making [27, 59, 60], or women found it difficult to complete. There is debate about whether DAs interfere with intuitive forms of information processing, and exercises that encourage deliberative (slow and analytic) decision-making may not always lead to better decisions. Clearly, more research is needed as to explore the factors that influence people using values clarification exercises, who might benefit more from such methods, and whether information alone might be enough to clarify values.

We note that GPs were the only health professionals involved in the study. Including other health professionals (e.g. midwives, obstetricians, and genetic counsellors) would have been useful to explore the diversity of perspectives. One study observed that health professionals varied in their attitudes towards using prenatal screening DAs; midwives seemed more positive about using DAs compared to GPs and obstetricians [58].

At the time of the study, NIPT was on the cusp of being implemented into the Australian healthcare system, predominately in the private health care system with test results being sent to offshore laboratories on a user pays basis with no reimbursement. At present, NIPT is more widely available in both the private and public healthcare system, and although it is less expensive than it used to be, it is still offered with no reimbursement. It is possible that discussions with health care professionals about NIPT may have influenced women's knowledge and understanding about NIPT, and women may have paid less attention to the decision aid because NIPT was too expensive for women to consider a viable option. However, we note that some GPs in our study were not fully aware of the availability of NIPT and found the decision aid to be informative in improving their own knowledge. Further, our results showed that women's knowledge of NIPT increased after exposure to the decision aid and they were able to correctly answer questions about accuracy of the NIPT that would have required reading the decision aid.

This study has a few limitations. Firstly, despite efforts to recruit partners to the study we were not successful. However, most women in the current study reported showing the DA to their partners, indicating that they valued their involvement. Similarly, previous research has shown screening decisions are often made by couples together [27, 36, 61, 62]. Others have also highlighted the challenges of recruiting men to participate in health research. Strategies have been proposed to help overcome men's resistance to participation, these include; emphasising the personal benefits and altruistic elements of the research, simplifying technical information, and using humour [63]. Future research should consider these recruitment strategies to ensure partners' perspectives are taken into account.

Secondly, although we made efforts to recruit women with varying education levels to ensure the tool was acceptable to different education groups, we encountered difficulties recruiting women from lower education groups. The length of recruitment was extended due to difficulties recruiting this group. This is perhaps not surprising given that lower socioeconomic groups are generally under-represented in health and medical research [64]. In addition, we did not measure participants' health literacy skills. While educational attainment is associated with literacy and health literacy, they are not synonymous. Further testing with higher and lower health literacy groups would be an important next step to identify whether the decision aid is suitable and understandable to different health literacy groups.

Thirdly, given the aims of the study were to provide descriptive data on the acceptability of the DA, the results should therefore be considered as preliminary. The small sample size in each education group meant that we were underpowered to perform statistical analyses to detect any statistical differences between the two groups. At this stage, it is not possible to make conclusive statements about the actual effect of the decision aid without a randomised controlled trial with a larger sample, to evaluate the efficacy of the DA compared to standard information. This will provide valuable evidence on the effect of the decision aid on informed decision-making (knowledge, attitudes, uptake, values consistency and deliberation), and enable us to generalise the findings to populations with different education levels.

Finally, in line with previous work [65], there was a very low response rate from GPs creating problems of non-response bias. GPs who responded may have had a stronger interest in prenatal screening and reactions to the DA may have been different among GPs who did not respond. Furthermore, although we asked GPs to invite all eligible pregnant women to participate, GPs may have selected women whom they thought had the necessary health literacy skills to read and understand the DA. We had considerable difficulties recruiting women with lower education levels throughout the study which subsequently delayed recruitment.

Conclusion

The DA was found to be acceptable, comprehensible, and useful to women from different educational backgrounds and GPs. Women's knowledge about screening, including NIPT, increased after exposure to the DA. The next steps will be to further test the DA among women with different health literacy skills, and then evaluate the efficacy of the DA on informed decision-making (knowledge, attitudes, values-consistency, deliberation) compared to standard information in a larger sample. It would also be important to identify strategies for how the tool could be more broadly used and implemented by GPs and other health professionals.

Practice implications

This is one of the few prenatal screening DAs to provide information about NIPT. It has the potential to provide prospective parents with clear and easy-to-read information, and complement existing information presented by health care professionals. A formal evaluation of the efficacy of the tool (compared to standard information) is necessary before it is made available.

Although all participants spoke English, around one-third of participants were bilingual. If translated into different languages, the DA could provide culturally and linguistically diverse (CALD) populations with a tool that is accessible in their own language and help to address the potential communication challenges. Future work could also focus on translating the DA into different languages to address the needs of those from CALD backgrounds.

Future work is also needed to identify and overcome the barriers to implementing DAs, with studies focused on identifying the contextual and facilitative mechanisms that could influence the implementation of the DA [66]. The potential use of social marketing, (the use of commercial marketing strategies to enhance public health and well-being [67], has also been suggested [57]. Future work could be directed towards identifying social marketing strategies (e.g. social media) to support the long-term implementation of DAs. We also note that this DA was developed in the context of the Australian healthcare system and the risk information presented is based on Australian data. The DA would need modification if tested in other countries.

Abbreviations
DA: Decision aid; NIPT: Non-invasive prenatal testing

Acknowledgements
We thank the women who took the time to participate in the study, and the GPs who helped us to recruit women and provide feedback. Special thanks to Dr. Cecile Muller, Ms. Kate Talbot, Dr. Jane Lloyd, Dr. Kate Dunlop, Dr. Mona Saleh, Ms. Marilena Pelosi, and Assistant Professor Marie-Anne Durand for their useful comments on the DA. We acknowledge Fiona Katauskas for her illustrations and Relax Design for their assistance with the graphical design of the decision aids.

Funding
At the time of this study, Dr. Sian Smith was supported by an Early Career Research Fellowship from the Australian National Health and Medical Research Council (ID 1034912). Professor Bettina Meiser was supported through an NHMRC Senior Fellowship, Level B (ID 1078523). Dr. Michelle Peate is supported by an Early Career Fellowship from the National Breast Cancer Foundation (ECF-015). Prof Jane Halliday is supported by NHMRC Senior Fellowship, Level B (ID1021252). Ms. Yanes is supported by NHMRC Postgraduate Research Scholarship and National Breast Cancer Foundations (ID 1133049). The funders had no role in the design or conduct of the study, in the collection, analysis and interpretation of data, or in the preparation or approval of the manuscript.

Authors' contributions
SS conceived the study. All authors (SS, AC, MW, MS, MP, AW, BM, RK, JH, SL, LT, KBS, MB) contributed to the design and development of the prenatal screening decision aid. SS, TY, MW and AC coordinated data collection. SS analysed the data and all of the authors contributed to interpreting it. SS wrote the first draft of the manuscript. All authors participated in writing and revising the draft manuscript critically for important intellectual content. All authors approved the final version of the manuscript.

Ethics approval and consent to participate
Ethics approval for the study was obtained from the South Eastern and South Western Sydney Local Health District Human Research Ethics Committees (ref number: HREC 12/219). Written informed consent was obtained from all GPs before they took part in the study. Verbal informed consent was obtained from all women before they completed the pre-questionnaire and were sent a copy of the decision aid. Given that the pre and post questionnaires were administered over the telephone, the Ethics Committees gave approval for women to provide verbal informed consent. Verbal consent was obtained using a verbal consent script, which explained to participants that participation was voluntary and that they could withdraw at any time. The research team kept a verbal consent log of participants who verbally agreed to participate in the study.

Consent for publication
N/A

Competing interests
The authors declare that they have no competing interests.

Author details
[1]Psychosocial Research Group, Lowy Research Centre, C25, Prince of Wales Clinical School, Faculty of Medicine, UNSW Sydney, Corner High and Botany St, Kensington, Sydney New South Wales 2033, Australia. [2]Centre for Applied Nursing Research, School of Nursing and Midwifery, Western Sydney University, Ingham, Sydney, Australia. [3]South Western Sydney Local Health District, Institute for Applied Medical Research, Sydney, Australia. [4]Department of Obstetrics and Gynaecology, Royal Women's Hospital, University of Melbourne, Parkville, Australia. [5]School of Women's and Children's Health, UNSW Sydney, Sydney, Australia. [6]Department of Maternal-Fetal Medicine, Royal Hospital for Women, Sydney, Australia. [7]Murdoch Children's Research Institute, Royal Children's Hospital, Parkville, Victoria, Australia. [8]Department of Paediatrics, University of Melbourne, Parkville, Australia. [9]Sydney School of Public Health, The University of Sydney, Sydney, Australia. [10]School of Psychiatry, Faculty of Medicine, UNSW Sydney, Sydney, Australia. [11]Sydney Medical School, The University of Sydney, Sydney, Australia. [12]Women's Services, Liverpool Hospital, Sydney, Australia. [13]Western Sydney University, Parramatta, Sydney, Australia.

References
1. Benn P, Borrell A, Jea C. Aneuploidy screening: a position statement from a committee on behalf of the Board of the International Society for Prenatal Diagnosis. Prenat Diagn 2011. 2011;31:519–22.
2. Bouman K, Bakker MK, Birnie E, ter Beek L, Bilardo CM, van Langen IM, de Walle HEK. The impact of national prenatal screening on the time of diagnosis and outcome of pregnancies affected with common trisomies, a cohort study in the northern Netherlands. BMC Pregnancy and Childbirth. 2017;17(1):4.
3. Ward P, Soothill P. Fetal anomaly ultrasound scanning: the development of a national programme for England. The Obstetrician & Gynaecologist. 2011;13(4):211–7.
4. EUROCAT (2010), EUROCAT Special Report: Prenatal Screening Policies in Europe 2010, EUROCAT Central Registry, University of Ulster. http://www.eurocat-network.eu/content/Special-Report-Prenatal-Screening-Policies.pdf. Accessed 11 Dec 2018.
5. St-Jacques S, Grenier S, Charland M, Forest J-C, Rousseau F, Légaré F. Decisional needs assessment regarding Down syndrome prenatal testing: a systematic review of the perceptions of women, their partners and health professionals. Prenat Diagn. 2008;28(13):1183–203.
6. Lou S, Mikkelsen L, Hvidman L, Petersen OB, Nielsen CP. Does screening for Down's syndrome cause anxiety in pregnant women? A systematic review. Acta Obstet Gynecol Scand. 2015;94.

7. Lo YMD, Corbetta N, Chamberlain PF, Rai V, Sargent IL, Redman CWG, Wainscoat JS. Presence of fetal DNA in maternal plasma and serum. Lancet. 1997;350(9076):485–7.

8. McLennan A, Palma-Dias R, da Silva CF, Meagher S, Nisbet DL, Scott F. Noninvasive prenatal testing in routine clinical practice – an audit of NIPT and combined first-trimester screening in an unselected Australian population. Aust N Z J Obstet Gynaecol. 2016;56(1):22–8.

9. Nicolaides KH. Screening for fetal aneuploidies at 11 to 13 weeks. Prenat Diagn. 2011;31(1):7–15.

10. Gil MM, Akolekar R, Quezada MS, Bregant B, Nicolaides KH. Analysis of cell-free DNA in maternal blood in screening for aneuploidies: meta-analysis. Fetal Diagn Ther. 2014;35(3):156–73.

11. Taylor-Phillips S, Freeman K, Geppert J, Agbebiyi A, Uthman OA, Madan J, Clarke A, Quenby S, Clarke A. Accuracy of non-invasive prenatal testing using cell-free DNA for detection of Down, Edwards and Patau syndromes: a systematic review and meta-analysis. Brit Med J Open. 2016;6 http://bmjopen.bmj.com/content/6/1/e010002.

12. Lewis C, Hill M, Chitty LS. Women's experiences and preferences for service delivery of non-invasive prenatal testing for aneuploidy in a public Health setting: a mixed methods study. PLoS One. 2016;11(4):e0153147.

13. Hill M, Fisher J, Chitty LS, Morris S. Women/'s and health professionals/' preferences for prenatal tests for Down syndrome: a discrete choice experiment to contrast noninvasive prenatal diagnosis with current invasive tests. Genet Med. 2012;14(11):905–13.

14. Allyse M, Minear M, Berson E, Sridhar S, Rote M, Hung A, Chandrasekharan S. Non-invasive prenatal testing: a review of international implementation and challenges. Int J Womens Health. 2015;7:113–26. Published online 2015 Jan 2016. https://doi.org/10.2147/IJWH.S67124.

15. Oepkes D, Page-Christiaens GC, Bax CJ, Bekker MN, Bilardo CM, Boon EMJ, Schuring-Blom GH, Coumans ABC, Faas BH, Galjaard R-JH, et al. Trial by Dutch laboratories for evaluation of non-invasive prenatal testing. Part I—clinical impact. Prenatal Diagnosis. 2016;36(12):1083–90.

16. Johansen P, Richter SR, Balslev-Harder M, Miltoft CB, Tabor A, Duno M, Kjaergaard S. Open source non-invasive prenatal testing platform and its performance in a public health laboratory. Prenat Diagn. 2016;36(6):530–6.

17. Chitty LS, Wright D, Hill M, Verhoef TI, Daley R, Lewis C, Mason S, McKay F, Jenkins L, Howarth A, et al. Uptake, outcomes, and costs of implementing non-invasive prenatal testing for Down's syndrome into NHS maternity care: prospective cohort study in eight diverse maternity units. Brit Med J. 2016;354.

18. Woolcock J, Grivell R. Noninvasive prenatal testing. Aust Fam Physician. 2014;43:432–4.

19. HGSA/RANZCOG Joint Committee on Prenatal Screening and Diagnosis: Prenatal screening and diagnosis of chromosomal genetic conditions in the fetus in pregnancy. In.: The Royal Australian and New Zealand College of Obstetricians and Gynaecologists & Womens Health Committee; 2016.

20. Dondorp W, de Wert G, Bombard Y, Bianchi DW, Bergmann C, Borry P, Chitty LS, Fellmann F, Forzano F, Hall A, et al. Non-invasive prenatal testing for aneuploidy and beyond: challenges of responsible innovation in prenatal screening. Eur J Hum Genet. 2015;23(11):1438–50.

21. de Jong A, Dondorp WJ, de Die-Smulders CEM, Frints SGM, de Wert GMWR. Non-invasive prenatal testing: ethical issues explored. Eur J Hum Genet. 2009;18(3):272–7.

22. van den Berg M, Timmermans DRM, ten Kate LP, van Vugt JMG, van der Wal G. Informed decision making in the context of prenatal screening. Patient Educ Couns. 2006;63(1–2):110–7.

23. Stacey D, Légaré F, Lewis K, Barry MJ, Bennett CL, Eden KB, Holmes-Rovner M, Llewellyn-Thomas H, Lyddiatt A, Thomson R, et al. Decision aids for people facing health treatment or screening decisions. Cochrane Database Syst Rev. 2017;4:CD001431. https://doi.org/10.1002/14651858.CD001431.pub5.

24. Vlemmix F, Warendorf JK, Rosman AN, Kok M, Mol BWJ, Morris JM, Nassar N. Decision aids to improve informed decision-making in pregnancy care: a systematic review. BJOG Int J Obstet Gynaecol. 2013;120(3):257–66.

25. Leiva Portocarrero ME, Garvelink MM, Becerra Perez MM, Giguère A, Robitaille H, Wilson BJ, Rousseau F, Légaré F. Decision aids that support decisions about prenatal testing for Down syndrome: an environmental scan. BMC Medical Informatics and Decision Making. 2015;15(1):76.

26. Beulen L, van den Berg M, Faas BHW, Feenstra I, Hageman M, van Vugt JMG, Bekker MN. The effect of a decision aid on informed decision-making in the era of non-invasive prenatal testing: a randomised controlled trial. Eur J Hum Genet. 2016;24(10):1409–16.

27. Portocarrero MEL, Giguère AMC, Lépine J, Garvelink MM, Robitaille H, Delanoë A, Lévesque I, Wilson BJ, Rousseau F, Légaré F. Use of a patient decision aid for prenatal screening for Down syndrome: what do pregnant women say? BMC Pregnancy and Childbirth. 2017;17(1):90.

28. McCray AT. Promoting Health literacy. J Am Med Inform Assoc. 2005;12(2):152–63.

29. Nutbeam D. Defining and measuring health literacy: what can we learn from literacy studies? Int J Public Health. 2009;54(5):303–5.

30. ABS: Adult Literacy and Life Skills Survey, Summary Results. Canberra: Australian Bureau of Statistics: Australian Government Publishing Service. Cat No. 4228.0; 2006.

31. Nagle C, Gunn J, Bell R, Lewis S, Meiser B, Metcalfe S, Ukoumunne OC, Halliday J. Use of a decision aid for prenatal testing of fetal abnormalities to improve women's informed decision making: a cluster randomised controlled trial [ISRCTN22532458]. BJOG: An International Journal of Obstetrics & Gynaecology. 2008;115(3):339–47.

32. Smith S, Sousa M, Essink-Bot ML, Halliday J, Peate M, Fransen M. Socioeconomic differences in informed decisions about Down syndrome screening: a systematic review and research agenda. J Health Commun. 2016;21(8):868–907.

33. Nagle C, Lewis S, Meiser B, Metcalfe S, Carlin JB, Bell R. Evaluation of a decision aid for prenatal testing of fetal abnormalities: a cluster randomised trial [ISRCTN22532458]. BMC Public Health. 2006;6:96.

34. Volk RJ, Llewellyn-Thomas H, Stacey D, Elwyn G. Ten years of the international patient decision aid standards collaboration: evolution of the core dimensions for assessing the quality of patient decision aids. BMC Medical Informatics and Decision Making. 2013;13(2):S1.

35. NSW Health's Centre for Genetics Education: Prenatal testing - Special tests for your baby during pregnancy. Edited by www.genetics.edu.au. 2013.

36. Willis AM, Smith SK, Meiser B, Muller C, Lewis S, Halliday J. How do prospective parents prefer to receive information about prenatal screening and diagnostic testing? Prenat Diagn. 2015;35(1):100–2.

37. Doak CCD, L. G, Root JH. Teaching patients with low literacy skills. 2nd ed. Philadelphia: J.B. Lippincott; 1996.

38. Clerehan R, Buchbinder R, Moodie J. A linguistic framework for assessing the quality of written patient information: its use in assessing methotrexate information for rheumatoid arthritis. Health Educ Res. 2005;20(3):334–44.

39. McCaffery K, Holmes-Rovner M, Smith S, Rovner D, Nutbeam D, Clayman M, Kelly-Blake K, Wolf M, Sheridan S. Addressing health literacy in patient decision aids. BMC Med Inform Decis Mak. 2013;13(Suppl 2):S10.

40. Houts PS, Doak CC, Doak LG, Loscalzo MJ. The role of pictures in improving health communication: a review of research on attention, comprehension, recall, and adherence. Patient Educ Couns. 2006;61(2):173–90.

41. South Western Sydney Local Health District. Health Profile of Local Communities. In: 3. Sydney: Local Health District. Accessed 4 July 2018, https://www.swslhd.health.nsw.gov.au/planning/content/pdf/SWSLHD%20Community%20Profile%20Summary%20070814.pdf; 2014.

42. The Royal Australian and New Zealand College of Obstetricians and Gynaecologists: Shared maternity care obstetric patients In., edn. Melbourne, Australia: Training, Accreditation and Recertification (TAR) Subcommittee of the Conjoint Committee for the Diploma of Obstetrics and Gynaecology (CCDOG) and approved by the RANZCOG Board and Council.; 2016.

43. Health NSW. Prenatal testing/screening for Down syndrome and other chromosomal abnormalities. Sydney, NSW: Australia: NSW Health, Ministry of Health; 2013.

44. Wakefield CE, Meiser B, Homewood J, Peate M, Kirk J, Warner B, Lobb E, Gaff C, Tucker K. Development and pilot testing of two decision aids for individuals considering genetic testing for Cancer risk. J Genet Couns. 2007;16(3):325–39.

45. Wakefield CE, Watts KJ, Meiser B, Sansom-Daly U, Barratt A, Mann GJ, Lobb EA, Gaff CL, Howard K, Patel MI. Development and pilot testing of an online screening decision aid for men with a family history of prostate cancer. Patient Educ Couns. 2011;83(1):64–72.

46. Hyett J, Mogra R, Sonek J. First trimester ultrasound assessment for fetal aneuploidy. Clin Obstet Gynecol. 2014;57(1):142–58.

47. Smith SK, Dixon A, Trevena L, Nutbeam D, McCaffery KJ. Exploring patient involvement in healthcare decision making across different education and functional health literacy groups. Soc Sci Med. 2009;69(12):1805–12.

48. Reyna VF. A theory of medical decision making and health: fuzzy trace theory. Medical Decis Making. 2008;28:850–65.

49. Setton R, Wilhelms E, Weldon B, Chick C, Reyna V. An overview of judgment and decision making research through the Lens of fuzzy trace theory. Xin li ke xue jin zhan. 2014;22(12):1837–54.

50. Schoonen H, van Agt HME, Essink-Bot M-L, Wildschut HI, Steegers EAP, de Koning HJ. Informed decision-making in prenatal screening for Down's syndrome: what knowledge is relevant? Patient Educ Couns. 2011;84(2):265–70.

51. Smith SK, Trevena L, Simpson JM, Barratt A, Nutbeam D, McCaffery KJ. A decision aid to support informed choices about bowel cancer screening among adults with low education: randomised controlled trial. Brit Med J. 2010;341:c5370.

52. Michie S, Dormandy E, Marteau TM. Increasing screening uptake amongst those intending to be screened: the use of action plans. Patient Educ Couns. 2004;55(2):218–22.

53. Lee PY, Khoo EM, Low WY, Lee YK, Abdullah KL, Azmi SA, Ng CJ. Mismatch between health-care professionals' and patients' views on a diabetes patient decision aid: a qualitative study. Health Expect. 2016;19(2):427–36.

54. Legare F, Stacey D, Briere N, Fraser K, Desroches S, Dumont S, Sales A, Puma C, Aube D. Healthcare providers' intentions to engage in an interprofessional approach to shared decision-making in home care programs: a mixed methods study. J Interprof Care. 2013;27.

55. Elwyn G, Laitner S, Coulter A, Walker E, Watson P, Thomson R. Implementing shared decision making in the NHS. Brit Med J. 2010;341.

56. Harrison JD, Masya L, Butow P, Solomon M, Young J, Salkeld G, Whelan T. Implementing patient decision support tools: moving beyond academia? Patient Educ Couns. 2009;76(1):120–5.

57. Stevens G, Thompson R, Watson B, Miller YD. Patient decision aids in routine maternity care: benefits, barriers, and new opportunities. Women and Birth. 2015;29(1):30–4.

58. Lépine J, Leiva Portocarrero ME, Delanoë A, Robitaille H, Lévesque I, Rousseau F, Wilson BJ, Giguère AMC, Légaré F. What factors influence health professionals to use decision aids for Down syndrome prenatal screening? BMC Pregnancy and Childbirth. 2016;16(1):262.

59. Garvelink MM, ter Kuile MM, Stiggelbout AM, de Vries M. Values clarification in a decision aid about fertility preservation: does it add to information provision? BMC Medical Informatics and Decision Making. 2014;14(1):68.

60. Peate M, Watts K, Wakefield CE. The 'value' of values clarification in cancer-related decision aids. Patient Educ Couns. 2013;90:281–3.

61. Carroll FE, Al-Janabi H, Flynn T, Montgomery AA. Women and their partners' preferences for Down's syndrome screening tests: a discrete choice experiment. Prenat Diagn. 2013;33(5):449–56.

62. Carroll FE, Owen-Smith A, Shaw A, Montgomery AA. A qualitative investigation of the decision-making process of couples considering prenatal screening for Down syndrome. Prenat Diagn. 2012;32(1):57–63.

63. Joseph G, Kaplan CP, Pasick RJ. Recruiting Low-income healthy women to research: an exploratory study. Ethnicity & health. 2007;12(5):497–519.

64. Bonevski B, Randell M, Paul C, Chapman K, Twyman L, Bryant J, Brozek I, Hughes C. Reaching the hard-to-reach: a systematic review of strategies for improving health and medical research with socially disadvantaged groups. BMC Med Res Methodol. 2014;14(1):42.

65. Cottrell E, Roddy E, Rathod T, Thomas E, Porcheret M, Foster NE. Maximising response from GPs to questionnaire surveys: do length or incentives make a difference? BMC Med Res Methodol. 2015;15:3.

66. Stetler CB, Damschroder LJ, Helfrich CD, Hagedorn HJ. A guide for applying a revised version of the PARIHS framework for implementation. Implement Sci. 2011;6:99.

67. Evans WD. How social marketing works in health care. Brit Med J. 2006; 332(7551):1207–10.

15

Acceptability of option B+ among HIV positive women receiving antenatal and postnatal care services in selected health centre's in Lusaka

Bridget Chomba Chanda[1,2*], Rosemary Ndonyo Likwa[2], Jessy Zgambo[3], Louis Tembo[4] and Choolwe Jacobs[3]

Abstract

Background: In 2013, Zambia accepted the immediate operationalization of Option B+, a policy used to try and eliminate mother to child transmission. This policy requires all HIV-positive pregnant and breastfeeding women to initiate antiretroviral treatment for life regardless of CD4 count. However, not all HIV positive women accept treatment for life. This study aimed to investigate acceptability of lifelong ART (Option B+) among HIV positive women receiving antenatal and postnatal services at the university teaching hospital and Lusaka urban city clinics.

Methods: This was a cross sectional study conducted in November, 2016 to March 2017. The study population comprised of HIV positive women in their reproductive age (15–49 years). A Structured questionnaire was used to collect data in a face to face interview with the participants. Data was entered in EpiData version 3.1 and analysed using Stata version 13. Multivariate logistic regression analysis was performed to determine predictors of acceptability.

Results: Overall, 427 women participated in this study. Their mean age was 30 years. Of the 427, over half (54%) had inadequate knowledge and about 30% of the women in the study still experience stigma and discrimination. 63.2% of the women had good attitude towards Option B+ and overall, the majority (77.8%) were willing to accept antiretroviral therapy for life. Multivariate analysis showed that only women with good attitude were 9.4 times more likely to accept Option B+ than those with a bad attitude [OR: 9.4: 95%CI, 5.8–15.2)].

Conclusion: This study showed that in general, women accepted initiation of Option B+. However, there is still a gap in the level of knowledge of Option B+ as well as stigma and discrimination in some communities, hence there is need to intensify programs that are aimed at educating the community on the importance of ART for life, combat stigma and discrimination and consequently promote acceptability of Option B+.

Keywords: Acceptability, Antiretroviral therapy, Option B +, Prevention of mother to child transmission; knowledge, Attitude, Discrimination

* Correspondence: chandabridget@gmail.com
[1]Department of Paediatric and Child Health, University Teaching Hospital-HIV/AIDS Program, P.O Box, 50440 Lusaka, Zambia
[2]Department of population studies and Nutrition, School of Public Health, University of Zambia, Geneva, Switzerland
Full list of author information is available at the end of the article

Background

About 160,000 new HIV infections among children aged 0–14 occurred in 2016, dramatically declining from 300,000 in 2010. Progress in reducing mother-to-child transmission of HIV has been dramatic since the introduction in 2011 of the 'Global Plan towards the Elimination of New HIV Infections among Children, and Keeping their Mothers Alive', largely because of increased access to PMTCT-related services and increased number of pregnant women living with HIV being initiated on lifelong antiretroviral medicines [1]. But it has not been fast enough to reach the 2020 targets set by UNAIDS and partners as part of the Super-Fast-Track Framework to end AIDS. Acceleration of treatment for all pregnant and breastfeeding women living with HIV is still needed to achieve elimination of new infections among children and halve HIV-related deaths among pregnant women and new mothers [1].

Under WHO's 2010 PMTCT ARV guidance, countries had the option to choose between two prophylaxis regimens for pregnant women living with HIV with CD4 greater than 350cells/mm3. Option A and Option B. Under Option A, women received antenatal and intrapartum antiretroviral prophylaxis along with an antiretroviral postpartum "tail" regimen to reduce risk of drug resistance, while infants receive postpartum antiretroviral prophylaxis throughout the duration of breastfeeding [2].

Option B, on the other hand, has a simpler clinical flow in which all pregnant and lactating women with HIV initially are offered ART – beginning in the antenatal period and continuing throughout the duration of breastfeeding. At the end of breastfeeding those women who do not yet require ART for their own health would discontinue the prophylaxis and continue to monitor their CD4 count, eventually re-starting ART when the CD4 falls below 350cells/mm3. Along with these two options a third approach is now being used, Option B+, in which all pregnant women living with HIV are offered life-long ART, regardless of their CD4 count [2].

To achieve the goal of elimination of mother to child transmission (eMTCT), in 2013, the Zambian government accepted the immediate operationalization of Option B+ [3]. This is done with the understanding that all HIV positive women are to be initiated on antiretroviral therapy (ART) for life. Antiretroviral therapy offers women the best chance of preventing mother to child transmission, however, not all HIV positive women are willing to accept ART for life.

Katirayi et al. [4] found that women reported difficulty around learning their HIV status and initiating ART on the same day. They needed time to think about ART initiation and wanted to first discuss with their partners before committing to lifelong treatment. A study conducted in Zimbabwe found that pregnant and lactating women find it easy to accept lifelong therapy because it is similar to taking medication for diabetes or birth control [5].

Other studies have identified attitudes towards lifelong treatment [6], knowledge of prevention of mother to child transmission [7], social demographic [8] and cultural characteristics [9] as factors that determine acceptability of Option B+. However, the impact of these factors may vary depending on the study setting and study population.

Overall, the evidence regarding how women's experiences in PMTCT option B+ services affect their subsequent care-seeking behaviour remains sparse. This appears particularly true with regard to the uptake of both long-term HIV care and treatment for the woman's own HIV infection and infant HIV testing and related services. However, women's experiences of and perspectives on current and proposed interventions and how these influence subsequent care-seeking behaviour need to be better understood to ensure that an appropriate and acceptable package of services could be offered and that the virtual elimination of mother-to-child HIV transmission become an attainable goal [10].

A study on acceptability of Option B+ among HIV positive pregnant and breastfeeding women is of supreme value in understanding the factors that inhibit enrolment on lifelong ART. During the implementation of different regimens for PMTCT, the efficacy of a regimen is not the only important aspect to consider but the way in which the people accept it will determine how well or how poorly it will work.

Study findings on the acceptability of Option B+ among Zambian women are limited. This study was conducted to determine acceptability of Option B+ and associated factors among HIV positive women receiving antenatal and postnatal care services at UTH and Lusaka Urban City Clinics. The information generated may be used to aid policy makers and HIV care givers in improving programmes aimed at encouraging the uptake of ART for life among pregnant and breastfeeding women and improve maternal health.

Methods
Study design and study setting

This was a cross sectional study conducted in five health centers in Lusaka from November, 2016 to March 2017. In Lusaka district, Maternal Child Health (MCH) and PMTCT services are offered in 24 of the 28 health centers and in all the health posts. The study sites (UTH, Matero Ref, Chawama, Kalingalinga and Chilenje) were chosen because they are in high density areas, offer antenatal, postnatal and PMTCT services.

Sample size determination

A single population proportion formula was used to determine the study sample size with 95% confidence interval, 50% proportion, a precision of 5 and 10% non-response rate. The overall estimated sample size was 427. The study population comprised of HIV positive women who were attending antenatal and postnatal care services at the selected health centres and the target age group were women in the reproductive age (15–49). Exclusion criteria were HIV positive women with inability to communicate, HIV positive women who did not consent to take part in the study and all HIV negative women.

Sampling method

This study used Stratified Random Sampling. Drawing from a total of 12 government owned delivery health facilities that reported their 2015 PMTCT annual program results to PEPFAR Zambia, five health facilities were selected. The chosen clinics and hospital were treated as strata's. The number of women to be included in each health facility was worked out in proportion to the population of HIV positive women in each facility. Simple random sampling (SRS) was then used to select the study participants. The target population was selected from each health facility using a sampling list (PMTCT Register), taking into account the inclusion and exclusion criteria. The women were identified by their hospital numbers. These numbers were written on separate pieces of paper, folded and mixed into a box to conduct a lottery.

Data collection and analysis

A structured interviewer administered questionnaire was used to collect data. Prior to administration of the questionnaire, a pilot study was conducted to check for appropriateness and consistency. The questionnaire was translated into Nyanja for those that did not understand or speak English. The questionnaire was divided into four sections namely, a) Socio-demographic factors, b) Knowledge of Option B+, c) Attitudes towards Option B + and D) Socio-cultural factors.

Data was entered into EpiData version 3.1 and analyzed using Stata IC 13–64-bit (STATA Corporation, College Station, TX, USA) for analysis. Frequencies and proportions were used to describe the study participants. The statistical significance in this study was set at 5% (0.05) and confidence interval at 95%. Acceptability was the main outcome variable in this study and was binary. Independent variables associated with acceptability of Option B+ were analysed using logistic regression analysis. Univariate and multivariate logistic regression analysis were employed. The level of knowledge was measured from a score of five questions from the questionnaire, a score of four and five was graded as

adequate knowledge and any score from 0 to 3 was graded as inadequate knowledge [6, 10]. Attitude was also measured using scores. A score of 3 was graded as good attitude and any score of 2 questions or less was graded as bad attitude [6, 10]. All variables found to be significantly associated with acceptability were included for multivariate logistic regression analysis to control for confounders.

Ethics and consent

Ethical approval of the study was obtained from the University of Zambia Biomedical Research and Ethics Committee (IRB00001131 of IORG0000774, Reference number 022–06-16). Written consent was obtained from all the participants as well as parental consent for participants under the age of 16.

Results

Socio-demographic and cultural characteristics of participants

Table 1 shows the socio-demographic and cultural characteristics of the participants; most of them (48.7%) were

Table 1 Socio-demographic and cultural characteristics of participants

Demographic Factors		Frequency	Percent
Age	15–24	36	8.4
	25–34	208	48.7
	35–44	167	39.1
	45–49	16	3.7
Marital status	single	77	18
	married	320	74.9
	divorced	16	3.7
	widowed	14	3.3
Occupation	employed	108	25.3
	unemployed	319	74.7
Education	primary	115	26.9
	secondary	236	55.3
	tertiary	73	17.1
	none	3	0.7
Cultural Factors			
Religion	Christianity	421	98.6
	Other	6	1.4
Denomination	Pentecostal	126	29.9
	Catholic	82	19.4
	Adventist	57	13.5
	UCZ	51	12.1
	Jehovah's Witness	28	6.6
	other	78	18.5
Fear of partner discrimination	Yes	152	35.6
	No	275	64.4
Fear of family discrimination	Yes	134	31.4
	No	293	68.6
Permission to begin ART	Yes	134	31.4
	No	293	68.6
	Total	427	100

within the age of 25–34 years with a mean age of 30. Majority (74.9%) were married at the time of the study and were not in formal employment. The educational levels of the respondents showed that 55.3% had reached secondary school while very few (17.1%) attained tertiary education. Regarding the socio-cultural factors, this study showed that most of the participants were Christian (98.6%) belonging to different Christian denominations. Thirty five percent (35%) of the participants expressed that their partners would discriminate them if they found out that they were on ART and most of them (68.6%) said they would not need permission from their partners or family members before initiating ART.

Acceptability, level of knowledge and attitudes towards option B+

Table 2 shows that out of the 427 participants, only 45.9% had adequate knowledge of Option B+. Despite the level of knowledge found, most of them (63.2%) had good attitude towards Option B+ and overall, majority (77.8%) were willing to be on ART for life.

Predictors of acceptability using logistic regression analysis

Table 3 shows the results of the logistic regression analysis. The univariate model showed that women who feared partner or family discrimination were less likely to accept Option B+ than those that believed that they would not be discriminated. Those with adequate knowledge were 2 times more likely to accept Option B+ than those with inadequate knowledge [OR: 2.1 (95%CI, 1.3–3.3)]. Attitude of women was observed to be statistically associated with acceptability with those with good attitude being 9 times more likely to accept Option B+ than those with a bad attitude [OR: 9.4 (95%CI, 5.8–15.2)].

All factors that were found to be significant in the univariate model were put in the multivariate model. The results show that attitude was the only factor significantly

Table 2 Level of knowledge and attitudes towards Option B+ among participants

	Frequency	Percent
Knowledge level		
Adequate Knowledge	196	45.9
Inadequate knowledge	231	54.1
Specific attitudes towards Option B+		
Good attitude	270	63.2
Bad attitude	157	36.8
Overall Acceptability		
yes	332	77.8
no	95	22.2
Total	427	100

associated with acceptability of Option B+ [AOR: 9.2 (95%CI, 5.7–15.1)]. Participants with good attitude were 9 times more likely to accept Option B+ than those that had a bad attitude.

Discussion

The majority of HIV positive women receiving antenatal and postnatal care services in this study accepted life-long treatment. Similarly, studies from Malawi and Zimbabwe on the acceptability of Option B+ among pregnant and breastfeeding women showed that women accepted ART for life [4, 11].

While the women in this study generally accepted Option B+, there is still a gap in the knowledge levels. The study showed that over half (54.1%) of the participants had inadequate knowledge of Option B+. These findings were consistent with a study conducted in Tanzania which showed inadequate knowledge on treatment and prevention for HIV infected pregnant women: only 34% knew that HIV-infected pregnant woman could be on ART and 47% did not know that antiretroviral (ARVs) should be used throughout life [7]. A similar study from Ethiopia shows contradicting results, which was; most of the participants (58%) had adequate knowledge of PMTCT Option B+ [6]. The results of this study highlight a clear need for proving more information on Option B+ to the general population, women who attend antenatal and postnatal visits at health facilities as well as the benefits of being initiated on Option B+ early.

Regarding the socio-cultural factors, no association was observed between religion and denomination with willingness to accept option B+. The differences in the denominations among the women in this study did not affect acceptability. This is in line with a study that was conducted in Tanzania which showed that belief in the healing power of prayer was not significantly associated with a person's hypothetical willingness to begin ARV treatment if they became HIV infected [12]. On the contrary, a study conducted in Ghana indicates that some respondents still held the opinion that HIV is a spiritual disease and therefore there is the need to seek spiritual interventions. Some defaulters cited "use of alternative medicines" as a reason for not going for antiretrovirals and others sleep in prayer camps. This causes them to default most often. However as disease progression among these groups becomes rapid they return to the health facility to continue treatment with ARVs [8].

This study also revealed that about 30% of the women still experience HIV related stigma and discrimination from their partners and families which may affect the acceptability of life-long treatment. Those who stated that their partner and family would discriminate them were less likely to accept Option B+ compared to those that believed they would not be discriminated. Research has

Table 3 Logistic regression analysis on acceptability of Option B+ in relation to potential predictors

Predictor variable	COR (95% CI) P-Value		AOR (95% CI) P-Value	
Employment status				
Employed	1		–	–
Unemployed	0.8(0.5–1.4)	0.427		
Marital status				
Single	1			
Married	1.9(1.1–3.2)	0.028		
Divorced	2.1(0.5–8.0)	0.284		
Widowed	6.25(0.8–50.5)	0.086	1.0(0.6–1.7)	0.903
Education level				
None	1			
Primary	1.4 (0.1–16.2)	0.779		
Secondary	1.86(0.17–20.9)	0.615	–	–
Tertiary	2.1(0.18–24.9)	0.554		
Age				
>=35	1			
15–34	0.6(0.3–1.1)	0.099	–	–
Religion				
Other	1		–	–
Christianity	3.6(0.7–18.0)	0.122		
Christian Denomination				
Catholics	1		–	–
Protestants	1.1(0.6–2.0)	0.794		
Fear of partner discrimination				
No	1			
Yes	0.7(0.2–1.2)	0.003	1.0(0.5–2.0)	0.901
Fear of family discrimination				
No	1			
Yes	0.5(0.02–1.0)	0.041	0.7(0.4–1.4)	0.308
Permission to begin ART				
No	1		–	–
Yes	1.2(0.7–2.0)	0.481		
Knowledge				
Inadequate	1			
Adequate	2.1(1.3–3.3)	0.003	1.3(0.7–2.4)	0.356
Attitude				
Bad	1			
Good	9.4(5.8–15.2)	0.0001	9.3(5.7–15.2)	0.0001

shown that stigma and discrimination undermine HIV prevention efforts by making people afraid to seek HIV information, services and modalities to reduce their risk of infection and to adopt safer behaviour's lest these actions raise suspicion about their HIV status [13].

With regards to getting permission from partner or family, most women in this study said they would not need any permission from their partners or family members before initiating ART for life. This implies that most women would not reject ART for life due to failure to get consent from partner/family. A study conducted in Malawi on Acceptability of lifelong treatment (Option B+) found contradicting results. The women were overwhelmed with the information, needed time to think about ART initiation and wanted to first discuss with their partners before committing to lifelong treatment [4].

Women in this study generally had a good attitude towards Option B+. Though receiving ART for life can be a burden; most of the women felt that they would not have problems with initiating ART for life. The good attitude found among the women could be attributed to the hope that ART can help improve the quality of life, survival and also benefit their children. This hope has helped change the negative attitudes towards lifelong treatment. Furthermore, the women with good attitude were more likely to accept Option B+ than the women with a bad attitude. This simply shows that the more the women develop a good attitude towards Option B+, the more the willingness to accept it. These findings were consistent with other research findings that have also shown that majority of the study participants 199 (66.1%) had positive attitude about PMTCT option B+ service [10]. A similar study conducted in Ethiopia reviewed that 76.3% of participants had positive attitude while others had poor attitude [6]. In order to have more HIV positive women on Option B+, intensive counselling needs to be done to help change the negative behaviours of some women.

However, this study has potential limitations that should be noted. Firstly this study was based on a cross-sectional design which does not show causal relationships. Secondly, Women who had been receiving ART prior to 2013 when Option B+ was implemented were included in this study. Generalization of the study findings was limited to selected health facilities of Lusaka District hence future studies should involve health facilities across the country.

Conclusion

This study reveals that majority of the participants in this setting accepted the lifelong treatment of Option B +. Their attitudes towards it were generally good. However, we have found inadequacy on the level of knowledge of Option B+ which suggests need for efforts to help individuals and the broader communities have a better understanding of Option B+ as a preventive measure for HIV among women and their unborn children. Redesigning health educational strategies on PMTCT and ART for life into local language may reach both the literate and illiterate. There is also need to intensify sensitization programmes in order to successfully combat stigma and discrimination found in this study.

Abbreviations

ART: Antiretroviral Therapy; ARV: Antiretroviral; EMTCT: Elimination of mother-to-child transmission (of HIV); HIV: Human immunodeficiency virus; MTC: Mother to child transmission; PMTCT: Prevention of mother-to-child transmission of HIV; UNAIDS: Joint United Nations Program on HIV/AIDS; UNICEF: United Nations International Children's Emergency Fund; UTH: University Teaching Hospital; WHO: World Health Organisation

Acknowledgements

Special thanks go to the health institutions involved in this study, data collectors and all the study participant.

Funding

Not applicable.

Authors' contributions

BC designed the study, supervised data collection, analysed the data and drafted the paper. RL and CJ contributed in the design of the study. RL and CJ provided scientific advices on data analysis and throughout the preparation of the manuscript. JZ contributed to the designing and drafting of the manuscript. LT contributed to the analysing the data. All authors read and approved the final version of the manuscript.

Competing interests

The authors declare that they have no competing interests.

Author details

[1]Department of Paediatric and Child Health, University Teaching Hospital-HIV/AIDS Program, P.O Box, 50440 Lusaka, Zambia. [2]Department of population studies and Nutrition, School of Public Health, University of Zambia, Geneva, Switzerland. [3]Department of Epidemiology and Biostatistics, School of Public Health, University of Zambia, Lusaka, Zambia. [4]Department of Health Promotion and Education, School of Public Health, University of Zambia, Lilongwe, Malawi.

References

1. UNICEF: Monitoring the situation of women and children, EMTCT. 2017. https://data.unicef.org/topic/hivaids/emtct/. Accessed 17th October, 2017.
2. WHO: Consolidated Guidelines on the use of antiretroviral drugs for treating and preventing HIV infection. Recommendations for a public health approach. Second edition, 2016. http://www.who.int/hiv/pub/arv/arv-2016/en/. Accessed 2nd May, 2018.
3. PEPFAR: Zambia country operational plan, Strateg Dir summary. 2016. https://www.pepfar.gov/documents/organization/222188.pdf. Accessed 20th April, 2018.
4. Katirayi L, H. Namadingo, E. Bobrow, A. Yemaneberhan, M. Phiri, S. White, F. Chimbwandira, et al. Acceptability of lifelong treatment (Option B+) among HIV-positive pregnant and lactating women in Selected Sites in Malawi. 2014. EGPAF.
5. Tumbare E , Chadambuka A, Muchedzi A, Mushavi A, Mahomva A. Acceptability of Lifelong antiretroviral treatment (Option B+) among HIV-Positive Pregnant and Breastfeeding Women in Selected Sites in Zimbabwe. 2015. Elizabeth Glaser, Paediatric AIDS Foundation.
6. Tsegaye Delelegn. Level of adherence and associated factors to option b+ PMTCT programme among pregnant & lactating mothers in selected government health facilities of south Wzone, Amhara region, north East Ethiopia. 2016.
7. Agnarson AM, Levira F , Masanja H, Ekström AM, Thorson A Antiretroviral Treatment Knowledge and Stigma-Implications for Programs and HIV Treatment Interventions in Rural Tanzanian Populations. 2013. Tanzania.
8. Boateng D, Kwapong GD and Agyei-Baffour P. Knowledge, perception about antiretroviral therapy (ART) and prevention of mother-to-child transmission (PMTCT) and adherence to ART among HIV positive women in the Ashanti Region, Ghana. 2013.
9. Mhod M. Lived experiences of stigma and discrimination among

people on antiretroviral therapy: a qualitative study in ilala municipality, dares salaam. 2013.

10. Kahsay TG. Assessment of Knowledge and Attitude about Prevention of Mother to Child Transmission of HIV Option B+ and associated factors among ANC clients in Dessie town. Addis Ababa, Ethiopia; 2015.

11. Chadambuka A , Muchedzi A , Katirayi L , Tumbare E , Musarandega R , Nyamundaya T, Mutede B, Tachiwenyika E, et al. Acceptability of option B+ among pregnant and breastfeeding women in selected districts in Zimbabwe. 2016.

12. James Z, Yamanaka Y, John M, Watt M, Ostermann J, Thielman N. Religion and HIV in Tanzania: influence of religious beliefs on HIV stigma, disclosure, and treatment attitudes; 2008.

13. UNAIDS: Reduction of HIV-related stigma and discrimination. 2014.

16

Group B streptococci vaginal colonization and drug susceptibility pattern among pregnant women attending in selected public antenatal care centers in Addis Ababa, Ethiopia

Solomon Assefa[1*], Kassu Desta[2] and Tsehaynesh Lema[3,4]

Abstract

Background: Group B Streptococcus (GBS) is the leading cause of septicemia, meningitis, and pneumonia in neonates. Maternal colonization with GBS is the principal risk factor for early-onset disease in infants. Group B Streptococcus is now an important cause of maternal and neonatal morbidity and mortality in many parts of the world. In Ethiopia, few studies have been done on GBS colonization among pregnant women. The aim of this study was to determine the prevalence of GBS colonization, antimicrobial susceptibility patterns and assess risk factors among pregnant women.

Methods: A prospective cross-sectional study was conducted from May to August 2014 at selected public antenatal care (ANC) centers in Addis Ababa, Ethiopia. Clinical and socio-demographical data were collected using structured questionnaire after obtaining written informed consent. A total of 281 lower vaginal swabs were collected and inoculated into 1 ml Todd Hewitt Broth supplemented with gentamicin and nalidixic acid to prevent the growth of contaminants. After overnight incubation, all broths were subcultured on 5% sheep blood agar for isolation of GBS. Antimicrobial susceptibility testing was performed according to the criteria of the Clinical and Laboratory Standard Institute (CLSI) guidelines 2013 by disk diffusion method. Data were entered and analysed using SPSS version 20.0 software. Chi-square test and binary logistic regression analysis were used. P-value < 0.05 was considered statistically significant.

Results: The overall prevalence of GBS colonization among pregnant women was 14.6% (41/281). Group B Streptococcus colonization was significantly associated with health institutions ($P < 0.05$). All GBS isolates were susceptible to chloramphenicol. Resistance to tetracycline, cefotaxime, clindamycin, penicillin, vancomycin, ampicillin and erythromycin was 90.2%, 34.1, 26.8%, 19.5, 17%, 14.6 and 7.5% respectively. Multidrug resistance (MDR) ($\geq$ 2 drugs) was detected in 43.9% (18/41) of the isolates.

Conclusion: There was a high frequency of GBS colonization (14.6%) and resistance to the commonly used antibiotics which suggests the importance of the screening of GBS colonization in pregnant women at 35–37 weeks of gestation and testing their antimicrobial susceptibilities in order to provide antibiotic prophylaxis and minimize newborn infection and co-morbidity.

Keywords: Antimicrobial susceptibility testing, Group B streptococci, Prevalence, Risk factors

* Correspondence: sole.lab2000@yahoo.com; solomonas64@gmail.com
[1]Ethiopian Public Health Institute, P.O. Box 1242, Arbegnoch Street, Addis Ababa, Ethiopia
Full list of author information is available at the end of the article

Background

Group B Streptococcus emerged as the leading cause of neonatal morbidity and mortality in the United States in the 1970s [1–3], with a frequency of 2–3 cases per 1000 live vertical transmission births [4] and case-fatality ratios as high as 50% [3]. Group B Streptococcus is one of the most important causes of neonatal sepsis, meningitis, and pneumonia [5–7]. Group B Streptococcus neonatal infection could be early-onset GBS disease (EOGBSD), which occurs within the first week of life, and late-onset GBS disease (LOGBSD), which occurs between one week to 3 months of age [4, 5].

During pregnancy, approximately 10–30% of women are colonized with GBS in vagina [8, 9] and 60% of their infants acquire this organism through birth canal [6]. Maternal colonization with GBS in the genitourinary or gastrointestinal tract and transmission to the infant during the labor and delivery process is the principal risk factor for early-onset invasive GBS disease [2, 3, 9].

The widespread use of intrapartum antibiotic prophylaxis to prevent early-onset GBS disease has raised concern about the development of antibiotic resistance among GBS isolates [3]. In the absence of a licensed GBS vaccine [3], universal screening of mothers for vaginal or rectal GBS colonization at 35 to 37 weeks of gestation and selective intrapartum antibiotic prophylaxis (IAP) for all screen-positive women is the strategy currently recommended to reduce incidence of colonization in neonates and prevent early-onset GBS-related diseases [3, 9, 10].

Group B Streptococcus is now recognized to be an important cause of maternal and neonatal morbidity and mortality in many parts of the world [6, 7]; however, it has been little studied in Ethiopia [11, 12]. Therefore, this study was conducted to determine the prevalence of GBS colonization, antimicrobial susceptibility pattern and assess risk factors related to GBS among pregnant women attending in selected public ANC centers at Addis Ababa, Ethiopia.

Methods

Study design and setting

A prospective cross-sectional study was conducted among pregnant women attending ANC clinics of ALERT Center, Alem Bank, and Woreda 03 health centers, Addis Ababa, Ethiopia from May to August 2014. ALERT Center is one of the specialized tertiary referral hospitals in the country. While the two health centers are mainly engaged in routine antenatal care and delivery service in addition to other health routine care deliveries.

Study population, sample size, and sampling technique

A total of 281 pregnant women (from 35 to 37 weeks of gestation) attending the routine ANC follow up were

screened for GBS colonization at ALERT Center ($n = 141$), Alem Bank ($n = 88$) and Woreda 03 ($n = 52$) Health centers. Eligible study participants were enrolled in this study using consecutive sampling technique. The sample size was calculated based on the prevalence indicated in the previous study using single population proportion formula [12]. Expected margin of error (d) was 0.05 and confidence interval (z) was 95%. Contingency for the unknown circumstance was 10%. Pregnant women with a premature rupture of membranes (PROM) and history of antibiotic(s) use within two weeks prior to recruitment were excluded from this study.

Data collection

After obtaining written informed consent, socio-demographic and clinical data were collected using a structured questionnaire. Moreover, recent HIV result was taken from study participants' medical records. Data were collected by well-trained gynaecologist and midwives.

Specimen collection and transport

Vaginal swabs were taken from the lower vagina using sterile cotton swab according to the Center for Disease Control and Prevention (CDC) and American College of Obstetricians and Gynecologists (ACOG) guidelines [3, 13], and inoculated directly into Todd-Hewitt broth (THB) (Oxoid Ltd., Basingstoke, Hampshire, England) and immediately transported to the Microbiology Laboratory of ALERT Center for further analysis.

Culture and identification of group B streptococci

The vaginal swabs were placed into 1 ml THB (Oxoid Ltd., Basingstoke, Hampshire, England) supplemented with gentamicin (8 µg/ml) (Intas pharmaceutical Ltd., Matoda village, Ahmedabad, Gujarat, India) and nalidixic acid (15 µg/ml) (Sigma Aldrich, Italy) to prevent growth of contaminants [3]. The broth was incubated for 18–24 h at 35–37 °C and inoculated on 5% sheep blood agar (SBA) (Oxoid Ltd., Basingstoke, Hampshire, England) and incubated overnight in 5% CO_2 atmosphere for 18–24 h. Broth cultures showing no visible turbidity after overnight incubation were re-incubated for additional hours and then subcultured after 48 h on SBA. Suspected GBS colonies (pink colonies, with narrow beta-hemolysis) were confirmed by Gram stain, catalase test and Christie, Atkins, and Munch-Peterson (CAMP) test.

Antimicrobial susceptibility testing

Antimicrobial Susceptibility Testing was performed according to Clinical and Laboratory Standard Institute guidelines (CLSI) guidelines 2013 using Kirby-Bauer disk diffusion method [14]. Direct colony suspension in sterile saline, equivalent to 0.5 McFarland standard was done and inoculated on Muller-Hinton agar (MHA) (Oxoid Ltd., Basingstoke, Hampshire, England) with 5% sheep's blood using a sterile cotton swab. An antibiotic disk (Oxoid Ltd., Basingstoke, Hampshire, England) was placed on the agar with clindamycin and erythromycin disks placed 16 mm from each other in order to detect inducible resistance to clindamycin (D-zone test) and incubated at 35–37 °C with 5% CO_2 atmosphere for 18–24 h. The zone of growth inhibition was measured using the Oxoid ruler (Oxoid Ltd., Basingstoke, Hampshire, England) and Linex ruler (Linex 116, Denmark). The antibiotics used were penicillin (P) (10 μg), ampicillin (AMP) (10 μg), erythromycin (E) (15 μg), clindamycin (DA) (2 μg), vancomycin (30 μg), cefotaxime (CTX) (30 μg), chloramphenicol(C) (30 μg) and tetracycline (TE) (30 μg). The result was interpreted according to CLSI guidelines 2013 as susceptible, intermediate or resistant [14].

Quality control

The sterility of culture media was checked by incubating overnight at 35–37 °C without specimen inoculation. *Enterococcus faecalis* (ATCC 29212), *S. agalactiae* (ATCC 27956), *S. pyogenes* (ATCC 19615), *S. aureus* (ATCC 25923) and *E. coli* (ATCC 25922) strains were used as a quality control organisms for culture and antimicrobial susceptibility testing.

Data analysis

Data were coded, entered, cleaned and analyzed by using SPSS version 20.0 software. Frequency distribution, percentage, tables, and charts were used to present results. Explanatory variables were individually cross-tabulated with the outcome variable and statistical significance assessed using chi-square and logistic regression model. A *p*-value less than 0.05 was considered statistically significant.

Ethical consideration

This study was approved and ethically cleared by the Departmental Ethics and Research Committee (DERC) of Department of Medical Laboratory Science, College of Health Science, Addis Ababa University (AAU) (Ref.No.: MLS/501/14and protocol No.: DRERC 056/13/MLS), Armauer Hansen Research Institute / All African Leprosy, Tuberculosis, Rehabilitation and Training Center (AHRI/ALERT) Ethical Review Committee (AAERC) (Project Reg. No.:PO17/14), Institutional Review Board (IRB) of Addis Ababa Health Bureau (Ref.No.: AAHB/ 5900/227) and National Research Ethics Review Committee (NRERC) (Ref.No.: 3.10/796/06). Official permission from the study sites was obtained. Written informed consent was obtained from each study participant. All participants' results were kept confidentially.

Results

Socio-demographic characteristics

A total of two hundred eighty-one (281) pregnant women (from 35 to 37 weeks of gestation) were enrolled from May to August 2014. The age of the study participants ranged from 18 to 39 years with a mean age of 26. 46 (± 4.41) years. Most of the study the participants were between the ages of 25–29 years 120 (42.7%). Most of the study participants were married (97.5%). The majority of the study participants were housewives (68.3%) (Table 1).

Group B Streptococcus colonization

The overall prevalence of GBS colonization among pregnant women at 35–37 weeks of gestation was 14.6% (41/281). The prevalence of GBS in the three health institutions was 20 (22.7%), 17 (12.1%) and 4 (7.7%) in Alem Bank health center, ALERT center, and Woreda 03 health center respectively.

Antimicrobial susceptibility testing

The antimicrobial susceptibility testing results of GBS isolates are summarized in Table 2. All GBS isolates were 100% susceptible to chloramphenicol. Most isolates (80.5% to 92.5%) were susceptible to penicillin G, vancomycin, ampicillin, and erythromycin. Most GBS isolates (90.2%) were resistant to tetracycline (Table 2).

Table 1 Socio-demographic characteristics of pregnant women investigated for GBS at three health institutions (*n* = 281)

Socio-demographic characteristics	Frequency	Percentage
Health Institutions		
ALERT Center	141	50.2%
Woreda 03 Health Center	52	18.5%
Alem Bank Health Center	88	31.3%
Age groups		
15–19	8	2.8%
20–24	85	30.2%
25–29	120	42.7%
30–34	49	17.4%
≥ 35	19	6.8%
Marital status		
Married	274	97.5%
Single	4	1.4%
Divorced	2	0.7%
Widowed	1	0.4%
Occupation		
Civil Servant	35	12.5%
House Wives	192	68.3%
Business Women	54	19.2%

Table 2 Antimicrobial susceptibility pattern of GBS isolates from pregnant women recruited from three health institutions ($n = 41$)

Antibiotics	Disk Potency (µg)	Susceptible	Intermediate	Resistant
Chloramphenicol (C)	30	41(100%)	0	0
Erythromycin (E)	15	38(92.5%)	0	3(7.5%)
Ampicillin (AMP)	10	35(85.4%)	0	6(14.6%)
Vancomycin (VA)	30	34(83%)	0	7(17%)
Penicillin G (P)	10	33(80.5%)	0	8(19.5%)
Clindamycin (DA)	2	30(73.2%)	0	11(26.8%)
Cefotaxime (CTX)	30	27(65.9%)	0	14(34.1%)
Tetracycline (TE)	30	3(7.3%)	1(2.4%)	37(90.2%)

Multi-drug resistance pattern

Multidrug resistance (MDR) (≥ 2 drugs) was detected in 43.9% (18/41) of the isolates. Resistance to 2, 3, 4, 5 and 6 drugs was found to be 38.88%, 5.55, 27.77%, 11.11 and 16.66% respectively (Table 3).

Risk factors for group B streptococci
Socio-demographic factors

The association of socio-demographic variables with GBS colonization is summarized in Table 4. In univariate analysis, GBS colonization showed statistically significant association with health institutions ($P < 0.05$). However, there was no statistically significant association between GBS colonization and age group, marital status and occupation ($P > 0.05$). This study revealed a higher GBS colonization rate among pregnant women of age group 15–19 years (25%) than the age group ≥35 years (10.5%). However, the difference was not statistically significant ($P > 0.05$). In multivariable logistic regression analysis,

Table 3 Multi-drug resistance pattern of GBS isolated from pregnant women recruited from three health institutions ($n = 41$)

Drugs resistance pattern (Antibiogram)	No. of drug to which strains were resistant	No. of resistant strains (%)
CTX:TE	2	2 (11.11)
DA:TE	2	1 (5.55)
E: TE	2	1 (5.55)
TE: VA	2	3 (16.66)
CTX: DA: TE	3	1 (5.55)
AMP: CTX: E: TE	4	1 (5.55)
CTX: DA: P: TE	4	2 (11.11)
CTX:DA:P:VA	4	1 (5.55)
CTX:DA:TE:VA	4	1 (5.55)
AMP: CTX: DA: P:TE	5	2 (11.11)
AMP: CTX: DA: E: P: TE	6	1 (5.55)
AMP:CTX: DA: P: TE: VA:	6	2 (11.11)

TE Tetracycline, *CTX* Cefotaxime, *VA* Vancomycin, *DA*: Clindamycin, *E* Erythromycin, *P* Penicillin G, *AMP* Ampicillin

GBS colonization was significantly associated with health institutions (P < 0.05) (Table 4).

Obstetric factors

In univariate analysis, GBS colonization did not show statistically significant association with the number of antenatal visits, gravidity, history of spontaneous abortion and stillbirth ($P > 0.5$). Pregnant women with no history of stillbirth (14.9%) showed higher GBS colonization rates than those mothers with a history of stillbirth (7.7%). However, the difference was not statistically significant ($P > 0.05$) (Table 5).

HIV infection

Of 281 pregnant women screened for GBS colonization, 25 (8.9%) were HIV positive. Among the pregnant women with HIV infection, 6 (24%) were positive for GBS and among pregnant women with HIV negative, 35 (13.7%) were GBS positive. However, this difference was not statistically significant (P > 0.05) (Table 5). The Confounding effect of HIV infection was checked as its biological plausibility is expected with GBS colonization, but statistically failed to be found independently significantly associated.

Discussion

In this study, the overall prevalence of GBS among pregnant women was 14.6%. This finding was almost similar with reports from other developing countries; in Malawi (16.5%) and Nigeria (11.3%) [15, 16], but higher than those reported in Gondar, North Ethiopia (9%) and Mozambique (1.8%) [11, 17] and slightly lower than those reported in Hawassa, South Ethiopia (20.8%), Tanzania (23%) and Zimbabwe (21%) [6, 12, 18]. The finding of this study was also comparable to the studies done in some European countries; in North-Eastern Italy (17.9%) by Busetti M et al., Turin, Italy (18%) by Savoia D et al., and Poland (17.2%) [19–21], but higher than those reported in Northern Greece (6.6%) [22], and slightly lower than those reported in Switzerland (21%), UK (21.3%) and Netherlands (21%) [23–25].

Table 4 Association between socio-demographic factors and GBS colonization among pregnant women at three health institutions (n = 281)

Socio demographic factors	Total	GBS Culture		COR (95% C.I)	p-value [a]	AOR(95% C.I)	p-value[b]
		GBS negative N (%)	GBS positive N (%)				
Age group							
15–19	8	6(75)	2(25)	2.83(0.32–24.8)	0.35		
20–24	85	72(84.7)	13(15.3)	1.54(0.32–7.45)	0.59		
25–29	120	102(85)	18(15)	1.50(0.32–7.06)	0.61		
30–34	49	43(87.8)	6(12.2)	1.19(0.22–6.47)	0.84		
≥ 35	19	17(89.5)	2(10.5)	1			
Health Institutions							
ALERT Center	141	124(87.9)	17(12.1)	1		1	
Woreda 03 HC	52	48(92.3)	4(7.7)	0.61(0.20–1.90)	0.392	0.71 (0.22–2.27)	0.568
Alem Bank HC	88	68(77.3)	20(22.7)	2.15(1.05–4.37)	0.035*	2.63 (1.22–5.65)	0.013*
Marital Status							
Married	274	234(85.4)	40(14.6)	1			
Single	4	3(75)	1(25)	1.95(0.20–19.2)	0.57		
Divorced	2	2(100)	0(0.0)	0.000	0.99		
Widowed	1	1(100)	0(0.0)	0.000	1.00		
Occupation							
Civil servant	35	32(91.4)	3(8.6)	1			
House wife	192	163(84.9)	29(15.1)	1.9(0.55–6.61)	0.314		
Business women	54	45(83.3)	9(16.7)	2.13(0.54–8.51)	0.283		

*Significant at p-value< 0.05; [1] indicates logical reference group or constant; CI Confidence Interval, COR Crude odds ratio, AOR Adjusted odds ratio, [a] p-value obtained by binary; [b] p-value obtained by multiple logistic regression; HC: Health Center; N Number; % Percentage

The result of our study was also almost similar with the studies conducted in Texas, USA (12.2%) [26], and in Brazil ranging from 14.6% to 20.4 [27–29], but higher than those reported in Argentina (7.6%) [30].The finding of this study (14.6%) was higher than reports from some Asian countries; such as Taiwan (6.2%), India (2.3%), China (7.1%) and Korea (8.3%) [31–34]. The variations between countries could possibly be due to differences in the sample size and type of sites cultured, culture methods, socio-economic status, sexual behavior and geographic areas.

In this study, GBS colonization was significantly associated with health institutions (P < 0.05). This finding was consistent with reports from another study [34]. Those pregnant women who were managed in Alem Bank Health center were 2.6 times more likely to be colonized with GBS compared to those pregnant women who were managed in the ALERT center (AOR: 2.6, 95% C.I: 1.22–5.65). This difference might be due to specimen collection techniques of health care providers. Those providers in the centers with lower GBS rates may not have used proper hygienic sampling techniques including insertion of the swab into the vaginal. Therefore, it needs further investigation to confirm the

relationship between GBS colonization and health institutions.

Group B Streptococcus colonization in this study was higher in HIV infected pregnant women, though the association was not significant. GBS colonization and HIV infection (P > 0.05). This might probably be due to the small number of HIV infected pregnant women among the studied population. Similar findings have been reported in studies conducted in Tanzania and Malawi [6, 35]. However, a study conducted in the Democratic Republic of Congo, colonization rate was significantly associated with HIV infection [36].

In the present study, we observed that primigravida women were more often associated with GBS colonization, though it was not statistically significant (P > 0.05). Similar findings have been reported in Ethiopia (2012), Nigeria and Brazil [12, 15, 28]. However, in another study colonization rates were found to be significantly greater among multigravida women than primigravida women (P < 0.001) [32, 34, 37]. This might be due to geographical variation. Therefore, further studies are needed to confirm the correlation between gravidity and colonization by GBS from the different geographical location.

Table 5 Association between obstetric factors and GBS colonization among pregnant women at three health institutions ($n = 281$)

Obstetric Factors	Total	GBS culture		COR (95% C.I)	p-value[a]	AOR (95% C.I)	p-value[b]
		GBS negative N (%)	GBS positive N (%)				
ANC visit							
One times	6	5(83.3)	1(16.7)	1.12 (0.13–10.1)	0.917		
Two times	37	32(86.5)	5(13.5)	0.88 (0.31–2.51)	0.808		
Three times	99	85(85.9)	14(14.1)	0.93 (0.45–1.92)	0.836		
Four times	139	118(85.4)	21(14.6)	1			
Type of Gravida							
Primigravida	88	74(84.1)	14(15.9)	1.16 (0.58–2.35)	0.673		
Multigravida	193	166(86)	27(14)	1			
Still birth							
No	268	228(85.1)	40(14.9)	1			
Yes	13	12(92.3)	1(7.7)	0.48 (0.06–3.76)	0.480		
Abortion							
No	211	180(85.3)	31(14.7)	1			
Yes	70	60(85.7)	10(14.3)	0.97 (0.45–2.09)	0.934		
HIV Infection							
No	256	221(86.3)	35 (13.7)	1		1	
Yes	25	19 (76)	6 (24)	1.99 (0.75–5.34)	0.170	2.8 (0.97–8.11)	0.057

[1]logical reference; *CI* Confidence interval, *COR* Crude odds ratio, *AOR* Adjusted odds ratio, N Number; % Percentage; [a] p-value obtained by binary; [b] p-value obtained by multiple logistic regression; Adjusted for HIV status

In the present study, history of spontaneous abortion did not influence GBS colonization in pregnant women. Similar findings have been reported in studies conducted in Tanzania and India [6, 32]. However, in another studies history of spontaneous abortion showed significant association with GBS colonization [34, 36]. Therefore, further studies are needed to confirm the correlation between abortion and colonization by GBS. The previous history of stillbirth did not influence GBS colonization. The lack of association with this factor might be explained by the fact that the numbers of participants in this study with such risk factor were small. This finding was consistent with studies from Dar es Salaam, Tanzania (2009) by Joachim A et al. [6].

Penicillin and ampicillin are the drugs of choice for prevention or treatment of GBS infections, and clindamycin and erythromycin are the recommended alternatives for patients who are allergic to ß-lactam agents. The widespread use of these antibiotics to prevent early-onset GBS disease has raised concern about the development of antibiotic resistance among GBS isolates [3].

In this study, all GBS isolates were susceptible to chloramphenicol. In our study, we observed resistance to penicillin (19.5%) and ampicillin (14.6%) which are the first choice of drugs for intrapartum prophylaxis. This did not match with the CDC 2010 guidelines study, which did not find any resistance to penicillin. These findings were comparable to those reported in another study [15]. The expanded use of beta-lactam antimicrobials in the treatment of several infective clinical syndromes and the free accessibility of purchase over the counter might be the cause of the emergence of GBS resistance strains in this environment.

The CDC 2010 guideline recommends testing of GBS isolates for susceptibility to clindamycin and erythromycin, as they are the drugs of choice for penicillin-allergic women at high risk for anaphylaxis [3]. An increase in resistance of GBS to erythromycin has been reported [1, 15, 38–41]. In this study, we found that 7.5% of the isolates were resistant to erythromycin. This was consistent with reports from other studies [6, 7, 12, 42, 43]. This rate of erythromycin resistance in the GBS isolates strongly supports the current CDC recommendation that antibiotic susceptibility test should be performed if erythromycin therapy is needed to prevent neonatal GBS infection. With respect to resistance to clindamycin, the finding of this study (26.8%) was similar to those reports from other studies [6, 15, 38–41, 43, 44]. Since clindamycin is another alternative antibiotic recommended by the CDC for pregnant women who are allergic to penicillin, the resistance level underline the need of carrying out a susceptibility test. This might be due to the widespread use of the antibiotics.

Vancomycin is recommended for GBS-colonized mothers with a high risk of anaphylaxis to penicillin and if the isolate is resistant to clindamycin [3]. In this study, we found that 17% of the isolates were resistant to vancomycin. This finding was comparable to those reported in another study [15]. Since vancomycin is another alternative drug recommended by the CDC for pregnant women who are allergic to penicillin and clindamycin-resistant isolates, the resistance level underline the need of carrying out a susceptibility test. Most GBS isolates (90.2%) were resistant to tetracycline which showed consistency with reports from other studies [12, 32, 38, 42, 45]. This may probably be due to the widespread use of this antibiotics and ease of procurement of antibiotic and/or could be attributed to the indiscriminate use of antimicrobial drugs in this area. The cefotaxime resistance (34.1%) in this study was difficult to explain since cefotaxime was rarely used in Ethiopia. In contrast to this, high susceptibility to cefotaxime was observed in other studies [15, 42].

Conclusion

There was high isolation rate of GBS (14.6%) among pregnant women. The resistance of the isolates to the commonly used antibiotics including penicillin, ampicillin, and clindamycin in this study calls for screening of all pregnant women at 35–37 weeks of gestation. Performing susceptibility testing before administration of any of these antibiotics to provide antibiotic prophylaxis to GBS carrier is necessary. The finding of this study also signifies that GBS infection might be a silent clinical problem that is undiagnosed in the present study area, therefore, it requires advocacy work for awareness and concerted effort for preventive measures.

Abbreviations
ACOG: American college of obstetricians and gynecologists; AHRI: Armauer hansen research institute; ALERT: All african leprosy, tuberculosis, rehabilitation and training center; ANC: Antenatal care; ATCC: American type culture collection; CAMP Test: Christie, atkins, munch, peterson test; CDC: Center for disease control and prevention; CLSI: Clinical and laboratory standard institute; DRERC: Departmental research and ethics review committee; EOGBSD: Early-onset group B streptococcal disease; GBS: Group B streptococci; HIV: Human immunodeficiency virus; IAP: Intrapartum antibiotics prophylaxis; IRB: Institutional review board; LOGBSD: Late- onset group B streptococcal disease; MHA: Muller Hinton Agar; NRERC: National research ethics review committee; PROM: Premature rupture of membranes; SBA: Sheep blood agar; SPSS: Statistical package for social sciences; THB: Todd hewitt broth

Acknowledgements
We would like to acknowledge the School of Allied Health Sciences, College of Health Sciences, Department of Medical Laboratory Sciences, Addis Ababa University, for the remarkable efficiency of their service and dedication to duty. Next, we would like to express our sincere gratitude to all ethical approval committee. Our gratitude also extends to the study sites for their official permission and support during specimen collection. Special thanks go to all study participants for their participation, without them this study would not have been realized.

Funding
The fund for this research project was covered by the principal investigator.

Authors' contributions
AS and LT conceived and designed the study. AS wrote the study protocol, supervised the data collection, did the laboratory work, did the analysis and interpretation of data, wrote the first draft and participated in all revisions till the final version of this paper. DK & LT contributed to the analysis, interpretation of results, revising the manuscript critically for intellectual content. All authors read and approved the final version of the manuscript for publication.

Authors' information
AS: Assistant researcher II (BSc, MSc), TB focal person in National Laboratory Capacity Building Directorate, Ethiopian Public Health Institute, Addis Ababa, Ethiopia. DK: Lecturer, assistant professor (BSc, MSc, Ph.D. candidate) at the Department of Medical Laboratory Science, School of Allied Health Sciences, College of Health Sciences, Addis Ababa University, Addis Ababa, Ethiopia. LT: Medical Microbiologist (BSc, MSc, Ph.D. candidate) at ALERT Center Clinical Laboratory and Armauer Hansen Research Institute, ALERT Center, Addis Ababa, Ethiopia.

Competing interests
The authors declare that they have no competing interests.

Author details
[1]Ethiopian Public Health Institute, P.O. Box 1242, Arbegnoch Street, Addis Ababa, Ethiopia. [2]Department of Medical Laboratory Sciences, School of Allied Health Sciences, College of Health Sciences, Addis Ababa University, P.O. Box 1176, Addis Ababa, Ethiopia. [3]Armauer Hansen Research Institute, P.O. Box 1005, Jimma Road, Addis Ababa, Ethiopia. [4]All Africa Leprosy, Tuberculosis, Rehabilitation and Training Center, P.O. Box 165, Jimma Road, Addis Ababa, Ethiopia.

References
1. Phares CR, Lynfield R, Farley MM, Mohle-Boetani J, Harrison LH, Petit S, et al. Epidemiology of invasive group B streptococcal disease in the United States, 1999-2005. JAMA. 2008;299(17):2056–65. https://doi.org/10.1001/jama.299.17.2056.
2. Committee on Infectious Diseases and Committee on Fetus and Newborn, Baker CJ, Byington CL, Polin RA. Policy Statement - Recommendations for the prevention of perinatal group B streptococcal (GBS) disease. Pediatrics. 2011;128(3):611–6. https://doi.org/10.1542/peds.2011–1466.
3. Verani JR, McGee L, Schrag SJ. Prevention of perinatal group B streptococcal disease: Revised guidelines from CDC, 2010: Department of Health and Human Services, Centers for Disease Control and Prevention,2010 Nov 19 Contract No.: RR-10.
4. Faro S, Brehm B, Smith F, Mouzoon M, Greisinger A, Wehmanen O, et al. Screening for group B streptococcus: a private hospital's experience. Infect Dis Obstet Gynecol. 2010;2010:1–4. https://doi.org/10.1155/2010/451096.
5. Maisey HC, Doran KS, Nizet V. Recent advances in understanding the molecular basis of group B Streptococcus virulence. Expert Rev Mol Med. 2008;10:e27. https://doi.org/10.1017/S1462399408000811.
6. Joachim A, Matee MI, Massawe FA, Lyamuya EF. Maternal and neonatal colonisation of group B streptococcus at Muhimbili National Hospital in Dar

es salaam, Tanzania: prevalence, risk factors and antimicrobial resistance. BMC Public Health. 2009;9:437. https://doi.org/10.1186/1471-2458-9-437.

7. Ezeonu I, Agbo M. Incidence and anti-microbial resistance profile of group B Streptococcus (GBS) infection in pregnant women in Nsukka, Enugu state, Nigeria. Afr J Microbiol Res. 2014;8(1):91–5. https://doi.org/10.5897/AJMR12.2307.

8. El Beitune P, Duarte G, Maffei CM. Colonization by Streptococcus agalactiae during pregnancy: maternal and perinatal prognosis. Braz J Infect Dis. 2005; 9(4):276–82. doi:S1413–86702005000400002

9. El Aila NA, Tency I, Claeys G, Saerens B, Cools P, Verstraelen H, et al. Comparison of different sampling techniques and of different culture methods for detection of group B streptococcus carriage in pregnant women. BMC Infect Dis. 2010;10:285. https://doi.org/10.1186/1471-2334-10-285.

10. Cheng PJ, Chueh HY, Liu CM, Hsu JJ, Hsieh II, Soong YK. Risk factors for recurrence of group B streptococcus colonization in a subsequent pregnancy. Obstet Gynecol. 2008;111(3):704–9. https://doi.org/10.1097/AOG.0b013e318163cd6b.

11. Schmidt J, Halle E, Halle H, Mohammed T, Gunther E. Colonization of pregnant women and their newborn infants with group B streptococci in the Gondar College of Medical Sciences. Ethiop Med J. 1989;27(3):115–9.

12. Mohammed M, Asrat D, Woldeamanuel Y, Demissie A. Prevalence of group B Streptococcus colonization among pregnant women attending antenatal clinic of Hawassa health center, Hawassa, Ethiopia. Ethiop J Health Dev. 2012;26(1):36–42.

13. American College of O, Gynecologists Committee on Obstetric P. ACOG Committee Opinion No. 485: Prevention of early-onset group B streptococcal disease in newborns. Obstet Gynecol Annu. 2011;117(4):1019–27. https://doi.org/10.1097/AOG.0b013e318219229b.

14. Cockerill FR. Performance standards for antimicrobial susceptibility testing: twenty-third informational supplement. Clinical Laboratory Standards Institute; 2013.

15. Onipede A, Adefusi O, Adeyemi A, Adejuyigbe E, Oyelese A, Ogunniyi T. Group B streptococcus carriage during late pregnancy in Ile-Ife, Nigeria. Afr J Clin Exp Microbiol. 2012;13(3):135–43.

16. Dzowela T, Komolafe O, Igbigbi A. Prevalence of group B Streptococcus colonization in antenatal women at the queen Elizabeth central hospital, Blantyre–a preliminary study. Malawi Med J. 2006;17(3):97–9.

17. De Steenwinkel FD, Tak HV, Muller AE, Nouwen JL, Oostvogel PM, Mocumbi SM. Low carriage rate of group B streptococcus in pregnant women in Maputo, Mozambique. Tropical Med Int Health. 2008;13(3):427–9. https://doi.org/10.1111/j.1365-3156.2008.02018.x.

18. Mavenyengwa RT, Afset JE, Schei B, Berg S, Caspersen T, Bergseng H, et al. Group B Streptococcus colonization during pregnancy and maternal-fetal transmission in Zimbabwe. Acta Obstet Gynecol Scand. 2010;89(2):250–5. https://doi.org/10.3109/00016340903398029.

19. Busetti M, D'Agaro P, Campello C. Group B streptococcus prevalence in pregnant women from north-eastern Italy: advantages of a screening strategy based on direct plating plus broth enrichment. J Clin Pathol. 2007; 60(10):1140–3. https://doi.org/10.1136/jcp.2006.043489.

20. Savoia D, Gottimer C, Crocilla C, Zucca M. Streptococcus agalactiae in pregnant women: phenotypic and genotypic characters. J Inf Secur. 2008; 56(2):120–5. https://doi.org/10.1016/j.jinf.2007.11.007.

21. Strus M, Pawlik D, Brzychczy-Wloch M, Gosiewski T, Rytlewski K, Lauterbach R, et al. Group B streptococcus colonization of pregnant women and their children observed on obstetric and neonatal wards of the University Hospital in Krakow, Poland. J Med Microbiol. 2009;58(2):228–33. https://doi.org/10.1099/jmm.0.002865-0.

22. Tsolia M, Psoma M, Gavrili S, Petrochilou V, Michalas S, Legakis N, et al. Group B streptococcus colonization of Greek pregnant women and neonates: prevalence, risk factors and serotypes. Clin Microbiol Infect. 2003; 9(8):832–8.

23. Rausch AV, Gross A, Droz S, Bodmer T, Surbek DV. Group B streptococcus colonization in pregnancy: prevalence and prevention strategies of neonatal sepsis. J Perinat Med. 2009;37(2):124–9. https://doi.org/10.1515/JPM.2009.020.

24. Jones N, Oliver K, Jones Y, Haines A, Crook D. Carriage of group B streptococcus in pregnant women from Oxford, UK. J Clin Pathol. 2006; 59(4):363–6. https://doi.org/10.1136/jcp.2005.029058.

25. Valkenburg-van den Berg AW, Sprij AJ, Oostvogel PM, Mutsaers JA, Renes WB, Rosendaal FR, et al. Prevalence of colonisation with group B streptococci in pregnant women of a multi-ethnic population in the Netherlands. Eur J Obstet Gynecol Reprod Biol. 2006;124(2):178–83. https://doi.org/10.1016/j.ejogrb.2005.06.007.

26. Chohan L, Hollier LM, Bishop K, Kilpatrick CC. Patterns of antibiotic resistance among group B streptococcus isolates: 2001-2004. Infect Dis Obstet Gynecol. 2006;2006:57492. https://doi.org/10.1155/IDOG/2006/57492.

27. Zusman AS, Baltimore RS, Fonseca SN. Prevalence of maternal group B streptococcal colonization and related risk factors in a Brazilian population. Braz J Infect Dis. 2006;10(4):242–6.

28. Simoes JA, Alves VM, Fracalanzza SE, de Camargo RP, Mathias L, Milanez HM, et al. Phenotypical characteristics of group B streptococcus in parturients. Braz J Infect Dis. 2007;11(2):261–6.

29. Costa AL, Lamy Filho F, Chein MB, Brito LM, Lamy ZC, Andrade KL. Prevalence of colonization by group B Streptococcus in pregnant women from a public maternity of northwest region of Brazil. Rev Bras Ginecol Obstet. 2008;30(6):274–80.

30. Quiroga M, Pegels E, Oviedo P, Pereyra E, Vergara M. Antibiotic susceptibility patterns and prevalence of group B Streptococcus isolated from pregnant women in Misiones, Argentina. Braz J Microbiol. 2008;39(2):245–50. https://doi.org/10.1590/S1517-83822008000200009.

31. Yang MJ, Sun PL, Wen KC, Chao KC, Chang WH, Chen CY, et al. Prevalence of maternal group B streptococcus colonization and vertical transmission in low-risk women in a single institute. J Chin Med Assoc. 2012;75(1):25–8. https://doi.org/10.1016/j.jcma.2011.10.011.

32. Sharmila V, Joseph NM, Arun Babu T, Chaturvedula L, Sistla S. Genital tract group B streptococcal colonization in pregnant women: a south Indian perspective. J Infect Dev Ctries. 2011;5(8):592–5. https://doi.org/10.3855/jidc.1551.

33. Lu B, Li D, Cui Y, Sui W, Huang L, Lu X. Epidemiology of group B streptococcus isolated from pregnant women in Beijing. China Clin Microbiol Infect. 2014;20(6):370–3. https://doi.org/10.1111/1469-0691.12416.

34. Kim EJ, Oh KY, Kim MY, Seo YS, Shin JH, Song YR, et al. Risk factors for group B streptococcus colonization among pregnant women in Korea. Epidemiol Health. 2011;33:1–7. https://doi.org/10.4178/epih/e2011010.

35. Gray KJ, Kafulafula G, Matemba M, Kamdolozi M, Membe G, French N. Group B Streptococcus and HIV infection in pregnant women, Malawi, 2008-2010. Emerg Infect Dis. 2011;17(10):1932–5. https://doi.org/10.3201/eid1710.102008.

36. Mitima KT, Ntamako S, Birindwa AM, Mukanire N, Kivukuto JM, Tsongo K, et al. Prevalence of colonization by Streptococcus agalactiae among pregnant women in Bukavu, Democratic Republic of the Congo. J Infect Dev Ctries. 2014;8(9):1195–200. https://doi.org/10.3855/jidc.5030.

37. Orrett FA. Colonization with group B streptococci in pregnancy and outcome of infected neonates in Trinidad. Pediatr Int. 2003;45(3):319–23.

38. Wang H, Zhao C, He W, Zhang F, Zhang L, Cao B, et al. High prevalence of fluoroquinolone-resistant group B streptococci among clinical isolates in China and predominance of sequence type 19 with serotype III. Antimicrob Agents Chemother. 2013;57(3):1538–41. https://doi.org/10.1128/AAC.02317-12.

39. Capanna F, Emonet SP, Cherkaoui A, Irion O, Schrenzel J, Martinez de Tejada B. Antibiotic resistance patterns among group B Streptococcus isolates: implications for antibiotic prophylaxis for early-onset neonatal sepsis. Swiss Med Wkly. 2013;143:1–4. https://doi.org/10.4414/smw.2013.13778.

40. DiPersio LP, DiPersio JR. High rates of erythromycin and clindamycin resistance among OBGYN isolates of group B Streptococcus. Diagn Microbiol Infect Dis. 2006;54(1):79–82. https://doi.org/10.1016/j.diagmicrobio.2005.07.003.

41. Yook JH, Kim MY, Kim EJ, Yang JH, Ryu HM, Oh KY, et al. Risk factors associated with group B streptococcus resistant to clindamycin and erythromycin in pregnant korean women. Infect Chemother. 2013;45(3): 299–307. https://doi.org/10.3947/ic.2013.45.3.299.

42. Boswihi SS, Udo EE, Al-Sweih N. Serotypes and antibiotic resistance in group B streptococcus isolated from patients at the maternity hospital, Kuwait. J Med Microbiol. 2012;61(1):126–31. https://doi.org/10.1099/jmm.0.035477-0.

43. Castellano-Filho DS, da Silva VL, Nascimento TC, de Toledo Vieira M, Diniz CG. Detection of group B Streptococcus in Brazilian pregnant women and

antimicrobial susceptibility patterns. Braz J Microbiol. 2010;41(4):1047–55. https://doi.org/10.1590/S1517-838220100004000024.

44. Frohlicher S, Reichen-Fahrni G, Muller M, Surbek D, Droz S, Spellerberg B, et al. Serotype distribution and antimicrobial susceptibility of group B streptococci in pregnant women: results from a Swiss tertiary centre. Swiss Med Wkly. 2014;144:w13935; https://doi.org/10.4414/smw.2014.13935.

45. Hannoun A, Shehab M, Khairallah MT, Sabra A, Abi-Rached R, Bazi T, et al. Correlation between group B streptococcal genotypes, their antimicrobial resistance profiles, and virulence genes among pregnant women in Lebanon. Int J Microbiol. 2009;2009:1–6. https://doi.org/10.1155/2009/796512.

17

Male partner attendance at antenatal care and adherence to antenatal care guidelines: secondary analysis of 2011 Ethiopian demographic and health survey data

Faye Forbes[1*], Karen Wynter[1], Catherine Wade[2], Berihun M. Zeleke[3,4] and Jane Fisher[1]

Abstract

Background: Complications during pregnancy, childbirth and the postpartum period present a significant and complex public health problem in low income countries such as Ethiopia. One strategy endorsed by the World Health Organisation (WHO) to improve maternal and child health outcomes is to encourage male partner involvement in pregnancy care. This research aimed to explore the relationships between 1) male attendance at antenatal care and 2) socio-economic and women's empowerment factors and adherence to focused antenatal care guidelines among women receiving care in Ethiopia.

Methods: Secondary analysis of 2011 Ethiopian Demographic and Health Survey (DHS) data. A sub-sample of couples with a child aged 0–2 years old, for whom women attended at least one antenatal care (ANC) appointment was selected. Predictor variables on socio-economic position, demographic and women's empowerment factors, and male attendance at antenatal care were identified. Six outcome variables were constructed to indicate whether or not women: commenced ANC in the first trimester, attended at least four ANC appointments, received a urine test, received a blood test, were counselled on potential complications during pregnancy and met these focused antenatal care guidelines. Binary logistic regression was performed to estimate the relationship between the predictor and outcome variables.

Results: After controlling for other factors, women whose partners attended ANC were significantly more likely to receive urine and blood tests and be counselled about pregnancy complications compared to women who attended alone. Male attendance was not associated with women commencing care in the first trimester or attending at least four appointments. Although more women whose male partners had attended appointments received all recommended components of ANC than those who attended alone, this association was not significant.

Conclusions: The results revealed some benefits and did not detect harms from including male partners in focused antenatal care. Including men may require changes to maternal healthcare systems and training of healthcare workers, to adopt 'father inclusive' practices. Given the limited research in this area, large population studies including the DHS routinely carried out in Ethiopia could enhance knowledge by including more detailed indicators of male involvement in pregnancy, maternal and child healthcare and early child development.

Keywords: Male involvement, Male attendance, Fathers, Ethiopia, Focused antenatal care, Demographic and health survey

* Correspondence: faye.forbes@monash.edu
[1]Jean Hailes Research Unit, School of Public Health and Preventive Medicine, Monash University, 553 St Kilda Rd, Melbourne, VIC 3004, Australia
Full list of author information is available at the end of the article

Background

Complications during pregnancy, childbirth and the postpartum period present a significant and complex public health problem in low income countries. In 2015 approximately 303,000 women died of pregnancy-related causes, with 99% of these deaths occurring in low- and middle-income countries and the highest proportion in Africa [1]. Many of these deaths are potentially avoidable by timely access to healthcare to prevent, identify and treat pregnancy-related problems.

Maternal and child health (MCH) were a focus of the Millennium Development Goals (MDG) (2000–2015), and continue to be prioritised in the Sustainable Development Goals (SDG) (2016–2030) agreed upon by the United Nations and co-operating countries [2]. The World Health Organisation (WHO) antenatal care (ANC) guidelines suggest a focused antenatal care model (FANC) involving four consultations and including screening tests and counselling, commencing in the first trimester and extending until birth. The WHO focus includes strategies to encourage women to attend healthcare during pregnancy, birth and in the post-natal period [3, 4].

One strategy "strongly recommended" by the WHO in the *WHO recommendations for health promotion interventions for maternal and newborn health 2015* (pp 17, [5]), is to support male involvement in pregnancy, childbirth and the post-birth period. Male involvement include men's role in maternal health decision making, male attendance at antenatal care, male attitudes towards maternal healthcare and male participation in home visits from health extension workers [6–25]. Male involvement interventions evaluated by the WHO include: mass media campaigns, community-based outreach and education for men, home visits, counselling for couples, groups or men only, and workplace-based education [5].

The WHO encourages male involvement for diverse reasons, including that in many countries in which maternal and child health indicators do not meet international criteria, men have significant influence over maternal healthcare decisions [26, 27]. Engaging men in healthcare early in pregnancy is viewed as an opportunity to educate men about the importance of perinatal healthcare, and to help men support their partners effectively during pregnancy, birth preparation and in the postnatal period [28, 29]. This is also an appropriate time to address men's sexual and reproductive health and to position men as responsible partners to women and fathers to their children [5].

However, the WHO acknowledge that the quality of evidence about male attendance at antenatal care is currently very low and any estimate of the effect is uncertain [5]. Two systematic reviews of the evidence in low and middle income countries presented findings from research conducted over diverse geographic regions and a range of maternal health outcomes [6, 7]. Study designs included cross-sectional demographic studies, pre-post intervention studies, retrospective cohort designs and two randomised controlled trials. Appraisal revealed limited high quality evidence with only 2/7 [7] and 6/14 studies [6] in each review rated as high quality.

Nevertheless, this evidence does tentatively suggest that in low and middle income countries men's attendance at antenatal care consultations may be associated with a range of positive maternal outcomes [6, 7], including: birth preparedness [30, 31], birth in a medical facility rather than at home [32], access to a skilled birth attendant rather than unskilled support [7, 32–34], attendance at postnatal healthcare services and reduced postnatal depression [7, 30]. One of the few studies to produce evidence rated as high quality in Aguiar and Jennings' 2015 review [6], was a randomised controlled trial (RCT) conducted in Nepal allocating women to a 3-arm trial consisting of women-only pregnancy and birth education, no education or couple pregnancy and birth education. The study found that women who attended antenatal care as part of a couple were better prepared for birth and used more postnatal care than women allocated to women-only or no education conditions [35].

On the other hand, male attendance at antenatal care consultations was not associated with an increase in antenatal care attendance in the RCT in Nepal [35] or with lower rates of miscarriage or stillbirth, use of antenatal care or birth preparedness in a RCT conducted in South Africa allocating men to three counselling sessions during the maternity period compared to a control condition [36].

As recognised by the WHO, involving men in pregnancy care could also be disadvantageous to women in some circumstances, primarily because it may reinforce the role of men as decision makers and provide opportunity for male coercion and control over women's decisions [5, 37]. Women's empowerment, rated as the sum of nine items including measures of social, economic and legal empowerment in the 2010–2011 Demographic and Health Surveys, was evaluated in eight sub-Saharan African countries, and compared between women whose male partners attended and did not attend antenatal healthcare visits [37]. Results were mixed with male attendance associated with increased indicator scores of women's empowerment in Burkina Faso and Uganda, decreased likelihood of empowerment in Malawi and no differences detected in Burundi, Mozambique, Rwanda, Senegal, or Zimbabwe [37].

Ethiopia is a Sub-Saharan African country in which improving maternal and child health and increasing the use of healthcare during the perinatal period is a national priority [38]. Despite significant improvements to the healthcare system and maternal and child health indicators since the launch of the MDGs, the maternal mortality ratio in Ethiopia is substantially higher than international standards [38] with an estimated 350 maternal deaths per 100,000 live births, placing the country 31st on the rankings of maternal mortality ratios in a listing of 184 countries [39].

In Ethiopia, maternal healthcare is provided by government- and privately-funded primary health care facilities. Government facilities consist of a primary district hospital (serving 60,000–100,000 people), health centres (1 per 15,000–25,000 people) and Health Posts staffed by Health Extension Workers (HEW) (1 per 3000–5000 people). This is supplemented by non-government organisations and profit-based facilities [38]. In 2011 most women who received antenatal care accessed this in government facilities. From the total population 28.7% received care from a midwife /nurse, 5.4% from a doctor and 8.7% from a HEW. Only 19% received the recommended four visits, 10% had a skilled birth attendant and 10% gave birth in a health facility [40].

Despite the Ethiopian government's focus on maternal health and the WHO recommendations regarding male involvement [5], it is not clear that the strategy of involving men in antenatal care has been implemented beyond family planning and prevention of parent-to-child transmission of HIV [38]. There are few data about the role of men in pre or postnatal care or in relation to birth preparedness in Ethiopia. A broad search of Ethiopian peri-natal care research which included information about male partners, revealed 15 quantitative, one mixed methods and one qualitative study, with quantitative samples ranging from 310 to 1750 participants with an average sample size of 724. The studies were diverse: conducted in a range of regions in urban or rural Ethiopia, and with male partner involvement defined in different ways - including male attitudes towards maternal healthcare, male partner education, co-habitation, male emotional support, male role in maternal healthcare decision making and male participation in discussions with home visiting HEWs [6–25]. Most studies did not focus exclusively on the role of men, instead examining factors related to maternal healthcare overall and including some information on male partner involvement.

Collectively these studies suggest that male involvement in perinatal care may be associated with positive maternal health outcomes in Ethiopia. Five quantitative studies showed that male partner attitude towards perinatal healthcare, approval of antenatal care and birth in a health facility, and knowledge of benefits of birth in a facility, were significantly associated with increased odds of receiving antenatal care and giving birth in a facility

[9–11, 18, 20]. Two quantitative studies found that partners' active involvement in home visiting programs for birth preparedness and antenatal education increased performance on birth preparedness measures and satisfaction with HEWs [8, 21]. One survey and one mixed methods study found male partner involvement in decision making was associated with increased odds of birth in a health facility [14, 16, 41]. Qualitative research identified that understanding of maternal health issues and financial status of the male partner contributed towards maternal healthcare use [24].

As yet there are no population level studies of associations between male partner attendance at antenatal care and perinatal healthcare use in Ethiopia, nor specific indicators of focused antenatal care, defined as beginning in the first trimester, comprising at least four sessions, and including the necessary screening and counselling components [4].

This research aimed to explore the relationships between 1) male attendance at antenatal care and 2) socio-economic and women's empowerment factors and adherence to focused antenatal care guidelines among women receiving care in Ethiopia.

Method
Setting
This was a secondary analysis of data collected in the Ethiopian Demographic and Health Survey (EDHS) in 2011 [40]. The EDHS sampling procedure randomly selected discrete geographic areas or 'clusters' (groupings of households) across each region of Ethiopia. Regions included: Tigray, Afar, Amhara, Oromiya, Somali, Benishangul Gumuz, Southern Nations Nationalities and Peoples (SNNP), Gambella and Harari and two city administrations (Addis Ababa and Dire Dawa).

Data source for the Ethiopian demographic and health survey
The EDHS surveys for women and men included the following sections: Respondent's socio-demographic characteristics, Reproduction, Contraception, Marriage and Sexual Activity, Fertility Preferences, Employment and Gender Roles, HIV/AIDS and Other Health Issues. Women received additional sections: Pregnancy and Postnatal Care, Child Immunization, Health and Nutrition.

Procedure for the Ethiopian demographic and health survey
Within each cluster 20–25 households were selected randomly from a complete list. Each household was invited to participate in a survey. Women and men between the ages of 15–49 years were invited to participate in separate surveys. The 30–60 min structured surveys

comprised with fixed response options translated into Amharic, Tigrigna or Oromiffa. Interviews were conducted in the home by trained interviewers.

Data linking and selection

Data from men were linked to data from the woman they indicated was their "first wife" using a combination of the identification numbers for the household and the first wife. Data from polygamous couples were included in the DHS survey, but excluded from the analysis as the husband's most recent child may not be the first wife's most recent child (see Fig. 1). Data were selected for analysis if: the man responded to the question "How old is your youngest child?" by indicating that his youngest child was aged up to 2 years; if the woman responded "yes" to the question "Did you receive antenatal care for your youngest child?"; and if the man responded "Yes" or "No" to the question "Were you ever present for any of those check-ups?" (refers to antenatal care check-ups). Antenatal care was defined in the EDHS survey as "healthcare accessed during pregnancy that directly related to the woman's pregnancy".

Data management and analysis
Key variables
The study outcome and key predictor variables, related EDHS survey items and recoded categories (where relevant) are available in a Additional file 1: Table S1.

Secondary analysis was performed on EDHS data using IBM SPSS Statistics version 23.

Descriptive statistics were used to summarise the demographic and socio-economic characteristics of study participants. Data were recoded to reduce the number of categories and aid interpretation (see Additional file 1: Table S1). Significant differences between men who did and did not attend at least one antenatal care appointment with their partner were calculated using independent sample t-tests and chi-square tests. P-values of $p < 0.05$ are reported as significant in all analyses.

Bivariate analysis was used to identify associations between outcome and predictor variables. Binary logistic regression was performed to estimate the relationship between the predictor variables and outcomes, reporting the Adjusted Odds Ratio (AOR) and 95% confidence interval (CI). The relationships between each predictor variable and the antenatal care outcome variables were evaluated while controlling for the effect of other variables (residence, education, age, parity, location of ANC, male partner attendance, wealth, role in MCH decision, attitude towards "wife beating" and exposure to media) contained in the model. All variables in each model were significantly associated with the relevant outcome variable and male attendance at antenatal care. Only cases where data were available for each indicator were kept in the model. Nagelkerke score was used to compare goodness of fit between models.

It is possible that male attendance at antenatal appointments may have a negative impact on antenatal care outcomes for some women, for example those in relationships characterised by coercion, control or physical and sexual violence perpetrated by an intimate partner. As a sensitivity analysis, we conducted bivariate analyses of associations between the outcome variables and male attendance separately for two groups of women, according to their response to a question "In your opinion, is a husband justified in hitting or beating his wife in the following situations: If she goes out without telling him?, If she neglects the children?, If she argues with him?, If she refuses to have sex with him?, If she burns the food?". The latter was used as a proxy indicator for intimate partner violence. A series of 3-way cross-tabulations with chi-square tests was conducted. If significant associations between an outcome variable and male attendance exist for one group, according to response to this question, and not for the other group, then a significant interaction between male attendance and presence of intimate partner violence would be indicated, and would subsequently be tested in the models.

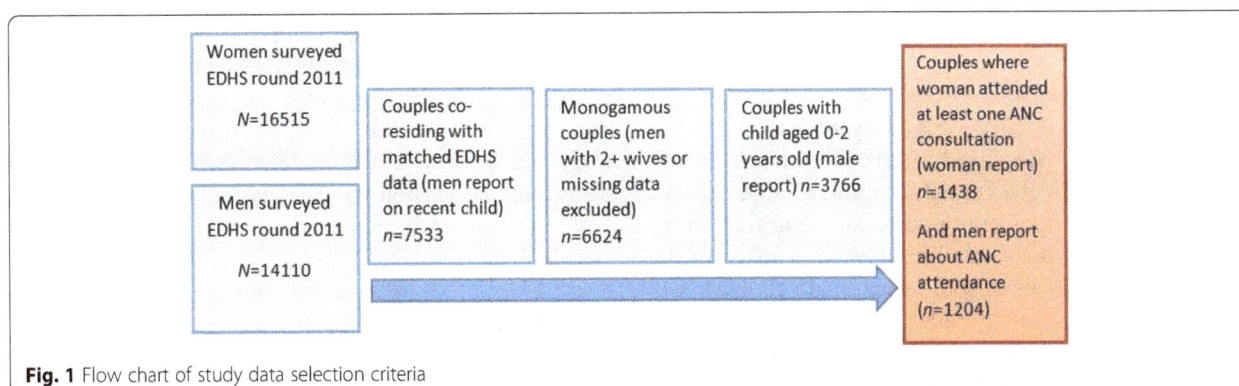

Fig. 1 Flow chart of study data selection criteria

Results

Sample characteristics

Complete data were available for 1204 couples who met inclusion criteria. The sample characteristics are presented in Table 1. Compared to men who did not attend, men who attended at least one antenatal care appointment with their partner were younger, had fewer children, were more educated, were wealthier, were more likely to live in an urban area, report partner or shared healthcare decision making, follow Ethiopian Orthodox religion and have exposure to media and were less likely to have a partner who reported, or to report themselves, that "wife beating" was acceptable in any circumstances.

Components of focused antenatal care compared on the basis of whether a woman's partner did or did not attend at least one antenatal care appointment are presented in Table 2. Women whose partner attended at least one antenatal care session were more likely to attend antenatal care in a private facility, to commence care in the first trimester of pregnancy, to attend four or more antenatal care sessions, to complete urine and blood screening tests during antenatal care and to be counselled about pregnancy complications than those who attended without a partner.

As described in the method section, associations between male attendance at antenatal care and outcome measures were compared between women who did and did not report that "wife beating" was acceptable. There were no differences.

Logistic regression analyses

Commencing antenatal care in the first trimester

Women in households classified by the DHS as being in the poorest, poor and middle wealth quintiles were approximately half as likely to begin care in the first trimester compared to those in households classified as being in the richest wealth quintile. Women receiving care in a government facility were less likely to commence care in the first trimester than those attending a private facility. After controlling for socio-economic and demographic factors, there was no significant association between male attendance at antenatal care and commencing ANC in the first trimester (see Table 3).

Number of antenatal visits

Women were significantly less likely to attend at least four ANC visits if they lived in urban centres and rural areas compared to the capital city, and if their partner had no education, primary or secondary education compared to higher education. The likelihood of receiving four ANC sessions increased as maternal age increased, but decreased as the number of children increased. Women in the poorest quintile were significantly less likely to commence care in the first trimester compared

to those in the wealthiest quintile. After controlling for socio-economic and demographic factors, there was no significant association between male attendance at ANC and receiving the recommended number of visits (see Table 3).

Urine sample and blood sample collected during ANC

Women attending antenatal care without a male partner were significantly less likely to receive both a urine and a blood test compared to those whose partners attended (Table 3). In addition, women were significantly less likely to provide both kinds of samples for screening tests if they lived in other urban or rural areas than those in the capital, and if they were in poorer wealth quintiles compared to the richest wealth quintile. Women who said "wife beating" was acceptable in some circumstances were significantly less likely to receive both kinds of tests, compared to those who said violence was never acceptable.

Women were less likely to report a urine sample if they attended a government facility for ANC compared to those receiving ANC at a private clinic. Women were more likely with increasing age to receive a blood test (see Table 3).

Counselled about pregnancy warning signs during antenatal care

Women attending antenatal care without a male partner were significantly less likely to report that they had been counselled about possible complications during pregnancy (Table 3). Women were significantly less likely to report being warned of complications if they lived in rural areas compared to those in Addis Ababa, if they were in the middle wealth quintile compared to the richest and if their partners had no education or only primary education compared to those with higher education (see Table 3).

All recommended components of focused antenatal care

Women were significantly less likely to receive all recommended components if they lived in rural areas compared to the capital city, and if their partner had only primary education compared to higher education. Women were also significantly less likely to receive all components if they attended a public health facility compared to a private facility. After controlling for socio-economic and demographic factors, there was no significant association between male attendance at ANC and receiving all recommended components of ANC (see Table 3).

Discussion

This is the first study examining male attendance at antenatal care and factors associated with meeting

Table 1 Characteristics of women and men in couples meeting inclusion criteria: n(%)

Characteristics n (%)	Men and women with children 0–2 with partners who attended at least one ANC session (included in study)			
	Women included in study	Men who attended ANC	Men who did not attend ANC	Sig differences between men
Age (Mean SD)	28.47 (6.72)	34 (7.37)	35.34 (8.02)	***
Number of children (Mean SD)	4.08 (2.62)	3.45 (2.74)	4.23 (2.76)	***
Education				
No school	776 (54%)	152 (27%)	228 (36%)	***
Primary	498 (35%)	263 (47%)	314 (49%)	NS
Secondary	103 (7%)	78 (14%)	57 (9%)	***
Higher	61 (4%)	69 (12%)	44 (7%)	***
Wealth Index				
Poorest quintile	217 (15%)	52 (9%)	104 (16%)	***
Poor quintile	217 (15%)	72 (13%)	97 (15%)	NS
Average quintile	241 (17%)	77 (14%)	109 (17%)	NS
Rich quintile	273 (19%)	100 (18%)	127 (20%)	NS
Richest quintile	484 (34%)	260 (46%)	206 (32%)	***
Residence				
Addis Ababa	121 (8%)	77 (14%)	44 (7%)	***
Other urban	308 (21%)	154 (27%)	136 (21%)	***
Rural	1009 (70%)	330 (59%)	463 (72%)	***
Healthcare decisions				
Woman alone	226 (16%)	108 (19%)	87 (14%)	*
Shared	939 (65%)	356 (64%)	445 (69%)	*
Man alone	271 (19%)	96 (17%)	110 (17%)	NS
Religion				
Orthodox	613 (43%)	276 (49%)	279 (43%)	***
Catholic	10 (1%)	3 (0%)	6 (1%)	NS
Protestant	256 (18%)	78 (14%)	106 (16%)	NS
Muslim	548 (38%)	199 (35%)	245 (38%)	NS
Traditional	9 (1%)	1 (0%)	1 (0%)	
Media exposure				
At least once per week	495 (34%)	416 (74%)	385 (60%)	***
Does not have access to TV, radio or newspaper	943 (66%)	145 (26%)	258 (40%)	***
Attitudes towards "wife beating" (women)				
Acceptable in at least one condition	944 (66%)	333 (59%)	436 (68%)	**
Never acceptable	494 (34%)	228 (41%)	207 (32%)	**

*** sig at $p < .001$ ** sig at $p < .01$ * sig at $p < .05$

WHO-recommended components of antenatal care in Ethiopia, a country with low rates of healthcare utilisation, high rates of maternal mortality and high rates of shared decision making [5, 40]. Strengths include the country-wide randomly selected sample of women already accessing care. It builds upon existing research which has focused mainly on Ethiopian women's involvement in *any* antenatal care [23–25], and examines for the first time, whether male attendance at antenatal care visits is associated with enhanced antenatal care, which includes screening tests, counselling and recommended timing of and amount of antenatal care. The data are from the first round of EDHS surveys to ask men about attendance at antenatal care [6]. Moreover an investigation of male attendance at antenatal care as a potential strategy for improving maternal and child health outcomes in Ethiopia has not previously been reported in published systematic reviews on the topic, [6, 7].

Table 2 Antenatal care variables for women whose partners did and did not attend antenatal care: n (%)

Antenatal care and pregnancy variables	Men who attended ANC $n = 561$	Men who did not attend ANC $n = 643$	Sig
Place woman received ANC			
Government facility	460 (84%)	595 (94%)	***
Private facility	78 (14%)	28 (5%)	***
Missing	15 (3%)	14 (2%)	NS
Trimester during which woman commenced antenatal care			
First trimester	196(35%)	181 (29%)	*
Second trimester	293(53%)	362 (57%)	NS
Third trimester	68 (12%)	93 (15%)	NS
Number of ANC consultations for woman			
< 4 ANC sessions	258 (46%)	340 (53%)	**
≥ 4 ANC sessions	300 (54%)	299 (47%)	**
Missing	3 (0%)	4 (1%)	
Screening tests during ANC woman			
Blood test	405 (72%)	380 (59%)	***
Urine test	331 (59%)	270 (42%)	***
Counselled about potential pregnancy complications			
Not told complications	394 (70%)	523 (82%)	***
Told complications	167 (30%)	119 (19%)	***

*** sig at $p < .001$ ** sig at $p < .01$ * sig at $p < .05$

Study limitations

Alongside the benefits of using rigorously collected population level data, there are limitations to secondary data analysis, specifically the study was limited to questions regarding male involvement already included in the Ethiopian Demographic and Health Survey. Further, the sample is representative of women accessing antenatal care, but does not allow generalisations to the entire population of women with children in Ethiopia many of whom do not access antenatal care.

Factors associated with comprehensive antenatal care

Consistent with previous research [14], these data suggest commencing care in the second or third trimester of pregnancy is common: only 32% of women included in the study had begun antenatal care in the first trimester (Table 3). Late presentation may be common across sectors of society because of lack of family planning, access to care or because of traditional views on healthcare during pregnancy, irrespective of urban or rural location, education, mother's age, empowerment, exposure to media or number of children. Wealth was the only significant factor in seeking care early – with women in the highest wealth quintile beginning before all other wealth groups. It is possible that the costs associated with healthcare (which may include lengthy transport) are prohibitive, or couples belonging to the wealthiest sub-cultures are more likely to plan for pregnancy, and thus detect the early signs and access antenatal care.

The study results are consistent with previous research across many low income countries, which indicate healthcare utilisation is positively associated with socioeconomic variables including wealth and education [42]. The findings are also similar to results of international research in which women were found to be less likely to attend antenatal care as they grow older and have more children [35]. Possibly this is associated with the growing demands of caring for an increasing number of children, resulting in difficulty attending healthcare, or growing familiarity with pregnancy and childbirth.

The most significant factor associated with attending the recommended amount of antenatal care, receiving screening tests and receiving all the components of antenatal care was where the woman lived. Living in the capital city significantly increased a woman's chance of receiving four antenatal care sessions and undergoing screening tests, independent of the influence of wealth, education or any other factor. Previous research using EDHS data has examined place of residence using an urban/rural dichotomy without presenting information on whether urban centres are different to the capital city [42, 43]. Our findings indicate the need for caution in interpreting urban antenatal statistics for Ethiopia, which may reflect indicators of health care in Addis Ababa (and possibly some regional capital cities), but not other urban centres. Residing in the capital city may be associated with system level factors (for example better equipped facilities and more accessible health centres)

Table 3 Multivariate logistic regression results for each outcome measure: Adjusted Odds Ratios (AOR) (95% Confidence Interval)

	First trimester (n = 1162)	Attended 4+ ANC (n = 1166)	Urine sample ANC (n = 1172)	Blood sample ANC (n = 1173)	Counselling ANC (n = 1168)	All components ANC (n = 1173)
Addis Ababa (reference)						
Urban	1.14(.71–1.83)	***.17(.08–.34)	***.07(.02–.31)	*.08(.01–.61)	.64(.40–1.02)	.68(.38–1.24)
Rural	.77(.42–1.40)	***.17(.08–.37)	***.03(.01–.13)	**.03(.00–.25)	*.57(.28–.96)	*.28(.09–.84)
Higher Education (reference)						
No Education	.84(.48–1.45)	***.32(.17–.59)	.64(.33–1.22)	1.08(.55–2.14)	*.57(.33–1.00)	.46(.18–1.17)
Primary Education	.79(.49–1.28)	***.35(.20–.61)	.57(.31–1.05)	.97(.51–1.86)	*.57(.36–.93)	**.34(.17–.65)
Secondary Education	1.32(.76–2.31)	*.49(.25–.93)	.91(.44–1.90)	1.31(.59–2.90)	.68(.39–1.17)	.75(.39–1.45)
Mother Age	1.03(.99–1.06)	**1.05(1.02–1.09)	.20(.96–1.04)	*1.04(1.0–1.08)	1.01(.97–1.05)	1.01(.95–1.07)
Number of Children	.91(.82–1.00)	**.87(.78–.94)	.92(.84–1.02)	.92(.84–1.02)	.98(.89–1.08)	.89(.73–1.08)
Private clinic ANC (reference)						
Public Health Service ANC	*.36(.23–.57)	.61(.37–1.01)	*.48(.26–.86)	1.21(.67–2.18)	.82(.52–1.31)	*.50(.28–.91)
Male Attendance (reference)						
No Male Attendance	1.05(.79–1.39)	1.06(.82–1.38)	*.73(.55–.97)	*.70(.53–.93)	**.64(.48–.86)	.65(.39–1.10)
Richest Wealth quintile (reference)						
Poorest Wealth quintile	**.43(.23–.80)	**.37(.21–.65)	***.34(.19–.60)	***.35(.20–.62)	.61(.32–1.19)	.20(.02–1.80)
Poor Wealth quintile	*.51(.28–.93)	.61(.35–1.04)	**.46(.26–.81)	**.42(.24–.74)	.60(.31–1.16)	.40(.07–2.24)
Middle Wealth quintile	*.54(.30–.97)	.62(.37–1.05)	**.41(.23–.70)	***.36(.21–.64)	*.50(.26–.96)	.36(.06–2.00)
Rich Wealth quintile	.61(.36–1.03)	.76(.47–1.24)	.66(.41–1.08)	**.49(.29–.82)	.69(.39–1.21)	.56(.16–1.94)
MCH Decision Woman (reference)						
MCH Decision Shared	.82(.56–1.18)	.97(.67–1.42)	.74(.49–1.11)	.80(.52–1.22)	1.18(.80–1.74)	1.21(.67–2.20)
MCH Decision Man	.86(.59–1.08)	.82(.60–1.30)	.71(.43–1.07)	.96(.58–1.58)	1.03(.61–1.72)	1.19(.48–2.94)
"Wife beating" not acceptable (reference)						
"Wife beating" acceptable	.80(.60–1.09)	.86(.64–1.14)	*.68(.50–.93)	*.69(.50–.94)	.76(.55–1.04)	.93(.55–1.59)
Media Weekly (reference)						
Media Less than weekly	.96(.68–1.35)	.91(.68–1.22)	.83(.61–1.14)	.81(.60–1.09)	.88(.60–1.28)	.43(.14–1.33)
Nagelkerke R2	.182	.229	.398	.284	.132	.330

*** sig at $p < .001$ ** sig at $p < .01$ * sig at $p < .05$

and individual level factors (for example more education about the importance of family planning and accessing healthcare during pregnancy) that facilitate meeting guidelines for focused antenatal care.

Variables which may indicate women's empowerment (participation in decision making and access to media) did not make a significant, independent contribution to any of the antenatal care outcomes when other factors were controlled. This is inconsistent with previous international research that found women's decision making and autonomy significantly impacted the likelihood of them accessing healthcare [27]. In previous studies, a greater proportion of women did not participate in healthcare decisions at all; thus the current study only included women receiving antenatal care and who had greater rates of participation in their own healthcare decisions – and may be considered more empowered. Which highlights the need for caution in generalising these results to the broader Ethiopian population.

Finally, after adjusting for socio-economic position, attending antenatal care from a private provider compared to the public health system was one of the few indicators that significantly increased a women's chance of receiving all recommended components of antenatal care. This might indicate that facility-related factors (such as equipment, training and caseload) and individual factors (such as attitude towards healthcare) are combined in women attending private clinics, and lead to these women being more likely to receive all components of antenatal care.

Associations with male attendance at antenatal care

Consistent with a growing body of international and Ethiopian research describing enhanced maternal health outcomes associated with male involvement in maternal healthcare [6–25], higher rates of screening tests (urine and blood samples) and counselling about potential pregnancy complications were significantly associated with male partner attendance at antenatal care. These associations remained significant after controlling for socio-economic factors, women's decision making power and location of antenatal care.

Men's attendance, combined with the fact that resources such as time and money have been made available, may indicate men's approval for care, which is associated with increased antenatal care use [9–11]. An alternative mechanism for the association between male attendance and antenatal care outcomes could be that male approval for care and understanding of the benefits of care led the couple to select better equipped facilities with better trained staff. Having a male partner present may also have elicited more comprehensive levels of care from the same facility, because the couple together were more capable of paying on the spot fees for screening tests, or able to ask more questions and elicit more in-depth counselling from health workers. Alternatively, health care provider behaviour may be different if a male partner is present. Due to cultural status of men as the head of a family, health workers may have been more likely to offer the necessary screening and counselling tests for couples than for women alone. On the other hand, differences in screening tests and counselling could also be related to factors unaccounted for in the model. For example, partner attendance could signal his anxiety about the pregnancy rather than approval of health services, which in turn prompts selecting the most equipped facility, the most skilled providers or all the necessary tests.

After controlling for socio-economic and demographic factors, women attending alone were only 35% as likely to receive all the necessary components of antenatal care compared to women who attended with a male partner. However in this sample the association was not statistically significant. Nevertheless the substantial AOR lends support to the argument there are benefits in antenatal care associated with male attendance in Ethiopia.

Contrary to previous international and Ethiopian research [9–11, 35] and different to the other indicators of best-practice antenatal care in this study, after controlling for socio-economic factors, neither commencing care in the first trimester nor attending at least four appointments was significantly associated between male attendance. The discrepancy with previous Ethiopian research is likely to be methodological, specifically due to differences between the samples of women in the studies along with differences in the criteria for defining antenatal care use. Previous research in Ethiopia used samples of women selected because of a recent birth, irrespective of whether they accessed any care [9–11], whereas the current study was limited to women who received at least one consultation. Other studies have defined antenatal care utilisation as either a binary variable (attending or not), or as a continuous variable

commencing at none, whereas the current study evaluated commencing care in the first trimester or attending at least four sessions. The definitions that include the option of no care appear more sensitive to male partner involvement.

Research from India and Nepal found male participation in antenatal care was associated with improvements in the use of skilled birth attendants and postnatal care use following targeted interventions [33, 35]. The current study did not incorporate consideration of whether the couple received systematically targeted information on any aspect of perinatal care. The results may suggest that male attendance at antenatal care without a targeted intervention beyond usual care is not associated with commencing care early or attending four sessions in women already attending care in Ethiopia.

Implications for practice, programmes, policy and future research

Including men in antenatal care is likely to entail changes to maternal healthcare systems and healthcare worker training, to adopt more 'father inclusive' practices, and as recommended by the WHO [5], may need specific attention to ensure women's autonomy is not compromised by male inclusion. Routine measurement of adherence to antenatal care protocols is also advised, regardless of whether women attend alone or with a male partner.

The results indicate that health promotion strategies relating to antenatal care attendance are best targeted outside the capital, focusing on other urban centres and rural areas to reach underserved populations. Given the importance of pregnancy complication warnings to large numbers of women giving birth at home, particular focus is needed on improving the counselling aspect of antenatal care for all women and their partners across Ethiopia. Focused antenatal care (FANC) guidelines emphasise the importance of counselling for women, and the FANC Ethiopian training module stresses a "shared responsibility for complication readiness and birth preparedness", stating that FANC should "alert the family in all pregnancies for potential complications which could occur at anytime" [4]. The finding that only a small proportion of women report being counselled on pregnancy complications is inconsistent with FANC guidelines and suggests antenatal care implementation has deviated from Ethiopian guidelines and WHO recommendations [4, 5].

Based on previous research male involvement may increase the likelihood of women attending ANC. This study examined whether it was associated with making women's care comprehensive enough to comply with WHO guidelines. As there were no associations between commencing care early or attending the minimum recommended number of ANC visits, caution should be applied in relying completely on male-focused strategies to encourage recommended antenatal care attendance.

Finally, future research on male involvement in antenatal care in Ethiopia is needed in order to understand women's, men's and health care workers attitudes towards male involvement to better understand the cultural context, potential harms, potential benefits, the barriers and the facilitators to accommodate changes in what is traditionally considered a woman's domain. In addition, there is need for controlled evaluation of targeted health promotion strategies aimed at men to examine the influence of specifically providing men with education on perinatal care. In addition, large population studies routinely carried out in Ethiopia could greatly enhance knowledge in this area if they included more detailed indicators of male involvement in pregnancy, maternal and child healthcare and early child development. Male involvement during pregnancy may have a range of additional benefits to maternal and child health, including post-natal care use, skilled birth attendance, improved partner support, maternal mental health and increased bonding between father and child [36]. Alternatively, there could be harms from male involvement not captured by existing research. Consequently, there is a need for greater exploration of the nature and role of male involvement in maternal and child health more broadly in Ethiopia.

Conclusions

In conclusion, consistent with WHO recommendations and previous research, the findings provide evidence that male attendance at antenatal care in Ethiopia may be associated with women receiving more comprehensive antenatal care. On balance the results revealed some benefits and did not detect harms from including male partners in antenatal care in Ethiopia. This is relevant to policy makers, practitioners and researchers working in public health in Ethiopia.

Abbreviations

ANC: Antenatal care; AOR: Adjusted odds ratio; DHS: Ethiopian demographic and health survey; EDHS: Ethiopian demographic and health survey; FANC: Focused antenatal care; HEW: Health extension workers; IRB: Institutional review board; MCH: Maternal and child health; MDG: Millennium development goals; RCT: Randomised controlled trial; SDG: Sustainable development goals; SNNP: Southern Nations nationalities and peoples; WHO: World health organisation

Authors' contributions

FF conceptualised and drafted the manuscript, KW guided analysis and result interpretation, CW reviewed and edited manuscript, BZ provided reviewed,

edited and provided country-specific policy expertise and JF provided overall conceptual guidance, reviewed and edited the manuscript. All authors read and approved the final manuscript.

Competing interests
The authors declare that they have no competing interests.

Author details
[1]Jean Hailes Research Unit, School of Public Health and Preventive Medicine, Monash University, 553 St Kilda Rd, Melbourne, VIC 3004, Australia. [2]Parenting Research Centre, 232 Victoria Parade, East Melbourne, VIC 3002, Australia. [3]School of Public Health and Preventive Medicine, Monash University, 553 St Kilda Rd, Melbourne, VIC 3004, Australia. [4]Institute of Public Health, College of Medicine and Health Sciences, University of Gondar, Gondar, Ethiopia.

References
1. World Health Organisation. Global health Observatory Data. Available from: http://www.who.int/gho/maternal_health/mortality/maternal_mortality_text/en/. Accessed 10 Sept 2016.
2. The United Nations. Millenium development goals report. 2015.
3. Ornella Lincetto SM-A, Patricia Gomez, Stephen Munjanja. Antenatal care. Opportunities for Africa's newborns: practical data, policy and programmatic support for newborn care in Africa: World Health Organisation; 2006.
4. The Open University. Antenatal Care: Module 13 Providing Focused Antenatal Care. Available from: http://www.open.edu/openlearnworks/mod/oucontent/view.php?id=44&printable=1. Accessed 10 Sept 2016.
5. Asefa F, Geleto A, Dessie Y. Male partners involvement in maternal ANC care: the view of women attending ANC in Hararipublic health institutions, eastern Ethiopia. Sci J Public Health. 2014;2(3):182–8.
6. World Health Organisation. WHO recommendations on health promotion interventions for maternal and newborn health. 2015.
7. Aguiar C, Jennings L. Impact of male partner antenatal accompaniment on perinatal health outcomes in developing countries: a systematic literature review. Matern Child Health J. 2015;19(9):2012–9.
8. Yargawa J, Leonardi-Bee J. Male involvement and maternal health outcomes: systematic review and meta-analysis. J Epidemiol Community Health. 2015;69(6):604–12.
9. Bitew Y, Awoke W, Chekol S. Birth preparedness and complication readiness practice and associated factors among pregnant women, Northwest Ethiopia. Int Scholarly Res Notices. 2016;2016:8727365.
10. Abosse Z, Woldie M, Ololo S. Factors influencing antenatal care service utilization in hadiya zone. Ethiopian J Health Sci. 2010;20(2):75.
11. Biratu BT, Lindstrom DP. The influence of husbands' approval on Woman's use of prenatal care: results from Yirgalem and Jimma towns, south West Ethiopia. Ethiopian J Health Development. 2007;20(2):85–92.
12. Birmeta K, Dibaba Y, Woldeyohannes D. Determinants of maternal health care utilization in Holeta town, Central Ethiopia. BMC Health Serv Res. 2013;13:256.
13. Habte D, Teklu S, Melese T, Magafu MG. Correlates of unintended pregnancy in Ethiopia: results from a national survey. PLoS One. 2013; 8(12):e82987.
14. Hailemichael F, Woldie M, Tafese F. Predictors of institutional delivery in Sodo town, southern Ethiopia: original research. Afr J Prm Health Care Fam Med. 2013;5(1):1–9.
15. Wilunda C, Quaglio G, Putoto G, Takahashi R, Calia F, Abebe D, et al. Determinants of utilisation of antenatal care and skilled birth attendant at delivery in south west Shoa zone, Ethiopia: a cross sectional study. Reprod Health. 2015;12:74.
16. Tebekaw Y, James Mashalla Y, Thupayagale-Tshweneagae G. Factors influencing Women's preferences for places to give birth in Addis Ababa, Ethiopia. Obstet Gynecol Int. 2015;2015:439748.
17. Wassie L, Bekele A, Ismael A, Tariku N, Heran A, Getnet M, et al. Magnitude and factors that affect males' involvement in deciding partners' place of delivery in Tiyo District of Oromia region, Ethiopia. Ethiop J Heal Dev 2014; Volume 28(Special Issue):1–43.
18. Katiso NAAY. Male partners' involvement in institutional delivery in rural Ethiopia: community based survey. J Women's Health Care. 2015;4:1000239.
19. Godefay H, Byass P, Graham W, Kinsman J, Mulugeta A. Risk factors for maternal mortality in rural Tigray, northern Ethiopia: a case-control study. PLoS One. 2015;10(12):e0144975.

20. Habte F, Demissie M. Magnitude and factors associated with institutional delivery service utilization among childbearing mothers in Cheha district, Gurage zone, SNNPR, Ethiopia: a community based cross sectional study. BMC Pregnancy Childbirth. 2015;15:299.

21. Birhanu Z, Godesso A, Kebede Y, Gerbaba M. Mothers experiences and satisfactions with health extension program in Jimma zone, Ethiopia: a cross sectional study. BMC Health Serv Res. 2013;13:74.

22. Biratu A, Haile D. Prevalence of antenatal depression and associated factors among pregnant women in Addis Ababa, Ethiopia: a cross- sectional study. Reprod Health. 2015;12:89.

23. Tura G. Antenatal care service utilization and associated factors in Metekel zone, Northwest Ethiopia. Ethiopian J Health Sci. 2009;19(2):111–8.

24. Warren C. Care seeking for maternal health: challenges remain for poor women. Ethiop J Health Dev. 2010;24(Special No. 1):100–104.

25. Alemayehu T, Haidar J, Habte D. Utilization of antenatal care services among teenagers in Ethiopia. a cross sectional study. Ethiop J Health Dev. 2010;24(3):221–5.

26. Jackson R, Tesfay FH, Godefay H, Gebrehiwot TG. Health extension workers and mothers attitudes to maternal health service utilization and acceptance in Adwa Woreda, Tigray region, Ethiopia. PLoS One. 2016;11(3):e0150747.

27. Osamor PE, Grady C. Women's autonomy in health care decision- making in developing countries: a synthesis of the literature. Int J Women's Health. 2016;8:191.

28. Madhavan VHS. Data availability on men's involvement in families in sub-Saharan Africa to inform family-centred programmes for children affected by HIV and AIDS. J Int AIDS Soc. 2010;13(2):S5.

29. Ditekemena J, Koole O, Engmann C, Matendo R, Tshefu A, Ryder R, et al. Determinants of male involvement in maternal and child health services in sub-Saharan Africa: a review. Reprod Health. 2012;9:32.

30. Mullany BC, Becker S, Hindin MJ. The impact of including husbands in antenatal health education services on maternal health practices in urban Nepal: results from a randomized controlled trial. Health Educ Res. 2007; 22(2):166–76.

31. Varkey LC, Mishra A, Das A, Ottolenghi E, Huntington D, Adamchak S, et al. Involving men in maternity care in India. New Delhi: Population Council; 2004.

32. Mangeni JN, Mwangi A, Mbugua S, Mukthar V. Male involvement in maternal health care as a determinant of utilization of skilled birth attendants in Kenya. Calverton: Demographic and Health Survey (DHS) Working Paper. ICF International; 2013.

33. Chattopadhyay A. Men in maternal care: evidence from India. J Biosoc Sci. 2012;44:129–53.

34. Kalembo FW, Zgambo M, Mulaga AN, Yukai D, Ahmed NI. Association between male partner involvement and the uptake of prevention of mother-to-child transmission of HIV (PMTCT) interventions in Mwanza district, Malawi: a retrospective cohort study. PLoS One. 2013;8(6):e66517.

35. Mullany BC, Lakhev B, Shretha D, Hindin MJ, Becker S. Impact of Husbands' participation in antenatal health education services on maternal health knowledge. J Nepal Med Assoc. 2009;48(173):28–34.

36. Kunene B, Beksinska M, Zondi S, Mthembu N, Mullick S, Ottolenghi E, et al. Involving men in maternity care: South Africa. Durban: Population Council; 2004.

37. Jennings L, Na M, Cherewick M, Hindin M, Mullany B, Ahmed S. Women's empowerment and male involvement in antenatal care: analyses of demographic and health surveys (DHS) in selected African countries. BMC Pregnancy Childbirth. 2014;14:297.

38. Federal Democratic Republic of Ethiopia Ministry of Health. Health sector development Programme IV annual performance report. Addis Ababa: Federal Democratic Republic of Ethiopia Ministry of Health; 2013/2014.

39. Tessema GA, Laurence CO, Melaku YA, Misganaw A, Woldie SA, Hiruye A, et al. Trends and causes of maternal mortality in Ethiopia during 1990- 2013: findings from the global burden of diseases study 2013. BMC Public Health. 2017;17(1):160.

40. Central Statistical Agency/Ethiopia and ICF International. Ethiopia Demographic and Health Survey 2011. Addis Ababa: Central Statistical Agency/Ethiopia and ICF International; 2012. Available at http://dhsprogram.com/pubs/pdf/FR255/FR255.pdf.

41. Wassie Lingerh, Bekele Ababeye, Ismael Ali, Tariku Nigatu, Heran Abebe, Getnet Mitike, et al. Magnitude and factors that affect males' involvement in deciding partners' place of delivery in Tiyo District of Oromia Region, Ethiopia. The Ethiopian journal of health development. 2014;28(Special issue 1):6–13.

42. Fekadu M, Regassa N. Skilled delivery care service utilization in Ethiopia: analysis of rural-urban differentials based on national demographic and health survey (DHS) data. Afr Health Sci. 2014;14(4):974–84.

43. Muchie KF. Quality of antenatal care services and completion of four or more antenatal care visits in Ethiopia: a finding based on a demographic and health survey. BMC Pregnancy Childbirth. 2017;17(1):300.

18

Seroprevalence of HIV, HTLV, CMV, HBV and rubella virus infections in pregnant adolescents who received care in the city of Belém, Pará, Northern Brazil

Aubaneide Batista Guerra[1,2,3], Leonardo Quintão Siravenha[2,3], Rogério Valois Laurentino[2,3], Rosimar Neris Martins Feitosa[2], Vânia Nakauth Azevedo[2], Antonio Carlos Rosário Vallinoto[2,3], Ricardo Ishak[2,3] and Luiz Fernando Almeida Machado[2,3*]

Abstract

Background: Prenatal tests are important for prevention of vertical transmission of various infectious agents. The objective of this study was to describe the prevalence of human immunodeficiency virus (HIV), human T-lymphotropic virus (HTLV), hepatitis B virus (HBV), cytomegalovirus (CMV), rubella virus and vaccination coverage against HBV in pregnant adolescents who received care in the city of Belém, Pará, Brazil.

Methods: A cross-sectional study was performed with 324 pregnant adolescents from 2009 to 2010. After the interview and blood collection, the patients were screened for antibodies and/or antigens against HIV-1/2, HTLV-1/2, CMV, rubella virus and HBV. The epidemiological variables were demonstrated using descriptive statistics with the G, χ^2 and Fisher exact tests.

Results: The mean age of the participants was 15.8 years, and the majority (65.4%) had less than 6 years of education. The mean age at first intercourse was 14.4 years, and 60.8% reported having a partner aged between 12 and 14 years. The prevalence of HIV infection was 0.3%, and of HTLV infection was 0.6%. Regarding HBV, 0.6% of the participants had acute infection, 9.9% had a previous infection, 16.7% had vaccine immunity and 72.8% were susceptible to infection. The presence of anti-HBs was greater in adolescent between 12 and 14 years old (28.8%) while the anti-HBc was greater in adolescent between 15 and 18 years old (10.3%). Most of the adolescents presented the IgG antibody to CMV (96.3%) and rubella (92.3%). None of the participants had acute rubella infection, and 2.2% had anti-CMV IgM.

Conclusions: This study is the first report of the seroepidemiology of infectious agents in a population of pregnant adolescents in the Northern region of Brazil. Most of the adolescents had low levels of education, were susceptible to HBV infection and had IgG antibodies to CMV and rubella virus. The prevalence of HBV, HIV and HTLV was similar to that reported in other regions of Brazil. However, the presence of these agents in this younger population reinforces the need for good prenatal follow-up and more comprehensive vaccination campaigns against HBV due to the large number of women susceptible to the virus.

Keywords: Pregnant adolescents, Brazil, HIV, HTLV, HBV, CMV, Rubella, Seroepidemiology

* Correspondence: lfam@ufpa.br
[2]Virology Laboratory, Institute of Biological Sciences, Federal University of Pará, Augusto Correa 1, Guamá, 66, Belém, Pará 075-110, Brazil
[3]Biology of Infectious and Parasitic Agents Graduate Program, Federal University of Pará, Belém, Pará, Brazil
Full list of author information is available at the end of the article

Background

Some infectious agents, including human immunodeficiency virus (HIV), human T-lymphotropic virus (HTLV), human cytomegalovirus (CMV), hepatitis B virus (HBV) and rubella virus, are of great importance in the context of pregnancy due to the possibility of transmission from the woman to the baby during the gestational period, at the time of delivery and through breastfeeding [1–4]. Therefore, knowledge of the serological statuses of women is fundamentally important for the provision of good prenatal care to ensure that the necessary measures are taken to avoid the vertical transmission of these agents.

In Brazil, 99,804 pregnant women were infected with HIV as of June 2016, of whom 7.4% were residents of the northern region. The state of Pará showed an increasing trend in HIV detection rates in pregnant women between 1995 and 2015 and reported 2980 cases by 2016. In Brazil, the majority of pregnant women living with HIV/AIDS are between 20 and 24 years of age, and only 15.5% are between 10 and 19 years of age [5].

Approximately 20 million people worldwide are estimated to be infected with HTLV-1 or HTLV-2 [6]. In Brazil, the prevalence rates of HTLV-1/HTLV-2 infections in pregnant women are generally low. The prevalence is approximately 0.1% in the state of Mato Grosso do Sul [7, 8], approximately 0.1% in the city of Botucatu, São Paulo [9, 10], approximately 0.66% in Rio de Janeiro [10], approximately 0.3% in the state of Maranhão and approximately 1.5% in Bahia, which is the area with the highest prevalence in the country [11]. In the northern region of Brazil, the prevalence of HTLV-1/HTLV-2 infection varies from 0% in the state of Amazonas [12] to 0.3% in the state of Pará [13].

The prevalence of anti-CMV IgG antibodies in pregnant women is high in Brazil (97.0%) [14] and various regions of the world (91.3–99.5%) [15, 16]. However, CMV infection is still one of the most common causes of congenital malformation [17]. In Brazil, the diagnosis of acute rubella infection in pregnant women is very low [7, 18] due to the efficacy of the vaccine [19] and periodic vaccination campaigns.

Vertical transmission of HBV is also an important public health problem, mainly due to the increased risk of chronification of infection in children, especially if the mother has the HBV e antigen (HBeAg) and HBV surface antigen (HBsAg) markers during pregnancy or at the time of delivery [20, 21]. Thus, knowledge of the serological status for the virus has great relevance for the clinical management of these women during the gestational period.

In Brazil, several studies have reported the prevalence rates of HIV, HTLV, CMV, HBV and rubella in general populations of pregnant women [12, 18, 22, 23]. However, epidemiological information about these agents is still scarce in Brazil. No data are available for pregnant adolescents in the northern region of Brazil. Thus, an evaluation of the seroprevalence of these pathogens in pregnant adolescents is important to assess their early circulation and the rate of vaccine coverage against rubella and HBV.

The aim of the present study was to describe the seroprevalence rates of HIV, HTLV, HBV, CMV and rubella virus infections and to determine the vaccination coverage against HBV in pregnant adolescents who received care in the city of Belém, capital of the state of Pará, Brazil.

Methods

Type of study and ethical aspects

The present study is descriptive, cross-sectional and observational. The study was approved by the Human Research Ethics Committee of the Instituto Evandro Chagas under number 13/2009. The participants and their legal guardians were informed about the study objectives. After the adolescents and their legal guardians agreed to participate in the research, they signed a consent form and then answered an epidemiological questionnaire via a confidential structured interview. The questionnaire contained questions regarding age, place of birth and current residence, years of education, school dropout, age at first intercourse, condom use and age of the partner. Additionally, the vaccination card of the pregnant adolescents was evaluated to determine whether they had received the HBV vaccine.

Sample size

The sample size determination was based on the estimated prevalence of viral infections in the general population. An estimated prevalence of 0.35% for HIV, 90% for CMV, 10% for HBV and 0.85% for HTLV resulted in a minimum sample size of 301 pregnant women. The sample error (ε) assumed in the present calculation was 5%, and a test power of 80% was established.

Study population

A total of 324 pregnant adolescents who underwent prenatal care at the Reference Unit Specialized in Maternal-Child and Adolescent Care (Unidade de Referência Especializada Materno-Infantil Adolescência - UREMIA) under the Executive Secretariat of Public Health of the State of Pará (Secretaria Executiva de Saúde Pública do Estado do Pará - SESPA) participated in the study from November 2009 to February 2010.

Adolescents ranging between 12 and 18 years of age at any stage of pregnancy and of any religion, ethnicity, and origin who agreed to participate in the study were included. Pregnant women under 12 and over 18 years of age were excluded, as were those who had known serology results for the agents studied or who did not agree to participate.

Serology

A 10-mL aliquot of peripheral blood was collected from each participant and placed in a tube containing ethyl-enediaminetetraacetic acid (EDTA) as an anticoagulant. The samples were transported to the Virology Laboratory of the Biological Sciences Institute (Instituto de Ciências Biológicas - ICB), Federal University of Pará (Universidade Federal do Pará - UFPA). Plasma and formed elements were separated by centrifugation at 8944 g for 10 min, transferred to an Eppendorf tube and frozen at − 20 °C prior to the serological and molecular biology analyses.

Anti-HIV antibody screening was performed using the ELISA method (Tetra Elisa kit, Biotest AG, Dreiech, Germany). The reactive samples were confirmed using the microparticle enzyme immunoassay method (MEIA, Abbott Axsym™ System, HIV-1/2, Abbott GmbH, Weisbaden, Delkenheim, Germany), followed by confirmation by indirect immunofluorescence (Bio-Manguinhos Fiocruz, Brazil).

Screening for anti-HTLV-1/HTLV-2 antibodies was performed using an ELISA immunoenzymatic assay (HTLV-1 + 2 Ab-Captures ELISA Test System; Ortho Clinical Diagnostic Inc., New Jersey, USA). Reactive samples were confirmed using nested PCR as previously described [24].

Serology for the HBsAg, HBV surface antibodies (anti-HBs) and total anti-HBc markers was performed by ELISA (ETI-AB-AUK-3, DiaSorin, Saluggia, Italy and ETI-MAK-2. PLUS, Diasorin, Italy). Samples that showed reactivity to total anti-HBc were tested for the presence of anti-HBc IgM. The detection of IgM and IgG for CMV and rubella virus was performed by ELISA (DiaSorin, Saluggia, Italy).

Statistical analysis

The Chi-square test (χ^2), G-test and Fisher's exact test were used to assess differences in proportions between the reactivity to the tested agents and the sociodemographic and epidemiological variables of the adolescents, including age, level of education, use of condoms during sexual intercourse and age of partner. Results with $p < 0.05$ were considered significant.

Results

The Table 1 presents the characteristics of pregnant adolescents. The mean age of the pregnant adolescents was 15.8 years (range from 12 to 18 years). The majority was between 15 and 18 years of age, lived in the capital of the state of Pará, had less than 6 years of education and continued to study. Regarding the onset of sexual

Table 1 Sociodemographic characteristics of the group of pregnant adolescents who received care in Belém, Pará, from November 2009 to February 2010

Demographic variable	Number	Percent
Age group		
12 to 14	52	16.1
15 to 18	272	83.9
Residence		
Capital	248	76.5
Interior	76	23.5
Years of education		
< 6	212	65.4
6–9	102	31.5
> 9	10	3.1
School dropout		
Yes	107	33.0
No	186	57.4
Did not attend school	31	9.6
Age at first intercourse		
9 to 11	6	1.9
12 to 14	197	60.8
15 to 17	121	37.3
Age of partner		
12 to 18	150	46.3
19 to 25	146	45.0
26 to 42	28	8.7
Condom use		
Sometimes	249	76.9
Never	75	23.1
Gestational age		
1 to 2 months	104	32.1
3 to 4 months	98	30.2
5 to 6 months	112	34.6
7 to 9 months	10	3.1
Vaccination against HBV		
No	228	70.4
Yes	87	26.8
Unknown	9	2.8

activity of the adolescents, the mean age at first intercourse was 14.4 years and the mean age of the partners at first intercourse was 19.8 years. The frequency of male condom use in sexual intercourse is low and few participants were previously vaccinated against HBV according vaccination cards of the adolescents.

The prevalence of HIV-1 infection was 0.3% (1/324). This adolescent was 17 years old, from the city of Belém, had 6 years of education and reported that she had dropped out of school when she found out about the pregnancy. Her first sexual intercourse was at age 14 without the use of a male condom and was with a 20-year-old sexual partner; both were users of non-injectable drugs. Regarding sexual practices, the adolescent reported a daily frequency of sexual intercourse and sporadic anal sex. She mentioned having had two sexual partners, one of whom was a non-injectable drug user from another state in Brazil. For HTLV, the prevalence of infection was 0.6% (2/324). These two adolescents were 15 and 16 years of age and in the first trimester of their first pregnancy. The younger woman resided in the municipality of Gurupá in the interior of the state of Pará, was married and had 8 years of education, whereas the other was single, had 6 years of education and resided in the city of Belém, also in Pará.

Regarding hepatitis B infection, 0.6% (2/324) of the adolescents presented recent infection (HBsAg and anti-HBc IgM positive), and only 16.7% (54/324) showed vaccine immunity to HBV (presence of isolated anti-HBs). A history of previous HBV infection was observed in 9.9% (32/324) of the adolescents (presence of total anti-HBc and anti-HBs); however, most of the adolescents (72.8%, 236/324) presented a serological profile of susceptibility to the virus. This finding was in agreement with the observations from the vaccination cards of the adolescents, which indicated that 70.4% of the participants were not previously vaccinated.

The statistical analysis showed no differences in proportions between the participants who were reactive and nonreactive for total anti-HBc according to the age group (Fisher's exact test; $p = 0.56$); however, we observed a difference in the proportions between the groups according to the age of the sexual partner (G test, $p = 0.01$) and the use of condoms in sexual intercourse ($p = 0.01$). We also observed that the age of the adolescents (χ^2, $p = 0.01$), the level of education (G test, $p = 0.02$) and the age of the sexual partner (G test, $p = 0.02$) were factors that influenced the proportion of adolescents who were positive and negative for anti-HBs (Table 2).

Regarding CMV, 2.2% of the adolescents had anti-IgM positive, 96.3% had only IgG antibodies, and only 1.5% did not present either of the two antibodies. Most of the participants presented rubella IgG (92.3%), and no acute infection by this agent was observed. No significant difference in any of the categorical variables assessed in the study was observed in the proportions of individuals who tested positive and negative for anti-CMV IgM (Table 2).

Table 2 Epidemiological characteristics in association with the presence of serological markers of CMV infection, HBV infection and HBV vaccine immunity of pregnant adolescents who received care in Belém, Pará, from November 2009 to February 2010

Variables	N (%)	Anti-CMV IgM		P value	Anti-HBc Total		P value	Anti-HBs		P value
		Pos (%)	Neg (%)		Pos (%)	Neg (%)		Pos (%)	Neg (%)	
Age Group										
12–14	52 (16.0)	3 (5.8)	49 (94.2)	0.08[a]	4 (7.7)	48 (92.3)	0.56[a]	15 (28.8)	37 (71.2)	0.01[b]
15–18	272 (84.0)	4 (1.5)	268 (98.5)		28 (10.3)	244 (89.7)		39 (14.3)	233 (85.7)	
Years of education										
< 6	212 (65.4)	4 (2.0)	198 (98.0)		20 (9.4)	192 (90.6)		22 (10.4)	190 (89.6)	
6–9	102 (31.5)	2 (2.0)	100 (98.0)	0.44[c]	10 (9.8)	92 (90.2)	0.62[c]	29 (28.4)	73 (71.6)	0.02[c]
> 9	10 (3.1)	1 (10.0)	9 (90.0)		2 (20.0)	8 (80.0)		3 (30.0)	7 (70.0)	
Age at first intercourse										
9 to 11	6 (1.8)	0 (0.0)	6 (100.0)		1 (16.7)	5 (83.3)		2 (33.3)	4 (66.7)	
12 to 14	197 (60.8)	3 (1.5)	194 (98.5)	0.9[c]	19 (9.6)	178 (90.4)	0.88[c]	32 (16.2)	165 (83.8)	0.62[c]
15 to 17	121 (37.3)	4 (3.3)	117 (96.7)		12 (9.9)	109 (90.1)		20 (16.5)	101 (83.5)	
Condom use										
Sometimes	249 (76.9)	5 (2.0)	244 (98.0)	0.9[a]	13 (5.2)	236 (94.8)	0.01[a]	41 (16.5)	208 (83.5)	0.86[c]
Never	75 (23.1)	2 (2.7)	73 (97.3)		19 (25.3)	56 (74.7)		13 (17.3)	62 (82.7)	
Age of partner (years)										
12 to 18	150 (46.3)	4 (2.7)	146 (97.3)		9 (6.0)	141 (94.0)		25 (16.7)	125 (83.3)	
19 to 25	146 (45.0)	3 (2.0)	143 (98.0)	0.5[c]	12 (8.2)	134 (91.8)	0.01[c]	19 (13.0)	127 (87.0)	0.02[c]
25 to 42	28 (8.7)	0 (0.0)	28 (100.0)		11 (39.3)	17 (60.7)		10 (35.7)	18 (64.3)	

[a]Fisher's exact test; [b]Chi-square test; [c]G test

Discussion

The present study reported for the first time the serological profiles for HTLV, HIV, HBV, CMV and rubella in pregnant adolescents who received care in the city of Belém, Pará, northern region of Brazil. Although the prevalence of HTLV in the study population (0.6%) was within the range previously observed in other populations in the state of Pará [24, 25], we considered the prevalence high compared to other studies performed in pregnant women in the state of Pará [13] and other locations in Brazil, including Manaus [12], Maranhão [26], Paraná [18] and Maceió [23]. This finding is worrying because it indicates early contact of young women with an agent whose screening is not included in the prenatal tests and whose main forms of transmission include breastfeeding. Notably, one of the adolescents resided in the capital and another in the interior of the state of Pará, which indicated a need for greater epidemiological surveillance of this agent in prenatal services throughout the state.

A different scenario was observed for HIV-1, since the prevalence of infection in pregnant adolescents in Pará (0.3%) was similar to the prevalence found in pregnant women in the state of Amazonas [12]; this result confirmed a low incidence of infection in the northern region of Brazil. Our results are in agreement with data from the Ministry of Health that note a higher number of cases of HIV-1 infection in women between the ages of 20 and 24 years [5]. In Brazil, other studies in non-adolescent pregnant women demonstrated a low seroprevalence of HIV-1 infection [7, 23, 27, 28], which differed from reports from other developing countries, where the prevalence of infection was greater than 5% [29–31].

Regarding serology for HBV, almost 10% of the adolescents in the present study had a profile of virus infection. This early contact with the virus has also been observed in several regions of Brazil [32]. The prevalence of recent HBV infection (0.6%) was low in the study population; however, most adolescents (83.3%) presented a serological profile of susceptibility to HBV infection, with an absence of anti-HBV antibodies. This finding indicates the need for greater epidemiological surveillance for HBV in this population of pregnant women. This surveillance should aim to increase vaccination coverage to avoid neonatal or vertical infection by this viral agent, which is associated with a greater probability of chronification of infection and the development of hepatic cirrhosis and hepatocellular carcinoma in infected children.

A low prevalence of HBV in the population of pregnant women has also been observed in several other regions of Brazil [18, 32–34] and other countries [35]. These prevalence rates were much lower than the prevalence rates found in pregnant women in Asian [36, 37] and African countries [38, 39]. No case of coinfection between HIV, HTLV and HBV was observed in the adolescents participating in the present study. Additionally, we observed that the presence of anti-HBs might be related to the age of the adolescent, the level of education and the age of the sexual partner, and the presence of anti-HBc was influenced by the non-use of condoms in sexual intercourse and the partner's age. In Brazil, few studies have associated epidemiological variables with serological markers of HBV infection other than HBsAg. In Maranhão, the presence of anti-HBc was associated with the level of education in pregnant women in general [40], but no association was observed in other Brazilian states, including Goiás [34] and Espírito Santo [41]. This finding indicates the need for better monitoring of these markers for the implementation of public policies to combat HBV. There are some limitations in this study specially in relation to hepatitis markers, such as anti-HBe, anti-HCV and anti-HDV which were not included in the present project due to lack of financial resources, however, in our future studies we will address these limitations.

Few studies have investigated the prevalence of CMV in the population of pregnant adolescents in Brazil. The present article is the first to report the high seroprevalence of anti-CMV IgG in pregnant adolescents from Pará (96.3%), which is similar to observations in pregnant women aged 12 to 19 years in Ribeirão Preto [14] and pregnant women in general from Mato Grosso do Sul [7], Espírito Santo [42] and developing countries [43, 44]. However, a higher percentage (2.2%) of pregnant adolescents in our study presented anti-CMV IgM (reactivation, reinfection or recent infection) compared to pregnant women from Mato Grosso do Sul (0.05%), where the age group was older [7]. This scenario is worrying, because CMV is one of the main infectious agents associated with congenital malformation. Thus, pregnancy at an early age carries a higher risk of infection and consequent vertical transmission of CMV.

No pregnant adolescent with acute rubella infection was detected, but 7.7% of the adolescents were susceptible to the virus, which reinforced the need for rubella vaccination campaigns to achieve greater coverage in Brazil and avoid the onset of congenital rubella syndrome. Similar results were reported in other regions of Brazil [7, 45, 46].

Our study had some limitations, such as the short time period for data collection and the impossibility of finding a statistical association between the presence or absence of infection with HIV or HTLV and acute infection with HBV or rubella virus based on epidemiological data, including the age, condom use and age at first intercourse, due to the low number of participants who presented positive serology for any of the evaluated markers. This shortcoming can most likely be overcome by increasing the sample size in future studies.

Conclusions

In conclusion, the prevalence of HIV, HTLV and HBV infection was similar to the prevalence rates reported in other states of Brazil and showed early contact of adolescents with some agents of parenteral transmission. Acute rubella infection was not observed; however, the occurrence of CMV infection (recent or reativaction) was higher than reported in pregnant women in general in Brazil, demonstrating the importance of prenatal follow-up from the beginning of pregnancy to reduce the onset of congenital cytomegalovirus. Finally, we found that the majority of adolescents were susceptible to HBV infection, which reinforced the need for public policies aimed at intensifying the immunization of this specific population against HBV due to the high rate of infection chronicity in children infected at birth or in the first year of life.

Abbreviations

anti-HBc: Antibody to hepatitis B core antigen; anti-HBe: Antibody to hepatitis B e antigen; anti-HBs: Antibody to hepatitis B surface antigen; anti-HCV: Antibody to hepatitis C virus; anti-HDV: Antibody to hepatitis D virus; CMV: Cytomegalovirus; EDTA: Ethylenediaminetetraacetic acid; ELISA: Enzyme-linked immunosorbent assay; HBeAg: Hepatitis B e antigen; HBsAg: Hepatitis B surface antigen; HBV: Hepatitis B virus; HIV: Human immunodeficiency virus; HTLV: Human T-lymphotropic virus; ICB: Biological Sciences Institute; PCR: Polymerase chain reaction; SESPA: Executive Secretariat of Public Health of the State of Pará; UFPA: Federal University of Pará; UREMIA: Reference Unit Specialized in Maternal-Child and Adolescent Care; χ²: Chi-square test

Acknowledgements

The authors thank all the individuals who took part in the study and the Federal University of Para.

Funding

The study was sponsored by CNPq (Brazilian National Research Council) and Federal University of Para. The authors received funding of PROPESP/UFPA for the publication cost of this article. The funders had no role in study, decision to publish or preparation of the manuscript.

Authors' contributions

LFAM designed the study, analyzed, interpreted data, and wrote the paper. ABG, LQS, RNMF, VNA participated in the experiments and data collection. LFAM, RVL analyzed and interpreted data. ACRV, RI and LFAM analyzed data and revised the manuscript. All authors read and approved the final manuscript.

Competing interests

The authors declare that they have no competing interests.

Author details

[1]Reference Unit Specialized in Maternal-Child and Adolescent Care, Belém, Pará, Brazil. [2]Virology Laboratory, Institute of Biological Sciences, Federal University of Pará, Augusto Correa 1, Guamá, 66, Belém, Pará 075-110, Brazil. [3]Biology of Infectious and Parasitic Agents Graduate Program, Federal University of Pará, Belém, Pará, Brazil.

References

1. Margioula-Siarkou C, Kalogiannidis I, Petousis S, Prapa S, Dagklis T, Mamopoulos A, et al. Cytomegalovirus, toxoplasma gondii and rubella vertical transmission rates according to mid-trimester amniocentesis: a retrospective study. Int J Prev Med. 2015;6:32.
2. Mendes MS, Costa MC, Costa IM. Human T-cell lymphotropic virus-1 infection: three infected generations in the same family. Rev Soc Bras Med Trop. 2016;49(5):660–2.
3. Kang W, Li Q, Shen L, Zhang L, Tian Z, Xu L, et al. Risk factors related to the failure of prevention of hepatitis B virus mother-to-child transmission in Yunnan, China. Vaccine. 2017;35(4):605–9.
4. Nakamura KJ, Heath L, Sobrera ER, Wilkinson TA, Semrau K, Kankasa C, et al. Breast milk and in utero transmission of HIV-1 select for envelope variants with unique molecular signatures. Retrovirology. 2017;14(1):6.
5. Brasil. Boletim Epidemiológico AIDS e DST. Brasília: Ministério da Saúde, Secretaria de Vigilância em Saúde, PN de DST e AIDS, Ano V, n. 1, 1a à 26a semanas epidemiológicas, jan./jun; 2016.
6. Gessain A, Cassar O. Epidemiological aspects and world distribution of HTLV-1 infection. Front Microbiol. 2012;3:388.
7. Figueiró-Filho EA, Senefonte FR, Lopes AH, de Morais OO, Souza Júnior VG, Maia TL, et al. Frequency of HIV-1, rubella, syphilis, toxoplasmosis, cytomegalovirus, simple herpes virus, hepatitis B, hepatitis C, Chagas disease and HTLV I/II infection in pregnant women of state of Mato Grosso do Sul. Rev Soc Bras Med Trop. 2007;40(2):181–7.
8. Dal Fabbro MM, Cunha RV, Bóia MN, Portela P, Botelho CA, Freitas GM, Soares J, Ferri J, Lupion J. HTLV 1/2 infection: prenatal performance as a disease control strategy in state of Mato Grosso do Sul. Rev Soc Bras Med Trop. 2008;41(2):148–51.
9. Olbrich Neto J, Meira DA. Soroprevalence of HTLV-I/II, HIV, siphylis and toxoplasmosis among pregnant women seen at Botucatu - São Paulo - Brazil: risk factors for HTLV-I/II infection. Rev Soc Bras Med Trop. 2004;37(1):28–32.
10. Monteiro DL, Taquette SR, Sodré Barmpas DB, Rodrigues NC, Teixeira SA, Villela LH, Bóia MN, Trajano AJ. Prevalence of HTLV-1/2 in pregnant women living in the metropolitan area of Rio de Janeiro. PLoS Negl Trop Dis. 2014; 8(9):e3146.
11. Mello MA, da Conceição AF, Sousa SM, Alcântara LC, Marin LJ, Regina da Silva Raiol M, Boa-Sorte N, Santos LP, de Almeida Mda C, Galvão TC, Bastos RG, Lázaro N, Galvão-Castro B, Gadelha SR. HTLV-1 in pregnant women from the southern Bahia, Brazil: a neglected condition despite the high prevalence. Virol J. 2014;11:28.
12. Machado Filho AC, Sardinha JF, Ponte RL, Costa EP, da Silva SS, Martinez-Espinosa FE. Prevalence of infection for HIV, HTLV, HBV and of syphilis and chlamydia in pregnant women in a tertiary health unit in the western Brazilian Amazon region. Rev Bras Ginecol Obstet. 2010;32(4):176–83.
13. Sequeira CG, Tamegão-Lopes BP, Santos EJ, Ventura AM, Moraes-Pinto MI, Succi RC. Descriptive study of HTLV infection in a population of pregnant women from the state of Pará, northern Brazil. Rev Soc Bras Med Trop. 2012;45(4):453–6.
14. Yamamoto AY, Castellucci RA, Aragon DC, Mussi-Pinhata MM. Early high CMV seroprevalence in pregnant women from a population with a high rate of congenital infection. Epidemiol Infect. 2013;141(10):2187–91.
15. El Sanousi SM, Osman ZA, Mohmed AB, Al Awfi MS. Cytomegalovirus infection in a cohort of pregnant women. Am J Infect Control. 2016;44(4):e41–3.
16. Numan O, Vural F, Aka N, Alpay M, Coskun AD. TORCH seroprevalence among patients attending obstetric Care Clinic of Haydarpasa Training and Research Hospital affiliated to Association of Istanbul Northern Anatolia Public Hospitals. North Clin Istanb. 2015;2(3):203–9.
17. Mussi-Pinhata MM, Yamamoto AY, Moura Brito RM, de Lima Isaac M, de Carvalho e Oliveira PF, Boppana S, et al. Birth prevalence and natural history of congenital cytomegalovirus infection in a highly seroimmune population. Clin Infect Dis. 2009;49(4):522–8.
18. Ferezin RI, Bertolini DA, Demarchi IG. Prevalence of positive serology for HIV, hepatitis B, toxoplasmosis and rubella in pregnant women from the

northwestern region of the state of Paraná. Rev Bras Ginecol Obstet. 2013; 35(2):66–70.

19. Robertson SE, Featherstone DA, Gacic-Dobo M, Hersh BS. Rubella and congenital rubella syndrome: global update. Rev Panam Salud Publica. 2003;14(5):306–15.

20. Degli Esposti S, Shah D. Hepatitis B in pregnancy: challenges and treatment. Gastroenterol Clin N Am. 2011;40(2):355–72. viii

21. Piratvisuth T. Optimal management of HBV infection during pregnancy. Liver Int. 2013;33 Suppl 1:188–94.

22. Maia MM, Lage EM, Moreira BC, Deus EA, Faria JG, Pinto JA, Melo VH. Prevalence of congenital and perinatal infection in HIV positive pregnant in Belo Horizonte metropolitan region. Rev Bras Ginecol Obstet. 2015;37(9): 421–7.

23. Moura AA, de Mello MJ, Correia JB. Prevalence of syphilis, human immunodeficiency virus, hepatitis B virus, and human T-lymphotropic virus infections and coinfections during prenatal screening in an urban northeastern Brazilian population. Int J Infect Dis. 2015;39:10–5.

24. Vallinoto AC, Pontes GS, Muto NA, Lopes IG, Machado LF, Azevedo VN, et al. Identification of human T-cell lymphotropic virus infection in a semi-isolated afro-Brazilian Quilombo located in the Marajó Island (Pará, Brazil). Mem Inst Oswaldo Cruz. 2006;101(1):103–5.

25. Santos EL, Tamegão-Lopes B, Machado LF, Ishak MO, Ishak R, Lemos JA, et al. Molecular characterization of HTLV-1/2 among blood donors in Belém, state of Pará: first description of HTLV-2b subtype in the Amazon region. Rev Soc Bras Med Trop. 2009;42(3):271–6.

26. Guimarães de Souza V, Lobato Martins M, Carneiro-Proietti AB, Januário JN, Ladeira RV, Silva CM, et al. High prevalence of HTLV-1 and 2 viruses in pregnant women in São Luis, state of Maranhão, Brazil. Rev Soc Bras Med Trop. 2012;45(2):159–62.

27. Domingues RM, Szwarcwald CL, Souza PR, Leal MC. Prenatal testing and prevalence of HIV infection during pregnancy: data from the " birth in Brazil" study, a national hospital-based study. BMC Infect Dis. 2015;15:100.

28. Lima KO, Salustiano DM, Cavalcanti AM, Leal ÉS, Lacerda HR. HIV-1 incidence among people seeking voluntary counseling and testing centers, including pregnant women, in Pernambuco state, Northeast Brazil. Cad Saude Publica. 2015;31(6):1327–31.

29. Manyahi J, Jullu BS, Abuya MI, Juma J, Ndayongeje J, Kilama B, et al. Prevalence of HIV and syphilis infections among pregnant women attending antenatal clinics in Tanzania, 2011. BMC Public Health. 2015;15:501.

30. Endris M, Deressa T, Belyhun Y, Moges F. Seroprevalence of syphilis and human immunodeficiency virus infections among pregnant women who attend the University of Gondar teaching hospital, Northwest Ethiopia: a cross sectional study. BMC Infect Dis. 2015;15:111.

31. Hokororo A, Kihunrwa A, Hoekstra P, Kalluvya SE, Changalucha JM, Fitzgerald DW, et al. High prevalence of sexually transmitted infections in pregnant adolescent girls in Tanzania: a multi-community cross-sectional study. Sex Transm Infect. 2015;91(7):473–8.

32. Brasil. Boletim Epidemiológico - Hepatites Virais. Brasília: Ministério da Saúde, Secretaria de Vigilância em Saúde, Departamento de DST, Aids e Hepatites Virais, Ano IV, n. 1; 2015.

33. Boa-Sorte N, Purificação A, Amorim T, Assunção L, Reis A, Galvão-Castro B. Dried blood spot testing for the antenatal screening of HTLV, HIV, syphilis, toxoplasmosis and hepatitis B and C: prevalence, accuracy and operational aspects. Braz J Infect Dis. 2014;18(6):618–24.

34. Fernandes CN, Alves Mde M, de Souza ML, Machado GA, Couto G, Evangelista RA. Prevalence of seropositivity for hepatitis B and C in pregnant women. Rev Esc Enferm USP. 2014;48(1):91–8.

35. Diale Q, Pattinson R, Chokoe R, Masenyetse L, Mayaphi S. Antenatal screening for hepatitis B virus in HIV-infected and uninfected pregnant women in the Tshwane district of South Africa. S Afr Med J. 2015;106(1):97–100.

36. Murad EA, Babiker SM, Gasim GI, Rayis DA, Adam I. Epidemiology of hepatitis B and hepatitis C virus infections in pregnant women in Sana'a, Yemen. BMC Pregnancy Childbirth. 2013;13:127.

37. Jutavijittum P, Yousukh A, Saysanasongkham B, Samountry B, Samountry K, Toriyama K, et al. High rate of hepatitis B virus mother-to-child transmission in Lao people's Democratic Republic. Southeast Asian J Trop Med Public Health. 2016;47(2):214–8.

38. Anaedobe CG, Fowotade A, Omoruyi CE, Bakare RA. Prevalence, sociodemographic features and risk factors of hepatitis B virus infection among pregnant women in southwestern Nigeria. Pan Afr Med J. 2015; 20:406.

39. Noubiap JJ, Nansseu JR, Ndoula ST, Bigna JJ, Jingi AM, Fokom-Domgue J. Prevalence, infectivity and correlates of hepatitis B virus infection among pregnant women in a rural district of the far north region of Cameroon. BMC Public Health. 2015;15:454.

40. Souza MT, Pinho TL, Santos MD, Santos A, Monteiro VL, Fonsêca LM, et al. Prevalence of hepatitis B among pregnant women assisted at the public maternity hospitals of São Luís, Maranhão, Brazil. Braz J Infect Dis. 2012;16(6): 517–20.

41. Figueiredo NC, Page-Shafer K, Pereira FE, Miranda AE. Serological markers for hepatitis B virus in young women attended by the family health program in Vitória, Espírito Santo, 2006. Rev Soc Bras Med Trop. 2008;41(6):590–5.

42. Spano LC, Gatti J, Nascimento JP, Leite JP. Prevalence of human cytomegalovirus infection in pregnant and non-pregnant women. J Inf Secur. 2004;48(3):213–20.

43. Alvarado-Esquivel C, Hernández-Tinoco J, Sánchez-Anguiano LF, Ramos-Nevárez A, Cerrillo-Soto SM, Estrada-Martínez S, et al. Seroepidemiology of cytomegalovirus infection in pregnant women in Durango City, Mexico. BMC Infect Dis. 2014;14:484.

44. Hamid KM, Onoja AB, Tofa UA, Garba KN. Seroprevalence of cytomegalovirus among pregnant women attending Murtala Mohammed specialist hospital Kano. Nigeria Afr Health Sci. 2014;14(1):125–30.

45. Inagaki AD, Oliveira LA, Oliveira MF, Santos RC, Araújo RM, Alves JA, et al. Seroprevalence of antibodies for toxoplasmosis, rubella, cytomegalovirus, syphilis and HIV among pregnant women in Sergipe. Rev Soc Bras Med Trop. 2009;42(5):532–6.

46. Avila Moura A, de Mello MJ, Correia JB. Serological statuses of pregnant women in an urban Brazilian population before and after the 2008 rubella immunization campaign. Vaccine. 2016;34(4):445–50.

Predictors of women's utilization of primary health care for skilled pregnancy care in rural Nigeria

Friday Okonofua[1,2,5*], Lorretta Ntoimo[1,3], Julius Ogungbangbe[4], Seun Anjorin[1], Wilson Imongan[1] and Sanni Yaya[6]

Abstract

Background: Although Primary Health Care (PHC) was designed to provide universal access to skilled pregnancy care for the prevention of maternal deaths, very little is known of the factors that predict the use of PHC for skilled maternity care in rural parts of Nigeria - where its use is likely to have a greater positive impact on maternal health care. The objective of this study was to identify the factors that lead pregnant women to use or not use existing primary health care facilities for antenatal and delivery care.

Methods: The study was a cross-sectional community-based study conducted in Esan South East and Etsako East LGAs of Edo State, Nigeria. A total of 1408 randomly selected women of reproductive age were interviewed in their households using a pre-tested structured questionnaire. The data were analyzed with descriptive and multivariate statistical methods.

Results: The results showed antenatal care attendance rate by currently pregnant women of 62.1%, and a skilled delivery of 46.6% by recently delivered women at PHCs, while 25% of women delivered at home or with traditional birth attendants. Reasons for use and non-use of PHCs for antenatal and delivery care given by women were related to perceptions about long distances to PHCs, high costs of services and poor quality of PHC service delivery. Chi-square test of association revealed that level of education and marital status were significantly related to use of PHCs for antenatal care. The results of logistic regression for delivery care showed that women with primary (OR 3. 10, CI 1.16–8.28) and secondary (OR 2.37, CI 1.19–4.71) levels education were more likely to receive delivery care in PHCs than the highly educated. Being a Muslim (OR 1.56, CI 1.00–2.42), having a partner who is employed in Estako East (OR 2.78, CI 1.04–7.44) and having more than five children in Esan South East (OR 2.00, CI 1.19–3.35) significantly increased the odds of delivery in PHCs. The likelihood of using a PHC facility was less for women who had more autonomy (OR 0.75, CI 0.57–0.99) as compared to women with higher autonomy.

Conclusion: We conclude that efforts devoted to addressing the limiting factors (distance, costs and quality of care) using creative and innovative approaches will increase the utilization of skilled pregnancy care in PHCs and reduce maternal mortality in rural Nigeria.

Keywords: Antenatal care, Delivery care, Primary health centres, Pregnant women, Edo State, Nigeria

* Correspondence: feokonofua@yahoo.co.uk
[1]Women's Health and Action Research Centre, Km 11 Benin-Lagos
Expressway, Benin City, Edo State, Nigeria
[2]The University of Medical Sciences, Ondo City, Ondo State, Nigeria
Full list of author information is available at the end of the article

Background

The high rate of maternal mortality is a major public health concern in Nigeria. Several studies have shown that pregnant women in rural areas of the country are at greater risk of dying during pregnancy or childbirth as compared to those that live in urban areas [1, 2]. This is largely due to limited access to maternal health care by rural women as health facilities are often located far from where they live, with the result that they rely more on use of traditional sources of care or to no care at all [3, 4].

The Nigerian health care system is founded on a tripod of Primary Health Care, Secondary Health Care and Tertiary Health Care. In compliance with global recommendations for optimal maternal health care [5], Primary Health Care provides Basic Emergency Obstetrics Care (BEOC) comprising skilled delivery care, administration of antibiotics, manual removal of the placenta, removal of retained products of conception, assisted vaginal delivery possibly with a vacuum extractor, and basic neonatal care including neonatal resuscitation. By contrast, Secondary and Tertiary Health facilities (consisting of General and Teaching Hospitals) provide Comprehensive Emergency Obstetrics Care (CEOC) that consists of all BEOC services as well as caesarean section, safe blood transfusion services and the treatment of the sick baby. The Federal Ministry of Health of Nigeria specifically recommends Primary Health Care as the entry point to the health care system in order to generate universal health coverage for all citizens [6].

There are currently 33,000 Primary Health Centres (PHCs) located in 774 Local Government Areas (LGAs) with a minimum of ten wards per LGA in Nigeria. Each ward has a population of between 5000 to 10,000 persons, with each expected to have a PHC that provides immediate point of entry to the health care system for pregnant women seeking skilled pregnancy care. Thereafter, women with complications are referred for CEOC provided in Secondary and Tertiary care facilities [6, 7].

Despite this organized system, available evidence suggests considerable under-utilization of available PHC facilities for care by women seeking antenatal and intrapartum care in rural areas of the country [8–11]. Data from the Nigeria Demographic and Health Survey [12] indicates that in 2013 whereas 86.0% of urban women in the country received antenatal care from a skilled birth attendant (doctor or midwife), only 46.5% of rural women received such skilled antenatal service. During the same period, only 21.9% of rural women were delivered by a skilled birth attendant, compared to 61.7% of urban women. By contrast, a large proportion of rural women (77%) throughout the country delivered at home or in the homes of traditional birth attendants, compared to 37% of urban women.

Clearly, the tendency for rural women not to receive skilled pregnancy care has been recognized as one of the most important social determinants of the high rate of maternal mortality in Nigeria. Universal health coverage for maternal health is currently lacking in the country largely due to poor use of available and affordable services in PHCs [13]. Efforts to reverse this trend will greatly boost current efforts to improve maternal health, improve women's access to skilled pregnancy care and prevent maternal deaths in the country.

Utilization of maternal healthcare services has been the subject of many descriptive and analytical studies in Nigeria [4, 14–19]. However, most studies did not disaggregate the analysis of the determinants by level of care (primary, secondary or tertiary) probably because many of the studies used secondary sources such as the National HIV/AIDS and Reproductive Health Surveys and Nigeria Demographic and Health surveys. Thus, little empirical evidence exists from primary sources on the reasons why women use or do not use primary healthcare facilities in Nigeria for maternal health care and the individual-level predictors of use or non-use. Analyses of utilization of primary health care facilities in Nigeria have been limited in their focus such as description of interventions [20, 21] quality of care and patients or community satisfaction, knowledge and use of partograph, adequacy of resources and providers, adequacy of antenatal care [9, 22–27]. Egbewale and Odu [8] described perceptions about PHC services and utilization highlighting reasons for use and non-use but this study was not specific on maternal healthcare. Ejembi et al. [11] presented utilization of PHC facilities for maternal care in two rural Hausa communities but it was a descriptive study limited to identifying the determinants.

The current analysis extends these past studies by engaging descriptive and analytical techniques to describe reasons for use and non-use of PHC facilities for maternal care and the individual-level predictors. The objective of this study was to identify the factors that lead pregnant women to use or not use existing primary health care facilities for antenatal and delivery care in two LGAs of Edo State. We believe the results would be useful for the design of interventions to improve women's access to existing skilled pregnancy care at the primary health care facilities and reduce maternal mortality in the LGAs, with potential for scale up for greater impact throughout the country.

Conceptual framework

This research is anchored on a behavioural model of health service use proposed by Andersen and Newman [28]. The framework was first developed in the 1960s and was designed to understand the conditions that predict utilization of health care services in the US. However, the framework has been adapted to research outside the US as described in a systematic review of studies using the model between 1998 and 2011 [29]. The model views utilization of health services as a form of individual behavior that is determined by individual characteristics of people which are influenced by societal and health systems determinants. The societal determinants (technology and societal norms such as health care financing) affect the individual determinants directly and through the health system determinants (resources - volume and distribution of labour and capital for health care, and organization - patient access to the medical care system, and structure- what happens after entry into the system). The individual characteristics that predict use of health services are classified into three: predisposition of an individual to use health services (predisposing factors), ability to secure services (enabling factors) and illness level (need factors). Predisposing factors include demographic characteristics such as age, sex, marital status, past illness, social structure (education, race, occupation, family size, ethnicity, religion, and residential mobility) and beliefs (values about health and illness, attitudes toward health services/providers, knowledge about disease). Previous research shows that the demographic characteristics of individuals predict their health behavior. For instance, being in a marital union is associated with better health and health-related behavior [30–32]. The past illness factor suggests that past experience of pregnancy and childbirth, parity, and experience of using a health care facility may affect the use of a primary health care facility for maternal care [28].

The enabling factors refer to the means available to individuals to achieve a need to use a health service. Enabling factors include family resources (income, level of health insurance coverage, or other source of third-party payment, type of regular source of care, the nature of that regular source of care, and accessibility of the source) and community characteristics (ratio of health personnel and facilities to population in a community, price of health services, region, urban-rural location). This implies that women's ability to use maternal health facilities will depend on the availability of such facilities and their possession of the means to access the facilities.

The need factors include perceived illness or the probability of its occurrence by the individual or her family (disability, symptoms, diagnosis, general state –such as number of days during which the individual is unable to do her usual work such as house chores, care of children, experience of symptoms, self-report of general state of health), and evaluation of the condition (symptoms and diagnosis – attempts to get at the actual illness and a clinical assessment of the severity). According to Andersen and Newman [28], these factors represent the most immediate determinants of health service utilization. The need component suggests that the utilization of maternal health services can be influenced by a woman's perception of the relative importance of modern health care services versus traditional methods of care. Added to this is a woman's perception and understanding of pregnancy complications and her desire to deliver safely and attain a healthy newborn baby.

Method
Study communities
The study was a cross-sectional community-based study conducted in Esan South East and Etsako East LGAs in Edo State in southern Nigeria. Edo State is one of Nigeria's 36 federating States located in the South-South geopolitical zone of the country. Both LGAs are located in the rural and riverine areas of the state, adjacent to River Niger, with Estako East in the northern part of the Edo State part of the river, while Esan South East is in the southern part. Administratively, each LGA comprises of 10 wards, with several communities located in each ward. The two LGAs have a total population of 313,717 persons, with Esan South East accounting for 167,721 and Etsako East LGA accounting for 145,996. The principal sources of maternity care in the two LGAs are Primary Health Centres (PHCs). However, Esan South East LGA has one General Hospital in Ubiaja (headquarters of the LGA) while Etsako East has one General Hospital in Agenebode (the LGA administrative headquarters) and another in nearby Fugar City. Several private hospitals also exist in both LGAs that offer maternal and child health services of various degrees of quality. These public and private facilities are used as additional to the existing PHCs or for referral maternal health services.

Sampling technique, data source and study population
The study was drawn from a survey conducted in July–August, 2017 as part of baseline data for the design of an on-going intervention research project to increase the access of rural women to skilled pregnancy care in 20 communities in Esan South East and Etsako East LGAs. A sample size of 1450 was derived for the project using the following formula:

$$n_1 = \{[p_1q_1 + p_oq_o]) \left(Z_{\alpha/2} + Z_\beta\right)^2\}/(p_1 - p_o)^2$$

p_0 = utilization of PHC for maternal and perinatal in the control arm (assumed to be – 5 reduction in the prevalence in the experiment site).

p_1 = utilization of PHC for maternal and perinatal care in the experimental arm.

z_α = Two-sided standard normal variate at 95% level of significance = 1.96.

z_β = Statistical power at 80% = 0.84;

$$n_1 = n_2$$

n_1 = no of study participants in the experimental group.

n^2 = no of study participants in the control group.

We assume 50% since there is no literature from the geographical location of the study which reported the prevalence of utilization of PHCs for maternal and perinatal health care. Thus:

$$n^1 = (0.50x1 - 0.50 + 0.45x1 - 0.45) (1.96/2 + 0.84)^2 / (0.50 - 0.45)^2$$
$$(0.25 + 0.2475) (3.3124) / 0.0025$$
$$n^1 = 659 n^2 = 659$$

Total sample size = 1318.

10% adjustment for non-response = 132.

Total = 1450 (725 respondents in the experiment LGA and 725 in the control LGA).

A multi-stage sampling technique was used to select communities and the respondents in each LGA. Two rural LGAs (Esan South East and Etsako East) were purposively selected from the 18 LGAs in Edo state. Each LGA is divided into 10 health/administrative wards, with each ward made up of communities. Twenty (20) communities were selected purposively for the study – 10 from each LGA. Five communities per LGA were selected from where a PHC facility is located, while the other five communities were those in areas where there are no PHC facilities. Particular communities were selected systematically. In Esan South East, PHCs are located in 24 communities, while 75 communities have no PHCs. In contrast, in Etsako East, PHC facilities are located in 27 communities, while 15 communities had no PHC facilities. A sample interval was generated and 5 communities were selected systematically from a list of communities with PHCs and 5 from communities without a PHC in each LGA.

Within communities, households were listed and the number of women of reproductive age in each household was obtained. All eligible women in each household were interviewed. The eligibility criteria were age 15–45 years, ever married, currently pregnant or have had a birth in the 5 years preceding the survey. In Etsako, 1487 households were listed and there were 1051 women of reproductive age in the households. Out of the 1051, 707 eligible women were interviewed with a non-response rate of 2.5%. In Esan South East, 1975 households were listed with 1084 women of reproductive age, 701 eligible women were interviewed with 3.3% non-response. A total of 1408 eligible women were interviewed in the two LGAs, with 2.9% overall non-response rate.

A questionnaire prepared by the investigators was used for data collection. The instrument (questionnaire) was pretested in a rural community with similar characteristics with the study locations. The questionnaire consisted of five sections. Section one contained the respondents' socio-demographic characteristics; section 2 was related to partners' and other family characteristics; section 3 contained questions on the respondents' reproductive history; section 4 was on antenatal, intrapartum and postnatal care experience for current pregnancy and births in the preceding 5 years; while section 5 contained questions on reasons for use and non-use of PHCs for maternal and child care.

Drawing from the literature, some reasons for use and non-use of a PHC facility for maternal health care were provided as multiple response options. The respondents selected as many options as are applicable to them. The following options of reasons for use were provided: cost not too much, no charges, facility is always open, provider is available, facility not far from my house, good quality service (subjective opinion of the respondent on the care provided in PHC facilities), husband wanted it, family wanted it, adequate security, other (specify). The reasons for non-use provided in the questionnaire were: cost too much, facilities not open, no provider in the facility, facility too far, no transport to facility, poor quality service (subjective view of the respondent on the care received), husband did not allow, family did not allow, no time because baby came suddenly, my culture forbids, no security, and other (specify). Additional reasons for use and non-use shown in the result tables were drawn from the other (specify) category.

The questionnaire was entered into Computer-Assisted Personal Interviewing (CAPI) using a Census and Survey Processing System (CSPro) software (CSentry). CSPro is a public domain software package developed by the US Census Bureau and ICF International. It is widely used for entering, editing, tabulating and disseminating census and survey data. The software runs on the Microsoft windows and Android families of operating systems [33]. Thus, instead of the paper and pen interviewing, the CAPI facilitated accuracy and speed in the data collection process. The questionnaire was administered through face-to-face interviewing by trained field assistants. The questions were fielded in English or in Pidgin English as appropriate, since all women in both communities either understand English or Pidgin English.

Variables and measures

The dependent variable for antenatal care was place of antenatal care: PHC facility coded 1 and other facilities/home coded 0. The dependent variable for delivery care was place of delivery; use of a PHC facility was coded 1 while other facilities and home was coded 0. Drawing on the model of health services utilization and past studies on utilization of facilities for maternal care in Nigeria, the following independent variables were included in the analyses: age, highest level of education, exposure to media, religion, employment (working and not working), marital status (married, living together, widowed, divorced, and separated), age at marriage, partner's age, partner's highest education, partner's employment, who pays for respondent's health care (respondent alone, husband alone or others, and respondent with husband), level of autonomy (less, more and much), number of living children, education difference between respondent and partner (both have no education, husband more educated than wife, wife more educated than partner, and same level of education but not none), and LGA.

Exposure to media was generated with frequency of listening to radio and watching television. The response options were everyday, at least once a week, less than once a week, and not at all. The responses were aggregated to generate a three-category measure of exposure to the media: high, moderate and no exposure. No exposure refers to neither listens to radio nor to television at all. An index for autonomy was generated with responses to 6 questions on ownership of land/house, participation in household decisions on respondent's health, major purchases, daily purchases, visits to family and friends, food to be cooked. Ownership of land or house was included because women in the study location are allowed to own land or a house if they wish. The response options were respondent alone, husband alone, respondent and husband, and others. These responses were further collapsed into two categories labeled respondent alone or respondent with husband indicating autonomy (coded 1) husband alone & others indicating no autonomy (coded 0) for participation in decisions. Ownership of land/house was categorized into respondent alone or with husband indicating autonomy (coded 1), owns no land/house and husband alone owns as no autonomy (coded 0). Using principal component analysis, a three-category index of autonomy was generated (less, more and much); scale reliability coefficient was 0.70. A response of 0 in all 6 questions and 1 in 1–2 questions was less autonomy; response of 1 in 3–4 questions was more autonomy, and a response of 1 in 5–6 questions was much autonomy. Women's participation in household decision-making, her health care, mobility, and ownership of land among others have been used in many previous studies as measures of women's autonomy [34–36].

Data analysis

The current analysis is based on antenatal care for currently pregnant respondents, and delivery or intrapartum care for the most recent births by the respondents. The data were extracted from the CAPI devise, cleaned and analyzed with STATA 12 for windows. To describe the characteristics of the respondents, univariate analysis using percentages and summary statistics was conducted. Reasons for use and non-use of a PHC facility for maternal care (antenatal care for current pregnancy and delivery care for the most recent births) were elicited from multiple response options. The results are presented as number of responses and percentages for each of the specified options and a few additional categories drawn from the other (specify) option. To compare proportions for each reason for use and non-use of a PHC for antenatal and delivery care between the two LGAs, a two-sample test of proportions was conducted.

Due to the small sample size for currently pregnant respondents who are receiving antenatal care ($n = 175$), a bivariate analysis using chi-squared test was conducted to test the relationship between the use of a PHC facility for antenatal care for currently pregnant respondents and selected characteristics of the respondents. Selection of the characteristics was based on their potential theoretical and practical influence on the use of a PHC facility for antenatal care. Binary logistic regression was conducted to determine the predictors of PHC facility use for delivery care during the most recent births by the respondents.

Some of the independent variables were re-coded for the chi-squared test and the multivariate analysis because of zero or few cases in some categories. The variables that were re-coded for the chi-squared test were age, level of education, religion (traditionalist and others were dropped because they had few cases and cannot be merged with any other category), marital status, (widowed, divorced, and separated were dropped because of few cases even after collapsing the three as formerly married). Others were partner's age, partner's level of education, payment for respondent's healthcare. In the multivariate analysis for delivery care, traditional and other religions were dropped due to few cases; age and partner's age was entered as a continuous variables. The variables included in the logistic regression model were either significant in a bivariate logistic regression model at 0.05 or 0.10 level of significance or conceptually important drawing from the behavioral model of health services utilization, past studies and the authors' knowledge of the study population. A Wald test was also conducted to test whether the explanatory variables in the logit model are simultaneously equal to zero. The test result was significant indicating that including these variables creates a statistically significant improvement in the fit of the model. The results of the logistic regression are presented as odds ratio (OR) with 95% confidence interval for the entire study population and for each LGA. Statistical significance for all the statistical analysis was set at 0.05.

Results

Characteristics of the study population

The study population is described in Table 1. The mean age of the respondents was 30 years with a standard deviation (SD) of 6.9 years. The mean age in Esan South East (31 years) was slightly higher than the overall

Table 1 Percent distribution of the respondents by personal, family and reproductive characteristics by LGA

Characteristic	All	Esan SE	Etsako East
Number of respondents	1408	701(49.8)	707(50.2)
Personal Characteristics			
Age			
Mean	30(SD 6.9)	31.5(SD 6.9)	28.6(SD 6.7)
16–19	64(4.5)	21(3.0)	43(6.1)
20–24	260(18.4)	87(12.4)	173(24.5)
25–29	354(25.1)	167(23.8)	187(26.4)
30–34	303(21.5)	175(24.9)	128(18.1)
25–39	249(17.7)	131(18.7)	118(16.7)
40–47	178(12.6)	120(17.1)	58(8.2)
Education			
No Education	206(14.6)	76(10.8)	130(18.4)
Primary	617(43.8)	253(36.1)	364(51.5)
Secondary	503(35.6)	316(45.1)	186(26.3)
Higher	83(5.9)	56(8.0)	27(3.8)
Exposure to media			
High exposure	420(29.8)	216(30.8)	204(28.8)
Moderate exposure	666(47.3)	392(55.9)	274(38.8)
No exposure	322(22.9)	93(13.3)	229(32.4)
Religion			
Catholic	369(26.2)	123(17.5)	246(34.8)
Other Christian	884(62.8)	551(78.6)	333(47.2)
Islam	145(10.3)	21(3.0)	124(17.6)
Traditionalist	8(0.6)	5(0.7)	3(0.4)
Other	1(0.1)	1(0.1)	0(0.0)
Employment			
Not working	287(20.4)	127(18.1)	160(22.6)
Working	1121(78.6)	574(81.9)	547(77.4)
Marital Status			
Married	926(65.8)	432(61.6)	494(69.9)
Living together	447(31.7)	248(35.4)	199(28.2)
Widowed	15(1.1)	11(1.6)	4(0.6)
Divorced	1(0.1)	1(0.1)	0(0.0)
Separated	19(1.3)	9(1.3)	10(1.4)
Age at marriage			
Mean (SD)	21.0(3.9)	21.8(4.2)	20.2(3.5)
14–17	235(16.7)	90(12.8)	145(20.5)
18–24	875(62.1)	415(59.2)	460(65.1)
25–29	249(17.7)	159(22.7)	90(12.7)
30–39	49(3.5)	37(5.3)	12(1.7)
Partner/Family Characteristics			
Partner's age			
Mean(SD)	39.4(9.2)	40.2(8.6)	38.5(9.6)
18–24	36(2.6)	13(1.9)	23(3.3)

Table 1 Percent distribution of the respondents by personal, family and reproductive characteristics by LGA *(Continued)*

Characteristic	All	Esan SE	Etsako East
25–29	142(10.2)	46(6.7)	96(13.7)
30–34	235(16.9)	104(15.1)	131(18.6)
35–39	255(18.3)	133(19.3)	122(17.3)
40–44	283(20.3)	160(23.2)	123(17.5)
45–49	239(17.2)	126(18.3)	113(16.1)
50–54	125(9.0)	73(10.6)	52(7.4)
55–82	78(5.6)	35(5.1)	43(6.1)
Partner's Education			
No Education	104(7.4)	62(8.8)	42(5.9)
Primary	348(24.7)	155(22.1)	193(27.3)
Secondary	737(52.3)	372(53.1)	365(51.6)
Higher	219(15.6)	112(16.0)	107(15.1)
Spousal education Difference			
Both have none	55(3.9)	24(3.4)	31(4.4)
Husband more	622(44.2)	239(34.1)	383(54.2)
Wife more	127(9.0)	91(13.0)	36(5.1)
Same but not none	604(42.9)	347(49.5)	257(36.3)
Partner's Employment			
Not working	82(5.8)	49(7.0)	33(4.7)
Working	1326(94.2)	652(93.0)	674(95.3)
Autonomy			
Less	507(36.0)	243(34.7)	264(37.3)
More	465(33.0)	220(31.4)	245(34.7)
Much	436(31.0)	238(33.9)	198(28.0)
Payment for respondent's health care			
Respondent alone	107 (7.6)	68(9.7)	39(5.5)
Partner alone	1140(81.0)	533(76.0)	607(85.9)
Respondent & partner	144(10.2)	92(13.1)	52(7.4)
Other	17(1.2)	8(1.1)	9(1.3)
Reproductive Characteristics			
Number of living children			
0–2	456(34.1)	230(33.2)	226(35.0)
3–4	415(31.0)	218(31.5)	197(30.5)
5+	466(34.9)	244(35.3)	222(34.4)
Currently pregnant			
Yes	277(19.7)	81(11.6)	196(27.7)
No	1120(79.5)	612(87.3)	508(71.9)
Unsure	11(0.8)	8(1.10	3(0.4)
Current Pregnancy (*n* = 277)			
Receiving antenatal care (ANC)			
Yes	172(62.1)	51(63.0)	121(61.7)
No	105(37.9)	30(37.0)	75(38.3)
Place of ANC			
Other govt. facility	11(6.3)	7(13.7)	4(3.2)

Table 1 Percent distribution of the respondents by personal, family and reproductive characteristics by LGA *(Continued)*

Characteristic	All	Esan SE	Etsako East
PHC	145(82.9)	39(76.5)	106(85.5)
Private Hospital	16(9.1)	4(7.8)	12(9.7)
Other	3(1.7)	1(2.0)	2(1.6)
Most recent birth (*n* = 1314)			
Antenatal care[a]			
Yes	168(91.8)	67(90.5)	101(92.7)
No	15(8.2)	7(9.5)	8(7.3)
Place of Antenatal care			
PHC	146 (84.9)	56 (84.9)	90 (84.9)
Other govt. hospital	14 (8.1)	5 (7.6)	9 (8.5)
Private hospital	10 (5.8)	5 (7.6)	5 (4.7)
Home	2 (1.2)	0 (0.0)	2 (1.9)
Place of delivery			
Other govt. facility	158(12.0)	96(13.9)	62(10.0)
PHC	612(46.6)	365(52.7)	247(39.8)
Private Hospital	218(16.6)	136(19.6)	82(13.2)
At home/other	326(24.8)	96(13.8)	230(37.0)

Note: [a]most of the respondents did not respond to the question on antenatal care for their most recent birth. The reported percentage of no antenatal care should be interpreted with caution

average whereas in Etsako East it was below the average (29 years). Most respondents had attained primary and secondary education, but in Etsako East, slightly more than half of the respondents had primary education unlike in Esan South East where the majority (45.1%) had secondary education. Exposure to media (listening to the radio and watching television) was moderate in both LGAs. Most respondents were Christians of non-Catholic affiliation. In both LGAs, the majority of the respondents were employed. An examination of the details of occupation showed that most were self-employed in the low-wage informal sector as traders, farmers, tailors, and hair stylists (not shown in the table).

Most respondents were in marital union. Slightly above 30% of those in union were living together with a partner (informal union). The proportion living together with a partner was higher in Esan South East (35.4%) than in Etsako East (28.2%). Mean age at first marriage was 21 years. The mean age of their partners was 39.4 years, slightly above 50% of the partners attained secondary education and most of them worked in formal and informal employments. With regard to gap in the level of education between the respondents and their partners, 44.2% had partners who were more educated, while 42.9% had the same level of education with their partners. In Esan South East, most of the respondents had same level of education with their partners (49.5%) whereas the majority in Etsako East had partners who were more educated (54.2%). Respondents with less autonomy were in higher proportion

in both LGAs; and for the majority of the respondents, partner alone pay for their health care.

Close to 20% (277) of the respondents were currently pregnant with a higher proportion in Etsako East. Among those who were currently pregnant, 62.1% were receiving antenatal care, and out of those who were receiving care, most of them were using a PHC facility. With regard to delivery care for the most recent births, 1314 respondents had a recent birth and only few reported receiving any antenatal care. Among the few, most (84.9%) received antenatal care in a PHC facility. Response to the question on place of delivery showed that 46.6% delivered in a PHC facility, while close to 25% delivered at home and with a Traditional Birth Attendant (TBA). In Esan South East, many respondents delivered in a PHC facility (52.7%) and in Etsako East, close to 40% delivered in a PHC. Unlike in Esan South East where 13.8% delivered at home and with a TBA, 37% of the respondents in Etsako East had their most recent births at home and with a TBA.

Reasons for use and non-use of a PHC facility

The respondents were asked to provide reasons why they used or did not use a PHC facility for antenatal care (current pregnancy) and delivery care for their most recent births.

Reasons for use

Reasons for use of PHC for antenatal and delivery care are presented in Table 2. The most frequently mentioned reasons for using a PHC facility for

Table 2 Percent distribution of reasons for using a PHC facility for antenatal and delivery - Number of responses (%)

Reason	Antenatal care			Delivery care		
	All	Esan South East LGA	Etsako East LGA	All	Esan South East LGA	Etsako East LGA
	(n = 533)	(n = 157)	(n = 376)	(n = 2294)	(n = 1303)	(n = 991)
Cost not too much	79(14.8)	24(15.3)	55(14.6)	386(16.8)	228(17.5)	158(15.9)
No charges	3(0.6)	2(1.3)	1(0.3)	20(0.9)	16(1.2)	4(0.4)
Facility is always open	43(8.1)	17(10.8)	26(6.9)	236(10.3)	161(12.4)	75(7.6)
Provider are available	75(14.1)	24(15.3)	51(13.6)	375(16.3)	220(16.9)	155(15.6)
Facility Not far from my house	145(27.2)	31(19.7)	114(30.3)	465(20.3)	208(16.0)	257(25.9)
Good quality service	106(19.9)	37(23.6)	69(18.4)	451(19.7)	259(19.9)	192(19.4)
Husband wanted it	54(10.1)	11(7.0)	43(11.4)	193(8.4)	96(7.4)	97(9.8)
Family wanted it	7(1.3)	5(3.2)	2(0.5)	63(2.7)	51(3.9)	12(1.2)
Adequate security	5(0.9)	5(3.2)	0(0.0)	43(1.9)	37(2.8)	6(0.6)
Baby's health/safety	7(1.3)	0 (0.0)	7(1.9)	14(0.6)	0(0.0)	14(1.4)
No other facility	–	–	–	10(0.4)	9(0.7)	1(0.1)
[a] Other	9(1.7)	1(0.6)	8(2.1)	38(1.7)	18(1.4)	20(2.0)
Test of proportions	$p = 0.0000$			$p = 0.0070$		

[a]Other includes reasons such as nothing, nice matron, works in a PHC, relative works there, to get birth certificate, and it is not necessary among others

antenatal care by currently pregnant respondents were that the facility is close to their residence (27.2%), good quality service (19.9%), and provider is available (14.1%). The least mentioned reasons were no charges (0.6%), and adequate security (0.9%). This pattern of response for antenatal care was similar across the two LGAs. The two-sample test of proportions for reasons for using a PHC for antenatal care indicates that the proportions differed significantly between the two LGAs. Particular reasons that were significantly different were cost too much, providers not available, facility not far from respondent's residence, good quality service, husband wanted it, family wanted it, adequate security, and other reason.

Reasons for using a PHC facility for delivery care were similar to the reasons for using a PHC facility for antenatal care: facility close to residence, good quality care and provider is available were the most frequently mentioned reasons. The least reasons were no charges, baby's safety/health and no other facility. The only variation for the LGAs was in Esan South East where good quality service was the most frequently mentioned reason, but Etsako East followed the general pattern of facility near residence, good quality care and provider available. Reasons for using a PHC for delivery care varied significantly between the two LGAs. Specific reasons that differed significantly were cost not too much, no charges, facility is always open, providers are available, facility not far from respondent's residence, good quality service, family wanted it and adequate security.

Reasons for non-use

The distribution of reasons for non-use of a PHC facility is shown in Table 3. Of the 97 responses elicited from currently pregnant respondents, no provider in the facility (17.5%), poor quality service (17.5%), and facility not open (12.3%) were the most commonly mentioned reasons. The least mentioned reasons were preference for home delivery/TBA, family did not allow and no PHC facility. Reasons such as my culture forbids and no security were not mentioned at all. In Esan South East, the most frequently mentioned reasons were poor quality service (47.6%), no provider in the facility (14.3%), and husband did not allow (14.3%), whereas in Etsako no provider in the facility featured prominently, followed by poor quality service and husband did not allow. There was a statistically significant difference between LGAs in all the reasons for non-use of a PHC for antenatal care except for husband and family wanted it.

The dominant reasons for not using a PHC for delivery care in the most recent births of the respondents were poor quality service (19.5%), no provider in the facility (12.0%), and facility is too far (11.7%). The least reasons were my culture forbids and no security. Distribution of responses in Esan South East showed poor quality service, facility too far and no provider as the common reasons whereas facility not open, no provider and poor quality service were the most frequently mentioned reasons in Etsako East. The reasons for non-use of a PHC for delivery care were not found to be statistically different between the LGAs. However, specific reasons such as cost too

Table 3 Percent distribution of reasons for non-use of a PHC facility for antenatal and delivery care - Number of responses (%)

Reason	Antenatal care			Delivery care		
	All	Esan South East LGA	Etsako East LGA	All	Esan South East LGA	Etsako East LGA
	(n = 97)	(n = 21)	(n = 76)	(n = 532)	(n = 243)	(n = 289)
Cost too much	7(7.2)	0(0.0)	7(9.2)	48(9.0)	14(5.8)	34(11.8)
Facility not open	12(12.3)	0(0.0)	11(14.5)	46(8.6)	4(1.6)	42(14.5)
No provider in the Facility	17(17.5)	3(14.3)	14(18.4)	64(12.0)	26(10.7)	38(13.1)
Facility too far	8(8.2)	2(9.5)	6(7.9)	62(11.7)	33(13.6)	29(10.0)
No transport to Facility	5(5.2)	0(0.0)	5(6.6)	21(3.9)	8(3.3)	13(4.5)
Poor quality service	17(17.5)	10(47.6)	7(9.2)	104(19.5)	67(27.6)	37(12.8)
Husband did not allow	10(10.3)	3(14.3)	7(9.2)	27(5.1)	10(4.1)	17(5.9)
Family did not allow	4(4.1)	2(9.5)	2(2.6)	9(1.7)	5(2.1)	4(1.4)
No time because baby came suddenly	–	–	–	33(6.3)	13(5.3)	20(6.9)
My culture forbids	0(0.0)	0(0.0)	0(0.0)	5(0.9)	0(0.0)	5(1.7)
No Security	0(0.0)	0(0.0)	0(0.0)	2(0.4)	1(0.4)	1(0.3)
No PHC facility	4(4.1)	0(0.0)	4(5.3)	20(3.8)	1(0.4)	19(6.6)
Prefer home delivery/TBA	2(2.1)	0(0.0)	2(2.6)	–	–	–
Choice	–	–	–	5(0.9)	5(2.1)	0(0.0)
Had complications	–	–	–	2(0.4)	2(0.8)	0(0.0)
Dislike PHC	–	–	–	8(1.5)	4(1.6)	4(1.4)
Referred	–	–	–	5(0.9)	5(2.1)	0(0.0)
[a]Other	12(12.4)	1(4.8)	11(14.5)	71(13.3)	45(18.5)	26(9.0)
Test of proportions	p = 0.0001			p = 0.3889		

[a]Other includes reasons such as dislike for injection/hospital, no money, nothing, and fear among others

much, facility not open, poor quality service, and culture forbids were significantly different.

Factors related to use of a PHC for antenatal care

The result of chi-squared test to examine the relationship between use of a PHC for antenatal care and selected characteristics of the respondents who were pregnant during the survey is presented in Table 4. The relationship between place of antenatal care and respondent's level of education was statistically significant. About 61% of those who had no education or primary education used a PHC compared to 38.6% of those who attained secondary and higher levels of education. This corresponds to a difference of 22.8%. Marital status was significantly associated with the use of a PHC facility for antenatal care. Close to 60% of the respondents who were married compared to 40.3% of those living together with a partner were using a PHC facility for antenatal care for their current pregnancy.

Predictors of use of PHC for delivery care

Results of the logistic regression model predicting the factors associated with utilization of a PHC for delivery care are presented in Table 5. Some of the predictors were significantly associated with the use of a PHC

facility for delivery care. Compared to the respondents who attained higher education (post-secondary), those who attained secondary (OR 2.37, CI 1.19–4.71), and primary education (OR 3.10, CI 1.16–8.28) were significantly more likely to use a PHC facility for delivery care. The odds of using a PHC for delivery care were significantly higher among Muslim respondents than Catholics (OR 1.56, CI 1.00–2.42). Respondents who had more autonomy were significantly less likely than those who had less autonomy to use a PHC facility for delivery care (OR 0.75, CI 0.57–0.99). The use of a PHC facility for delivery care in a respondent's most recent birth was 61% more likely for respondents who have 5 or more living children relative to those who had 0–2 children.

There was a statistically significant difference between the two LGAs in the use of a PHC facility. Utilising a PHC for delivery care was less likely in Etsako East than in Esan South East (OR 0.55, CI 0.42–0.71). Thus, a separate analysis was conducted for each LGA to determine what differences there might be between the LGAs in the predictors of PHC facility use for delivery care. In Esan South East, only number of living children predicted use of a PHC facility for delivery care. Respondents who have 5 or more living children were more likely than those who had 0–2 children to use a PHC for

Table 4 Association between Place of Antenatal Care and Selected Respondents' Characteristics

Characteristic	PHC facility	Other	Pearson Chi2/ p-value
LGA			
Esan South East	39(26.9)	12(40.0)	(1) = 2.0668
Etsako East	106(73.1)	18(60.0)	p = 0.151
Age			
16–30	108(74.5)	24(80.0)	(1) = 0.4083
31–47	37(25.5)	6(20.0)	p = 0.523
Level of education			
No education/primary	89(61.4)	11(36.7)	(1) = 6.1988
Secondary/higher	56(38.6)	19(63.3)	p = 0.013
Exposure to media			
High exposure	37(25.5)	10(33.3)	
Moderate exposure	65(44.8)	15(50.0)	(2) = 2.2397
No exposure	43(29.7)	5(16.7)	p = 0.326
Religion			
Catholic	32(22.2)	12(40.0)	
Other Christian	74(51.4)	13(43.3)	(2) = 4.3749
Islam	38(26.4)	5(16.7)	p = 0.112
Employment			
Not working	55(37.9)	7(23.3)	(1) = 2.3154
Working	90(62.1)	23(76.7)	p = 0.128
Marital status			
Married	86(59.7)	26(86.7)	(1) = 7.8589
Living together	58(40.3)	4(13.3)	p = 0.005
Age at marriage			
14–17	24(16.5)	2(6.7)	
18–24	100(69.0)	23(76.7)	
25–29	17(11.7)	4(13.3)	(3) = 1.9270
30–39	4(2.8)	1(3.3)	p = 0.588
Partner's age			
18–29	41(28.3)	6(20.0)	
30–34	29(20.0)	6(20.0)	
35–39	28(19.3)	7(23.3)	
40–44	25(17.2)	8(26.7)	(4) = 2.4716
45–82	22(15.2)	3(10.0)	p = 0.650
Partner's level of education			
None/primary	36(24.8)	5(16.7)	(1) = 0.9228
Secondary/higher	109(75.2)	25(83.3)	p = 0.337
Payment for respondents health care			
Husband alone/others	120(82.8)	29(96.7)	(1) = 3.8010
Respondent alone/with husband	25(17.2)	1(3.3)	p = 0.051
Autonomy			
Less	72(49.7)	12(40.0)	
More	34(23.4)	10(33.3)	(2) = 1.4493

Table 4 Association between Place of Antenatal Care and Selected Respondents' Characteristics *(Continued)*

Characteristic	PHC facility	Other	Pearson Chi2/ p-value
Much	39(26.9)	8(26.7)	p = 0.484
Number of living children			
0–2	56(53.9)		
3–4	28(26.9)	15(65.2)	
5+	20(19.2)	4(17.4)	(2) = 1.1485
		4(17.4)	p = 0.563
Spousal education difference			
Same but not none	60(41.4)	15(50.0)	
Wife more	6(4.1)	2(6.7)	
Husband more	61(42.1)	11(36.6)	(3) = 1.6735
Both none/either none	18(12.4)	2(6.7)	p = 0.643

delivery care in their most recent birth (OR 2.00, CI 1.19–3.35). In Etsako East, use of a PHC facility for delivery care was positively associated with Islamic religious affiliation compared to Catholics (OR 1.87, CI 1.13–3.10), and respondents whose partners worked were more likely to use a PHC facility than those whose partners did not work (OR 2.78, CI 1.04–7.44).

Discussion

The study was designed to investigate why women use or do not use PHCs for antenatal and delivery care in rural parts of Edo State in Southern Nigeria. We based the study on the premise that PHCs offer the best opportunity for rural women in Nigeria to enter the health care system to receive the most optimal evidence-based and cost-effective access to skilled delivery care [37, 38]. PHCs are not only located closest to rural women within the current health care system in the country; they also provide opportunity for health workers to offer personalized care that address the cultural and social realities of rural women.

We used different approaches to determine why women use or do not use PHCs for antenatal and delivery care. First, we asked pregnant women and recently delivered women where they are receiving or previously received antenatal care in their previous pregnancies. The results were more accurate for currently pregnant women, while we believe that the difficulty with recall of antenatal events hindered the ability of recently delivered women to provide reliable answers to the question. With currently pregnant women, we found that a large proportion in both LGAs (> 60%) were receiving antenatal care in PHCs. This was not unexpected since the women were drawn from communities that have PHCs as their primary sources of health care.

We then asked women who received antenatal care from PHCs the reasons they choose the facilities.

Table 5 Logistic Regression model predicting the likelihood of using a PHC facility for delivery care

Variable	Odds Ratio (95% Confidence Interval)		
	All respondents	Esan South East	Etsako East
Age	0.96(0.94–0.99)*	0.97(0.93–1.01)	0.97(0.93–1.01)
Education			
Higher (Ref)	1.00	1.00	1.00
Secondary	2.37(1.19–4.71)*	1.69(0.67–4.26)	2.74(0.90–8.32)
Primary	3.10(1.16–8.28)*	2.17(0.53–8.88)	3.32(0.75–14.6)
No Education	2.36(0.70–7.93)	1.69(0.30–9.54)	2.35(0.38–14.2)
Exposure to media			
High (Ref)	1.00	1.00	1.00
Moderate	1.14(0.87–1.50)	1.14(0.79–1.65)	1.11(0.73–1.71)
None	1.35(0.96–1.91)	1.43(0.82–2.50)	1.30(0.82–2.08)
Religion			
Catholic (Ref)	1.00	1.00	1.00
Other Christian	1.20(0.91–1.58)	1.37(0.90–2.08)	1.02(0.70–1.48)
Islam	1.56(1.00–2.42)*	0.56(0.20–1.55)	1.87(1.13–3.10)*
Partner's age	0.99(0.97–1.01)	0.97(0.94–1.00)	1.00(0.97–1.02)
Partner's Education			
No Education (Ref)	1.00	1.00	1.00
Primary	0.76(0.33–1.76)	0.70(−.26–1.88)	1.07(0.20–5.80)
Secondary	0.99(0.34–2.83)	0.71(0.18–2.73)	1.45(0.20–10.5)
Higher	1.05(0.28–3.95)	0.49(0.08–3.04)	2.11(0.21–20.8)
Partner's Employment			
Not working (Ref)	1.00	1.00	1.00
Working	1.62(0.95–2.77)	1.25(0.63–2.45)	2.78(1.04–7.44)*
Autonomy			
Less (Ref)	1.00	1.00	1.00
More	0.75(0.57–0.99)*	0.78(0.52–1.15)	0.76(0.51–1.15)
Much	1.11(0.83–1.47)	0.83(0.56–1.23)	1.51(0.98–2.33)
Number of children			
0–2 (Ref)	1.00	1.00	1.00
3–4	1.23(0.90–1.67)	1.18(0.76–1.83)	1.20(0.76–1.89)
5+	1.61(1.11–2.33)*	2.00(1.19–3.35)**	1.19(0.68–2.07)
Spousal Education Difference			
Both have none(Ref)	1.00	1.00	1.00
Husband more	1.12(0.35–3.59)	0.96(0.19–4.75)	1.08(0.13–8.65)
Wife more	1.84(0.68–5.00)	0.94(0.23–3.84)	2.23(0.41–11.9)
Same but not none	1.59(0.55–4.62)	1.06(0.25–4.51)	1.75(0.25–11.8)
LGA			
Esan South East (Ref)			
Etsako East	0.55(0.42–0.71)***		

*$p < 0.05$ **$p < 0.01$ ***$p < 0.001$

The most commonly proffered reasons (in order of frequency) were: facility near to place of residence, good quality service, cost not too much, and husband wanted it. On the other hand, when the 40% of women in both LGAs who had not received antenatal care in PHCs were asked the reasons why they did not, the most common reasons (in order of frequency) were: poor quality service, no provider in the facility, facility not open, facility too far, and costs too much.

Thus, it was evident that reasons for use and non-use of PHCs for antenatal were related to perceptions about distance of PHCs, quality of PHC service delivery (costs, availability of health personnel, etc.), and partners consent to use of the facilities.

As for skilled delivery care in PHCs, evidently only women who recently delivered could be relied on to provide information on this question. The result showed that more than 45.0% of women delivered in PHCs while up to 25% delivered at home or in the homes of traditional birth attendants. Reasons for use of PHCs for delivery (in order of frequency) included: nearness of PHC to place of residence, good quality service, costs not too much, provider available, and husband's desire. By contrast, the reasons given by women for not using PHCs for delivery were: poor quality service, provider not in facility, facility too far, costs too much, and facilities not open. Some of these reasons for non-use of a PHC facility for antenatal and delivery care have been identified in previous studies in Nigeria and other countries [8, 11, 39, 40]. Sustainable interventions that will specifically address these recurrent reasons, particularly among rural populations are imperative if Nigeria would achieve her developmental targets on maternal health.

Our bivariate analysis to determine how the use of PHCs is related to various socio-demographic variables showed that only women's education and marital status were associated with use of PHCs for antenatal care. Married women as well as women with no education and those with primary level education were more likely to use PHCs for antenatal care as compared to women living together with a partner and women with secondary and higher level education. Previous studies show that formal marital union is associated with better health seeking behavior than consensual union or cohabitation [30–32].

The results of binary logistic regression to determine the independent effects of socio-economic pre-disposing variables in predicting the likelihood of use of PHCs for delivery care showed that higher education reduced the odds of delivery in PHCs in both LGAs. By contrast, the odd of delivery in PHC was higher in Esan South East as compared to Etsako East. Also, being a Muslim and having a partner who was employed increased the odds of delivery in Estako East, but not in Esan South East, while having more than five existing children significantly predicted the likelihood of delivery in a PHC in Esan South East but not in Etsako East.

It was of interest that higher level education of women in this study was shown to reduce the likelihood of women utilizing PHCs for antenatal and delivery care. This is contrary to the results of several studies on maternal health

services utilization in Nigeria and other parts of Africa [41–44] which suggest that women with higher level education are more likely to utilize available health facilities. While such studies have addressed maternal health service utilization overall, very few have addressed service utilization at PHCs in rural communities. We believe that our result on education is attributable to the fact that women commonly identified poor quality care as the reasons for non-use of services in PHCs. Our sub-analysis showed that women with higher level education (secondary and tertiary) were more likely to use other facilities and to report poor quality care as reasons for non-use of PHCs. This is further supported by data showing that women with higher autonomy (but not those with better educated partners) were more likely not to use PHCs for antenatal and delivery care. Better educated women and women with higher levels of education are more likely to ignore the services in PHCs on account of perceptions about quality and presumably opt for services in private clinics or in secondary/tertiary care facilities [39].

We therefore recommend that improved quality service delivery would be an important and critical intervention to increase the access of rural women to antenatal and delivery care in PHCs. In this regard, attention needs to be paid by policymakers and health providers to addressing physical distance of PHCs, improving PHC infrastructure, availability of health personnel, reliability of drugs and equipment supplies, constancy of opening times and reduction in costs of services. Innovations and creativity around transportation of women to PHCs when in labor, community support for costs alleviation such as health insurance, community health education, and linkages to higher level care through the development of an effectiveness referral system would build confidence in the use of PHCs for antenatal and delivery care among rural women.

Contrary to our expectation, cultural preference for home births did not significantly feature as a reason for non-use of PHCs for antenatal and delivery care. Among the cohort of women, only two reported that they preferred traditional birth attendants while five reported that culture forbids the use of facility delivery. Also, the fact that being a Muslim in the LGAs (with multiple religious affiliations) increased the odds of PHC delivery suggests that religion is not an important deterrent, with all religious faiths in the two LGAs showing substantial use of health facilities. We believe that community health education can counter the effect of culture and tradition and increase the use of PHCs by rural women for skilled pregnancy care.

Strengths and limitations

The major strength of the study is its community design approach using a representative sample of women in 20 predominantly rural communities in a geographical zone of Nigeria. This ensures that the results can be generalized to the entire Nigerian healthcare system, especially for rural communities in the country. The study was also conducted by a trained research team that was embedded in the project communities over 17 days. This enabled confidence building with community members, ensuring accuracy and reliability of data collection. Our use of CAPI ensured further accuracy and speed in data collection, enabling the generation of the data and related statistics immediately after the field work. This ensures the currency of information needed to design interventions for improving the access of rural women to skilled pregnancy care.

The major limitation of the study is our inability to collect information from recently delivered women on use of antenatal care. This was possibly due to difficulty in recalling events related to antenatal care which predate the time of delivery. While women could recall delivery events, they were less able to recall antenatal care events possibly due to better inclination to recall the outcomes rather than the processes of pregnancy care.

Despite this limitation, we believe that the results of this study are useful for designing interventions to improve the delivery of PHCs for skilled pregnancy care in Nigeria. Incidentally, the Federal Ministry of Health and all States of the country have identified PHC as the primary instrument and target for improved universal coverage that would ensure skilled pregnancy care for the reduction of maternal mortality in the country [38]. We believe that the results of this study are useful for scaling evidence-based interventions for alleviating the demand and supply factors that hinder the access of rural women to skilled pregnancy care in the country.

Conclusion

We conclude that considerations for distance and costs, and perceptions relating to poor quality care are the factors that mostly hinder women's access to skilled pregnancy care in PHCs in rural Nigeria. Efforts devoted to addressing these factors using innovative approaches will likely increase pregnancy care utilization in PHCs and reduce maternal mortality in rural Nigeria.

Abbreviations
LGA: Local government area; NPC: National population commission; NPHCDA: National primary health care development agency; PHC: Primary health care; UNFPA: United Nations fund for population activities; WHO: World health organization

Acknowledgements
We thank Brian Igboin who supervised, collated and ensured data quality in Etsako East Local Government; Francis Igberaese, and Joab Oghene who coordinated the data collection in Esan South East and Etsako East respectively; and Michael Ekholuenetale, Michael Alli, Mary-Jane Emiowele, Precious Ntulu, Best Ojemhen, Jessy Ezebuihe, Peace Oppogen, Progress Emoitlotoga, Abubakar Zuleya Ogechukwu Onwuma who were data collectors in the two LGAs. We are also grateful to Evans Ejedenawe, Raphael Okpaire, Cynthia Okojie, Tayo Ozobo, Akingbe Aminat, Ebunu Fatimetu, who served as community focal persons in both LGAs. They were instrumental in helping the project teams to gain access to the project communities.

Funding
This study was funded by the International Development Research Centre (IDRC) under the Innovating for Maternal and Child Health in Africa (IMCHA) project. The content is solely the responsibility of the authors and does not necessarily represent the official views of the funding organizations.

Authors' contributions
FEO conceived and supervised the study and wrote sections of the paper and revised the final draft, NLFC supervised the data collection, analyzed the data and wrote sections of the paper; JO supervised the data collection and assisted in data analysis, SA supervised the data collection and contributed to the study design; WI supervised the study and contributed to the study design, SY contributed to the conception of the study and the development of the study questionnaire. All authors approved the final version of the paper.

Ethics approval and consent to participate
Ethical approval for the study was obtained from the National Health Research Ethics Committee (NHREC) of Nigeria – protocol number NHREC/01/01/2007–10/04/2017.
The communities were contacted through lead contact persons, and permission to undertake the study was obtained from the Heads (Odionwere) of the communities. Consent was also obtained from the Heads of individual Households identified for the study. The participating women were informed of the purpose of the study, and individual written informed consent was obtained from them to conduct the study. They were assured of confidentiality of information obtained, and also that such information would only be used for the study and not for other purposes. No names or specific contact information were obtained from the study participants. Only women that agreed to participate in the fully explained study were enlisted in the study.

Competing interests
The authors declare that they have no competing interests.

Author details
[1]Women's Health and Action Research Centre, Km 11 Benin-Lagos Expressway, Benin City, Edo State, Nigeria. [2]The University of Medical Sciences, Ondo City, Ondo State, Nigeria. [3]The Federal University, Oye-Ekiti, Ekiti State, Nigeria. [4]the Federal Bureau of Statistics, Abuja, Nigeria. [5]the Centre of Excellence in Reproductive Health Innovation (CERHI), University of Benin, Benin City, Nigeria. [6]the University of Ottawa, Ottawa, Canada.

References
1. Azuh DE, Azuh AE, Iweala EJ, Adeloye D, Akanbi M, Mordi RC. Factors influencing maternal mortality among rural communities in southwestern Nigeria. Int J Women's Health. 2017;9:179–88.
2. Yar'zever SI. Temporal analysis of maternal mortality in Kano state, northern Nigeria: a six-year review. Am J Public Health Res. 2014;2: 62–7.
3. Odetola TD. Health care utilization among rural women of child-bearing age: a Nigerian experience. Pan Afr Med J. 2015;20:151.
4. Ononokpono DN, Odimegwu C, Imasiku ENS, Adedini SA. Contextual determinants of maternal health care service utilization in Nigeria. Women Health. 2013;53:647–68.
5. UNFPA. Setting standards for emergency obstetric and neonatal care – basic and comprehensive care. http://www.unfpa.org/resources/setting-standards-emergency-obstetric-and-newborn-care/. Accessed 24 Dec 2017.
6. NPHCDA. National primary health care development agency: minimum standards for primary health Care in Nigeria. Abuja, Nigeria: Department of Planning, Research and Statistics, National Primary Health Care Development Agency; 2012. www.nphcda.gov.ng.
7. NPHCDA. Institutionalization of the primary health care planning and reviews in Nigeria: progress and status. Abuja, Nigeria; 2013.
8. Egbewale B, Odu O. Perception and utilization of primary health Care Services in a Semi-Urban Community in south-western Nigeria. J Community Med Prim Health Care. 2013;24:11–20.

9. Nkwo PO. Poor availability of skilled birth attendants in Nigeria: a case study of Enugu state primary health care system. Ann Med Health Sci Res. 2015;5:20–5.

10. Babatunde OA, Aiyenigba E, Awoyemi OA, Akande TM, Musa OI, Salaudeen AG, et al. Primary health care consumers' perception of quality of care and its determinants in north-Central Nigeria. J Asian Sci Res. 2013;3:775–85.

11. Ejembi C, Alti-Muazu M, Chirdan O, Ezeh H, Sheidu S, Dahiru T. Utilization of maternal health services by rural Hausa women in Zaria environs, northern Nigeria: has primary health care made a difference? J Community Med Prim Health Care. 2004;16:47–54.

12. NPC, ICF International. Nigeria demographic and health survey 2013. Abuja and Rockville: National Population Commission, Nigeria and ICF International; 2014.

13. Mimiko O. Experiences with universal health coverage of maternal health care in Ondo state, Nigeria, 2009-2017. Afr J Reprod Health. 2017;20:1–18.

14. Aremu O, Lawoko S, Dalal K. Neighborhood socioeconomic disadvantage, individual wealth status and patterns of delivery care utilization in Nigeria: a multilevel discrete choice analysis. Int J Womens Health. 2011;3:167–74.

15. Babalola S, Fatusi A. Determinants of use of maternal health services in Nigeria-looking beyond individual and household factors. BMC Pregnancy Childbirth. 2009;9:43.

16. Dahiru T, Oche OM. Determinants of antenatal care, institutional delivery and postnatal care services utilization in Nigeria. Pan Afr Med J. 2015;21:321–37.

17. Dairo M, Owoyokun K. Factors affecting the utilization of antenatal care services in Ibadan, Nigeria. Benin J Postgrad Med. 2010;12:3–13.

18. Fagbamigbe AF, Idemudia ES. Barriers to antenatal care use in Nigeria: evidences from non-users and implications for maternal health programming. BMC Pregnancy Childbirth. 2015;15:95.

19. Fawole OI, Adeoye IA. Women's status within the household as a determinant of maternal health care use in Nigeria. Afr Health Sci. 2015;15:217–24.

20. Okoli U, Morris L, Oshin A, Pate MA, Aigbe C, Muhammad A. Conditional cash transfer schemes in Nigeria: potential gains for maternal and child health service uptake in a national pilot programme. BMC Pregnancy Childbirth. 2014;14:408.

21. Samuel FO, Olaolorun FM, Adeniyi JD. A training intervention on child feeding among primary healthcare workers in Ibadan municipality. Afr J Prim Health Care Fam Med. 2016;8:1–6.

22. Oyekale AS. Assessment of primary health care facilities service readiness in Nigeria. BMC Health Serv Res. 2017;17:172.

23. Nnebue CC, Ebenebe UE, Adogu PO, Adinma ED, Ifeadike CO, Nwabueze AS. Adequacy of resources for provision of maternal health services at the primary health care level in Nnewi, Nigeria. Niger Med J. 2014;55:235.

24. Ajayi IO, Osakinle DC. Socio demographic factors determining the adequacy of antenatal care among pregnant women visiting Ekiti state primary health centers. Online J Health Allied Sci. 2013;12:1–6.

25. Oladapo OT, Iyaniwura CA, Sule-Odu AO. Quality of antenatal Services at the Primary Care Level in Southwest Nigeria. Afr J Reprod Health. 2008;12:71–92.

26. Uzochukwu B, Onwujekwe O, Akpala C. Community satisfaction with the quality of maternal and child health services in Southeast Nigeria. East Afr Med J. 2004;81:293–9.

27. Fawole A, Adekanle D, Hunyinbo K. Utilization of the partograph in primary health care facilities in southwestern Nigeria. Niger J Clin Pract. 2010;13:200–4.

28. Andersen R, Newman JF. Societal and individual determinants of medical care utilization in the United States. Milbank Q. 2005;83:1–28.

29. Babitsch B, Gohl D, von Lengerke T. Re-visiting Andersen's behavioral model of health services use: a systematic review of studies from 1998-2011. GMS Psycho-Soc-Med. 2012;9:Doc 11.

30. Ross CE, Mirowsky J, Goldsteen K. The impact of the family on health: the decade in review. J Marriage Fam. 1990;52:1059–78.

31. Musick K, Bumpass L. Reexamining the case for marriage: union formation and changes in well-being. J Marriage Fam. 2012;74:1–18.

32. Waite LJ. Does marriage matter? Demography. 1995;32:483–507.

33. United States Census Bureau. https://www.census.gov/data/software/cspro.html. Accessed 1 Jan 2018.

34. Dyson T, Moore M. On kinship structure female autonomy and demographic behavior in India. Popul Dev Rev. 1983;9:35–60.

35. Jejeebhoy SJ, Sathar ZA. Women's autonomy in India and Pakistan: the influence of religion and region. Popul Dev Rev. 2001;27:687–712.

36. Bamiwuye SO, De Wet N, Adedini SA. Linkages between autonomy, poverty and contraceptive use in two sub-Saharan African countries. Afr Popul Stud. 2013;27:164–73.

37. World Health Organization. Declaration of Alma-Ata: International Conference on Primary Health Care, Alma-Ata, USSR, 6–12 September 1978. Retrieved Febr. 1978;14:2006.

38. Federal Government of Nigeria. Integrating primary health care governance in Nigeria (PHC under one roof): implementation manual. National Health Care Development Agency; 2013.

39. Ensor T, Cooper S. Overcoming barriers to health service access: influencing the demand side. Health Policy Plan. 2004;19:69–79.

40. Hounton S, Menten J, Ouédraogo M, Dubourg D, Meda N, Ronsmans C, et al. Effects of a skilled care initiative on pregnancy-related mortality in rural Burkina Faso. Tropical Med Int Health. 2008;13:53–60.

41. Banda PC, Odimegwu CO, Ntoimo LF, Muchiri E. Women at risk: gender inequality and maternal health. Women Health. 2016;57:405–29.

42. Jacobs C, Moshabela M, Maswenyeho S, Lambo N, Michelo C. Predictors of antenatal, skilled birth attendance and postnatal care utilization among the remote and poorest rural communities in Zambia: a multi-level analysis. Front Public Health. 2017;5:11.

43. Okafor IP, Sekoni AO, Dolapo DC. Predictors of maternal health service utilization: a community-based, rural-urban comparison in Nigeria. East Afr J Public Health. 2014;11:45–65.

44. Rustaremwa G, Wandera SO, Jhamba T, Akiror E, Kiconco A. Determinants of maternal health services utilization in Uganda. BMC Health Serv Res. 2015;12:271.

Permissions

The contributors of this book come from diverse backgrounds, making this book a truly international effort. This book will bring forth new frontiers with its revolutionizing research information and detailed analysis of the nascent developments around the world.

We would like to thank all the contributing authors for lending their expertise to make the book truly unique. They have played a crucial role in the development of this book. Without their invaluable contributions this book wouldn't have been possible. They have made vital efforts to compile up to date information on the varied aspects of this subject to make this book a valuable addition to the collection of many professionals and students.

This book was conceptualized with the vision of imparting up-to-date information and advanced data in this field. To ensure the same, a matchless editorial board was set up. Every individual on the board went through rigorous rounds of assessment to prove their worth. After which they invested a large part of their time researching and compiling the most relevant data for our readers.

The editorial board has been involved in producing this book since its inception. They have spent rigorous hours researching and exploring the diverse topics which have resulted in the successful publishing of this book. They have passed on their knowledge of decades through this book. To expedite this challenging task, the publisher supported the team at every step. A small team of assistant editors was also appointed to further simplify the editing procedure and attain best results for the readers.

Apart from the editorial board, the designing team has also invested a significant amount of their time in understanding the subject and creating the most relevant covers. They scrutinized every image to scout for the most suitable representation of the subject and create an appropriate cover for the book.

The publishing team has been an ardent support to the editorial, designing and production team. Their endless efforts to recruit the best for this project, has resulted in the accomplishment of this book. They are a veteran in the field of academics and their pool of knowledge is as vast as their experience in printing. Their expertise and guidance has proved useful at every step. Their uncompromising quality standards have made this book an exceptional effort. Their encouragement from time to time has been an inspiration for everyone.

The publisher and the editorial board hope that this book will prove to be a valuable piece of knowledge for researchers, students, practitioners and scholars across the globe.

List of Contributors

R. Geurtzen, Arno Van Heijst, Jos Draaisma and Marije Hogeveen
Amalia Children's Hospital, Department of Pediatrics, Radboud university Medical Center, 6500HB Nijmegen, The Netherlands

Rosella Hermens
Scientific Institute for Quality of Care, Radboud university medical center, Nijmegen, The Netherlands

Hubertina Scheepers
Department of Gynecology, Maastricht UMC+, Maastricht, The Netherlands

Mallory Woiski
Amalia Children's Hospital, Department of Gynecology, Radboud University Medical Center, Nijmegen, The Netherlands

Evelyn Sakeah, Raymond Aborigo, Maxwell Dalaba, Ernest Kanyomse, Daniel Azongo, Dominic Anaseba, Samuel Oladokun and Abraham Rexford Oduro
Navrongo Health Research Centre, Post Office Navrongo, Upper East Region, Ghana

James Kotuah Sakeah
Department of Medicine, University of Calgary, Alberta, Canada

Jianyuan Huang
School of Public Administration, Hohai University, Nanjing, China

Xiaoming Sun, Jingshu Mao and Xingyu Shu
School of Sociology and Population Sciences, Nanjing University of Posts and Telecommunications, Nanjing, China

Norman Hearst
Department of Family and Community Medicine, University of California, San Francisco, CA, USA

Zhanhong Zong
School of Public Administration, Hohai University, Nanjing, China

School of Sociology and Population Sciences, Nanjing University of Posts and Telecommunications, Nanjing, China

Espen Bjertness
Department of Community Medicine, Institute of Health and Society, Faculty of Medicine, University of Oslo, Postboks 1130 Blindern, 0318 Oslo, Norway

Dina Sami Khalifa
Department of Community Medicine, Institute of Health and Society, Faculty of Medicine, University of Oslo, Postboks 1130 Blindern, 0318 Oslo, Norway
Faculty of Health Sciences, Ahfad University for Women, Khartoum, Sudan

Kari Glavin
VID Specialized University, Oslo, Norway

Lars Lien
National Advisory Board on Dual Diagnosis, Innlandet Hospital Trust, Hamar, Norway
Department of Public Health, Hedmark University College, Elverum, Norway

Wondwosen Teklesilasie
School of Public and Environmental Health, College of Medicine and Health Sciences, Hawassa University, Hawassa, Ethiopia
Department of Reproductive Health and Health Service Management, School of Public Health, College of Health Sciences, Addis Ababa University, Addis Ababa, Ethiopia

Wakgari Deressa
Department of Preventive Medicine, School of Public Health, College of Health Sciences, Addis Ababa University, Addis Ababa, Ethiopia

Fen-Fang Chung
Department of Nursing, College of Nursing, Chang Gung University of Science and Technology, Taoyuan, Taiwan
Department of Nursing, Linkuo Chang Gung Memorial Hospital, Taoyuan, Taiwan

Gwo-Hwa Wan
Department of Respiratory Therapy, College of Medicine, Chang Gung University, 259, Wen-Hwa 1st Road, Kwei-Shan, Taoyuan 333, Taiwan, Republic of China
Department of Obstetrics and Gynecology, Taipei Chang Gung Memorial Hospital, Taipei, Taiwan
Department of Respiratory Care, Chang Gung University of Science and Technology, Chiayi, Taiwan

Su-Chen Kuo
Department of Midwifery and Women Health Care, National Taipei University of Nursing and Health Sciences, Taipei, Taiwan

Kuan-Chia Lin
Institute of Hospital and Health Care Administration, Community Research Center, National Yang-Ming University, Taipei, Taiwan

Hsueh-Erh Liu
Department of Nursing, College of Nursing, Chang Gung University of Science and Technology, Taoyuan, Taiwan
School of Nursing, College of Medicine, Chang Gung University, 259, Wen-Hwa 1st Road, Kwei-Shan, Taoyuan 333, Taiwan, Republic of China
Department of Rheumatology, Linkuo Chang Gung Memorial Hospital, Taoyuan, Taiwan

Michael W. Seward, Denise Simon and Emily Oken
Division of Chronic Disease Research Across the Lifecourse, Department of Population Medicine, Harvard Medical School and Harvard Pilgrim Health Care Institute, Boston, MA, USA

Martha Richardson
Obstetrics & Gynecology, Harvard Vanguard Medical Associates, Boston, MA, USA

Matthew W. Gillman
Division of Chronic Disease Research Across the Lifecourse, Department of Population Medicine, Harvard Medical School and Harvard Pilgrim Health Care Institute, Boston, MA, USA
Environmental Influences on Child Health Outcomes (ECHO) Program, Office of the Director, National Institutes of Health, Bethesda, MD, USA

Marie-France Hivert
Division of Chronic Disease Research Across the Lifecourse, Department of Population Medicine, Harvard Medical School and Harvard Pilgrim Health Care Institute, Boston, MA, USA
Diabetes Unit, Massachusetts General Hospital, Boston, MA, USA

Nancy F. Berglas and Sarah C. M. Roberts
Advancing New Standards in Reproductive Health, Department of Obstetrics, Gynecology and Reproductive Sciences, University of California, San Francisco, 1330 Broadway, Suite 1100, Oakland, CA 94612, USA

Valerie Williams
Department of Obstetrics and Gynecology, Louisiana State University Health Sciences Center New Orleans, 1542 Tulane Avenue, New Orleans, LA 70112, USA

Katrina Mark
Department of Obstetrics, Gynecology and Reproductive Sciences, University of Maryland School of Medicine, 655 W. Baltimore Street, Baltimore, MD 21201, USA

Jennifer Hatfield and Reginald S. Sauve
Department of Community Health Sciences, Cumming School of Medicine, University of Calgary, 3280 Hospital Drive, NW, Calgary, AB, Canada

Eveline Thobias Konje
Department of Biostatistics & Epidemiology, School of Public Health, Catholic University of Health and Allied Sciences, Bugando Area, Mwanza, Tanzania
Department of Community Health Sciences, Cumming School of Medicine, University of Calgary, 3280 Hospital Drive, NW, Calgary, AB, Canada

Moke Tito Nyambita Magoma
Options Tanzania Ltd 76 Ali Hassan, Mwinyi Road, Dar es Salaam, Tanzania

Susan Kuhn
Department of Paediatrics, University of Calgary, 2888 Shaganappi Tr. NW, Calgary, AB, Canada

Deborah Margret Dewey
Department of Community Health Sciences, Cumming School of Medicine, University of Calgary, 3280 Hospital Drive, NW, Calgary, AB, Canada
Department of Paediatrics, University of Calgary, 2888 Shaganappi Tr. NW, Calgary, AB, Canada
Owerko Centre at the Alberta Children's Hospital Research Institute, Cumming School of Medicine, University of Calgary, 2500 University Dr. NW, Calgary, AB, Canada

Samuel Ginja
School of Psychology, Ulster University, Cromore Road, Coleraine, Co., Londonderry BT52 1SA, UK

Jane Coad, Elizabeth Bailey and Samantha Nightingale
Centre for Innovative Research Across the Life Course (CIRAL), Faculty of Health & Life Sciences, Coventry University, Priory Street, Coventry CV1 5FB, UK

Sally Kendall
Centre for Health Services Studies, University of Kent, Canterbury, Kent CT2 7NF, UK

Trudy Goodenough and Toity Deave
Centre for Child & Adolescent Health, University of the West of England Bristol, Oakfield House, Oakfield Grove, Clifton, Bristol BS8 2BN, UK

Jane Smiddy
Nursing, Midwifery and Health, Health and Life Sciences, Northumbria University, Coach Lane Campus, Benton, Newcastle upon Tyne NE7 7XA, UK

Crispin Day
Department of Psychology, Child & Adolescent Mental Health Service Research Unit, King's College London, Institute of Psychiatry, Psychology and Neuroscience, De Crespigny Park, London SE5 8AB, UK

Raghu Lingam
Population Child Health Research Group, Women's and Children's Health, University of New South Wales, Sydney, Australia

Honghui Yu
Department of Anesthesiology, Tongji Hospital affiliated Tongji Medical College, Huazhong University of Science and Technology, Wuhan 430030, China

Xueyan Jiang and Min Shen
Department of Maternal and Child Health, School of Public Health, Tongji Medical College, Huazhong University of Science and Technology, Wuhan 430030, China

Wei Bao
Department of Epidemiology, College of Public Health, University of Iowa, Iowa City, IA 52242, USA

Guifeng Xu
Department of Epidemiology, College of Public Health, University of Iowa, Iowa City, IA 52242, USA
Center for Disabilities and Development, University of Iowa Stead Family Children's Hospital, Iowa City, IA 52242, USA

Rong Yang
Wuhan Children's Hospital (Wuhan Maternal and Child Healthcare Hospital), Tongji Medical College, Huazhong University of Science & Technology, Wuhan 430015, China

Yu-Mi Im
Department of Nursing, Seoul Women's College of Nursing, Seoul, South Korea

Tae-Jin Yun
Division of Pediatric Cardiac Surgery, Asan Medical Center, University of Ulsan College of Medicine, Seoul, South Korea

Il-Young Yoo
College of Nursing, Yonsei University, Seoul, South Korea

Sanghee Kim and Sue Kim
College of Nursing, Mo-Im Kim Nursing Research Institute, Yonsei University, 50 Yonsei-ro, Seodaemun-gu, Seoul 03722, Korea

Juhye Jin
Department of Nursing, College of Health and Life Science, Korea National University of Transportation, Jeungpyeong-gun, South Korea

Serawit Lakew
Department of Nursing and Midwifery, Arbaminch University, Arba Minch, Ethiopia

Alaso Ankala
Department of Nursing and Midwifery, Arba Minch College of Health Sciences, Arba Minch, Ethiopia

Fozia Jemal
Department of Obstetrics and Gynecology, Tikur Anbesa Specialized Hospital, Addis Ababa University, Addis Ababa, Ethiopia

Sian Karen Smith, Antonia Cai, Michelle Wong, Bettina Meiser and Rajneesh Kaur
Psychosocial Research Group, Lowy Research Centre, C25, Prince of Wales Clinical School, Faculty of Medicine, UNSW Sydney, Corner High and Botany St, Kensington, Sydney New South Wales 2033, Australia

Mariana S. Sousa
Psychosocial Research Group, Lowy Research Centre, C25, Prince of Wales Clinical School, Faculty of Medicine, UNSW Sydney, Corner High and Botany St, Kensington, Sydney New South Wales 2033, Australia
Centre for Applied Nursing Research, School of Nursing and Midwifery, Western Sydney University, Ingham, Sydney, Australia
South Western Sydney Local Health District, Institute for Applied Medical Research, Sydney, Australia

Michelle Peate
Department of Obstetrics and Gynaecology, Royal Women's Hospital, University of Melbourne, Parkville, Australia

Alec Welsh
School of Women's and Children's Health, UNSW Sydney, Sydney, Australia
Department of Maternal-Fetal Medicine, Royal Hospital for Women, Sydney, Australia

Sharon Lewis
Murdoch Children's Research Institute, Royal Children's Hospital, Parkville, Victoria, Australia

Jane Halliday
Murdoch Children's Research Institute, Royal Children's Hospital, Parkville, Victoria, Australia
Department of Paediatrics, University of Melbourne, Parkville, Australia

Lyndal Trevena
Sydney School of Public Health, The University of Sydney, Sydney, Australia

Tatiane Yanes
School of Psychiatry, Faculty of Medicine, UNSW Sydney, Sydney, Australia

Kristine Barlow-Stewart
Sydney Medical School, The University of Sydney, Sydney, Australia

Margot Barclay
Women's Services, Liverpool Hospital, Sydney, Australia
Western Sydney University, Parramatta, Sydney, Australia

Bridget Chomba Chanda
Department of Paediatric and Child Health, University Teaching Hospital-HIV/AIDS Program, Lusaka, Zambia
Department of population studies and Nutrition, School of Public Health, University of Zambia, Geneva, Switzerland

Rosemary Ndonyo Likwa
Department of population studies and Nutrition, School of Public Health, University of Zambia, Geneva, Switzerland

Jessy Zgambo and Choolwe Jacobs
Department of Epidemiology and Biostatistics, School of Public Health, University of Zambia, Lusaka, Zambia

Louis Tembo
Department of Health Promotion and Education, School of Public Health, University of Zambia, Lilongwe, Malawi

Solomon Assefa
Ethiopian Public Health Institute, Arbegnoch Street, Addis Ababa, Ethiopia

Kassu Desta
Department of Medical Laboratory Sciences, School of Allied Health Sciences, College of Health Sciences, Addis Ababa University, Addis Ababa, Ethiopia

Tsehaynesh Lema
Armauer Hansen Research Institute, Jimma Road, Addis Ababa, Ethiopia
All Africa Leprosy, Tuberculosis, Rehabilitation and Training Center, Jimma Road, Addis Ababa, Ethiopia

Faye Forbes, Karen Wynter and Jane Fisher
Jean Hailes Research Unit, School of Public Health and Preventive Medicine, Monash University, 553 St Kilda Rd, Melbourne, VIC 3004, Australia

Catherine Wade
Parenting Research Centre, 232 Victoria Parade, East Melbourne, VIC 3002, Australia

Berihun M. Zeleke
School of Public Health and Preventive Medicine, Monash University, 553 St Kilda Rd, Melbourne, VIC 3004, Australia
Institute of Public Health, College of Medicine and Health Sciences, University of Gondar, Gondar, Ethiopia

Rosimar Neris Martins Feitosa and Vânia Nakauth Azevedo
Virology Laboratory, Institute of Biological Sciences, Federal University of Pará, Augusto Correa 1, Guamá, 66, Belém, Pará 075-110, Brazil

Aubaneide Batista Guerra
Reference Unit Specialized in Maternal-Child and Adolescent Care, Belém, Pará, Brazil
Virology Laboratory, Institute of Biological Sciences, Federal University of Pará, Augusto Correa 1, Guamá, 66, Belém, Pará 075-110, Brazil
Biology of Infectious and Parasitic Agents Graduate Program, Federal University of Pará, Belém, Pará, Brazil

Leonardo Quintão Siravenha, Rogério Valois Laurentino, Antonio Carlos Rosário Vallinoto, Ricardo Ishak and Luiz Fernando Almeida Machado
Virology Laboratory, Institute of Biological Sciences, Federal University of Pará, Augusto Correa 1, Guamá, 66, Belém, Pará 075-110, Brazil

Biology of Infectious and Parasitic Agents Graduate Program, Federal University of Pará, Belém, Pará, Brazil

Seun Anjorin and Wilson Imongan
Women's Health and Action Research Centre, Km 11 Benin-Lagos Expressway, Benin City, Edo State, Nigeria

Friday Okonofua
Women's Health and Action Research Centre, Km 11 Benin-Lagos Expressway, Benin City, Edo State, Nigeria
The University of Medical Sciences, Ondo City, Ondo State, Nigeria
the Centre of Excellence in Reproductive Health Innovation (CERHI), University of Benin, Benin City, Nigeria

Lorretta Ntoimo
Women's Health and Action Research Centre, Km 11 Benin-Lagos Expressway, Benin City, Edo State, Nigeria
The Federal University, Oye-Ekiti, Ekiti State, Nigeria

Julius Ogungbangbe
the Federal Bureau of Statistics, Abuja, Nigeria

Sanni Yaya
the University of Ottawa, Ottawa, Canada

Index